More Praise for
The Sexual Healing Journey

"*The Sexual Healing Journey* is a much needed resource for individuals and couples struggling to create healthy, joyous, safe, and loving sexual lives in the aftermath of abuse. Hopeful, clear, practical, and thorough, it makes the process of reclaiming the pleasure of healthy sexuality seem possible and accessible."

— ELLEN BASS, coauthor of *The Courage to Heal*
and coeditor of *I Never Told Anyone*

"Wendy Maltz is one of our most gifted healers, and she has written a beautiful book. Practical, useful, and long-needed, it will be a gift to many."

— PATRICK J. CARNES, PH.D., author of *Don't Call It Love*
and *Out of the Shadows*

"This book still stands as *the most important resource* available to survivors concerning sexual functioning and sexual healing. *The Sexual Healing Journey* offers essential hope and compassion in addition to understandable explanations and exercises that improve self-awareness, communication, touching, sexual contact, and sexual intimacy. I highly recommend it to all practitioners and I routinely suggest it to clients and their significant others as an indispensable resource."

— CHRISTINE A. COURTOIS, Ph.D., author of *Healing the Incest Wound*
and *Recollections of Sexual Abuse*

"This is *an excellent resource*! Wendy Maltz deals directly with the negative effects of sexual abuse while managing to stay a strong advocate for healthy sex."

— MITCHELL TEPPER, PH.D., M.P.H., Founder of the Sexual Health Network and
SexualHealth.com

"With the compassion and caring that bespeaks her own healing journey, Wendy Maltz has given us a treasure: her clinical anecdotes are poignant; her instructions are thoughtful and clear. *The Sexual Healing Journey* will always have a space on my bookshelf; it is a must-read for survivors, therapists, and those who care."

—CLYDE W. FORD, PH.D., author of *Where Healing Waters Meet*
and *Compassionate Touch*

"A *must-read* for any survivor who wants to experience the pleasures of a safe and loving sexual relationship. Thank you, Wendy, for providing this gentle, empowering guide!"

—MARYLIN VAN DERBUR, former Miss America, incest survivor,
named "Outstanding Woman Speaker in America"

"This book is a powerful and effective means of restoring and enhancing sexuality in the aftermath of sexual abuse. Wendy Maltz's practical, plain-spoken approach and specific exercises are a helpful adjunct to therapy, as well as a valuable guide for people who want to address these issues on their own."

—AL COOPER, PH.D., Director, San Jose Marital and Sexuality Centre
and staff psychologist at Stanford University

"This highly useful book provides much needed comfort, reassurance, and practical information for survivors of abuse who wish to reclaim healthy sexuality and for the people who care about them. . . . An *invaluable resource*."

—YVONNE DOLAN, M.A., author of *Resolving Sexual Abuse* and *One Small Step*

"*The Sexual Healing Journey* allows the sexual abuse survivor to let go of shame and pain from the past and embrace a healthy sexual self. It is a book of heart, hope, and answers, and I highly recommend it."

—CLAUDIA BLACK, PH.D., author of *It Will Never Happen to Me* and *Changing Course*

The
Sexual Healing
Journey

THE
SEXUAL
HEALING
JOURNEY

A Guide for Survivors
of Sexual Abuse

REVISED EDITION

WENDY MALTZ

Illustrations by Carol Arian

HARPER

NEW YORK • LONDON • TORONTO • SYDNEY

To inquire about scheduling Wendy Maltz for speaking engagements, you may write to her at the address below or e-mail her at: info@healthysex.com. Ms. Maltz welcomes your feedback and responses to *The Sexual Healing Journey* but regrets that she is unable to answer individual letters, phone calls, and e-mails requesting advice on personal situations. (Please refer to the organizations listed in the Resources section for referrals.)

Wendy Maltz and Associates
P.O. Box 648
Eugene, Oregon 97440

Her web site is http://www.HealthySex.com.

A previous edition of this book was published in 1991 by HarperCollins Publishers.

HarperCollins books may be purchased for educational, business, or sales promotional use. For information please write: Special Markets Department, HarperCollins Publishers Inc., 10 East 53rd Street, New York, NY 10022.

Library of Congress Cataloging-in-Publication Data is available.
ISBN 0-06-095964-9

First Perennial edition published 1992.
First Quill edition published 2001.

10 11 RRD   30 29 28 27 26 25 24 23

To LARRY,

In celebration of the sweet love we share

Contents

x

Contents

PART THREE

Getting There: Creating Positive Experiences

Acknowledgments

Many people have helped make this book a reality. I mention only some here by name, but I am very grateful to all who have helped me on this journey.

Foremost, I would like to express my heartfelt appreciation to the many survivors and intimate partners of survivors I have become acquainted with through counseling, research, conferences, and workshops. Their courage, persistence, and accomplishments have inspired me, professionally and personally. I am grateful that many of them chose to share their personal struggles and triumphs in this book. Their stories and words give the material emotional depth, immediacy, and rich meaning. This book is written in honor of them and of all people traveling on sexual healing journeys.

A special thank-you goes to Harriet Goldhor Lerner for recognizing the significance of my work and for providing me with valuable author-to-author counsel and affable support.

I am also grateful for the support of clinical colleagues who have been interfacing sexual abuse and sexuality. Their insights, knowledge, research, and writings have helped me in developing my own treatment strategies and techniques, which, in turn, generated material for this book. Several colleagues' work has been of particular importance in this new field, namely, Derek Jehu, Judith Becker, Peter Dimock, Barry McCarthy, Patrick Carnes, Joe LoPiccolo, Christine Courtois, Jan Hindman, and Mark Schwartz.

I also thank Felicia Eth, my literary agent, for her friendly, enthusiastic, direct, and competent representation, and my brother-in-law, Richard Garzilli, for his expert contract review and legal advice.

During the course of the writing, I was blessed with help from some extremely bright and competent people. In particular, I thank my editor, Janet Goldstein, for her superb editorial guidance in planning and developing the book from its inception. Janet's warmth, friendliness, intellect, and gifted editorial skills helped me realize my own ability as a writer who could produce a popular book. Her awareness of psychological processes and personal growth helped shape the book to be sensitive to the many different survivors for whom it is written. It was marvelous to have an editor who enthusiastically supported the project and believed in the social importance of my work.

In addition, I thank two very special, talented writers who provided "in the trenches" editorial consultation. Dean Baker, a Eugene writer, provided friendly and creative assistance in the early stages of preparing the manuscript. I am especially indebted to his keen ability to translate psychological jargon and concepts into everyday language. Suzie Boss, a Portland, Oregon, writer, provided essential help with the arduous task of revising the manuscript. Suzie's consistent encouragement, compassionate understanding, and outstanding writing abilities helped me keep an active pace through numerous drafts and made a valuable contribution to the final shape of the book.

I am also indebted to a number of people who read the first draft of the manuscript and gave helpful feedback, specifically, Larry Maltz, Karla Baur, Peter Dimock, Ellen Bass, Laura Davis, Norma Ragsdale, Susan and Dale Goodman, Bryan McCrea, and my father, Joe Becker. Their knowledge, perceptive insights, and sensitivities helped me acknowledge areas in the book that needed improvement and further development.

I am deeply grateful to my family and friends for providing continual, loving encouragement and support during the nearly two years this book was being written. Friends Sandy Solomon and Lucia Hardy helped me brainstorm the outline and focus for the book. My parents, Joe and Arlene Becker, who taught me the value of persistence and determination, provided loving support. And I thank my siblings, Jane Garzilli, Sara Nielsen, and Bill Becker, for their understanding and enthusiasm for this project. My sister-in-law, Suzanne Jennings, was especially kind, sending me cards and writings to lift my spirits during those inevitable times when I felt bogged down by all the work.

Larry, my husband, spent countless days and evenings taking care of our children and household so that I could work on the book. He discussed theories and ideas with me, and offered new insights. He cheered on my progress and comforted me when I felt discouraged. I do not believe I could have written this book were it not for his understanding, wisdom, tender reassurances, and nurturing love.

My children, Jules and Cara, showed tremendous support given how difficult it was for them, at times, to have their mother so preoccupied. They both helped me with the research: stamping envelopes, sorting mailers, and preparing the questionnaires. I was particularly moved by the sweet hugs, kisses, and words of encouragement they gave me after quietly entering the computer room when they missed me or wanted to show they cared. Given my family's personal sacrifices, contributions, and enduring support, this book is best described as a Maltz family production.

A special thank-you to Fiona Hallowell, Gail Winston, and Stephanie Small, editors at HarperCollins, for their friendly support and work on the ten-year-anniversary update of the book. I would also like to thank my son, Jules Maltz, for his excellent computer research and help revising the Resources section.

Preface

I cruise down to the Willamette River perched atop my shiny red bike. The sun warms my cheeks and I breathe in the startling beauty of the day. It's spring, and the riverfront surges with new life. Flowers paint yellow and pink light along the banks, animals sing and dance their annual mating dances, and the river swells with rushing water from melted snow. It was on a bike ride to this river back in 1989 that I first decided to write *The Sexual Healing Journey*. Today, I celebrate the book's ten-year anniversary and reflect on its history and importance as a healing resource for survivors.

I remember feeling compelled to write this book. It was as though I had discovered a new plant with medicinal properties in my own backyard and just had to share it. In my clinical practice, through academic research, and in my personal life, I was learning a lot about sexual healing that I knew would be of immense benefit to others. Few resources for healing existed at that time. And the ones that were available were limited in content and tone. I wanted to create an information-packed, compassionate resource that would empower and assist a wide range of survivors and their intimate partners. I was challenged by the dilemma facing many survivors: wanting to enjoy sexual intimacy but having difficulty addressing sexual issues directly.

When I decided to write *The Sexual Healing Journey* there weren't any resources that offered sex therapy techniques specifically designed for survivors. People with problems related to incest, rape, and sexual molestation were encouraged to use traditional approaches and techniques. These exercises were prescribed and prescripted. They were insensitive to the special needs of people with sexual trauma histories. Many survivors found them unappealing and, in some instances, retraumatizing. As one survivor told me, "They were too much, too soon, and too sexual!"

By contrast, the healing approaches I was learning about and developing in my work back in the late 1980s were proving to be very effective. My techniques were set up to teach basic skills first: rudimentary self-awareness, communication, and touching; the need to initiate and control sexual contact; the need to go slowly and build bridges from one experience to another.

My goal became to create a comprehensive healing guide beneficial to all survivors, regardless of how or when they were abused, the amount of sexual abuse recovery work they had already done, or their present lifestyles and sexual orientations. To extend the range of this book beyond what I had learned in my clinical practice as a therapist and in my early research, I interviewed a lot of survivors who had worked on sexual healing with other therapists. To reach even more people, I designed a lengthy questionnaire which I administered to more than 140 survivors, partners of survivors, and clinicians specializing in sexual healing.

I recall it being a very busy and exciting time, as I gathered and organized the information for this book. It was a great opportunity for me—both as a woman who has recovered from sexual abuse herself, and as a therapist who specializes in treating sexual problems. I learned more about effective healing techniques. And as the writing progressed, it was exhilarating to experience the book take on a life of its own.

I was blessed with the supportive input and assistance of many other people—colleagues, friends, family, and survivors. They became actively involved and kept reminding me how important the book would be to others. A male survivor wrote on the back of his questionnaire, "I'd be pleased if my story can help just one person, although I wish this kind of book were not necessary." Another survivor wrote, "I pray that people can realize abuse may have caused their sexual problems, and seek and get help." Their words kept the project flowing and kept me cognizant of how vital a role sexual healing plays in recovery from abuse.

While I brought professional wisdom to the project, the book was also very important to me on a personal level. I am what I call a "patchwork survivor"— one who has experienced different kinds of sexual abuse at different times in his or her life. When I was a little girl, I was touched inappropriately by an uncle who acted in a sexually seductive and flirtatious manner toward me. These experiences made me fear my own sexual energy and harmed my ability to select loving and caring partners in my early dating years.

When I was a junior at the University of Colorado, I was assaulted while walking on a heavily wooded campus path one afternoon. A man sprang out from behind some bushes, threw me up against a wall, fondled me, and tried to rape me. I defended myself with the book I was carrying: a treatise on Mahatma Gandhi's methods of nonviolent protest. For a long time, I joked about how funny it was that I hit him with such a book, preferring not to remember the terror and powerlessness I had felt then. It wasn't until he heard other people approaching on the path that he let me go and ran away.

Later, in graduate school, I went out with a law student I barely knew. He invited me to his apartment to listen to records. After a few kisses he suddenly changed. A faraway look came over him, and he seemed to become another person. He grabbed me, held me down, and raped me. I felt used, humiliated, and mad at myself. I never reported the event. It wasn't until years later when I read books about date rape that I admitted I had been a victim. I had to learn to call it rape and to release myself from feeling responsible for what had happened to me.

This patchwork of experiences, along with years of study and work as a sex therapist, has helped me understand the challenge of sexual healing. I know how hard it can be to overcome denial and feelings of responsibility. I know how long it can take to stop old patterns of behavior that continually re-create the abuse. I know how slowly one has to go to relearn touch and sexual responsiveness in a new way, free of the memories of abuse. And I know how important it is to respect and love oneself, embracing a new concept of what it means to be a sexual person.

One of the things that I enjoyed most about writing this book was the opportunity it gave me to share my hard-earned insights about sexual healing with others. I like the idea of breaking silence and reducing shame about important sexual issues. Too many times, people suffer unnecessarily—stuck in self-hatred, ignorance, and dissatisfaction—because they are denied accurate information about sex. It felt good to produce a resource which gives survivors and partners a crucial message: You are not alone. You can safely learn from the healing experiences of others who have gone before you.

The book also prompted me to go further in my own sexual healing. More memories of childhood abuse surfaced. I confronted my uncle about the covert type of incest I experienced as a child. He was furious and denied the abuse at first. A year later, after doing some counseling work of his own, he visited me in Eugene, Oregon, to work on family reconciliation. We met, and I told him what I remembered and how his actions had affected my life.

My uncle listened, shared more information, took responsibility for his actions, and offered a sincere apology. It was heart-wrenching to realize how much the past abuse had prevented an active, healthy uncle-niece relationship for many years. We both cried. Afterwards, I felt like I shed layers of unnecessary sexual shame I hadn't even been aware of carrying. I also gained a greater respect for the courage it takes for someone who perpetrated sexual abuse in the past to step forward and be accountable.

A year after I met with my uncle, I returned to Boulder, Colorado, to visit the path where I had been sexually assaulted twenty-five years earlier. I was amazed. First of all, I could hardly recognize the spot where the attack occurred because the school had cleared away the dense bushes where the assailant had hidden before jumping me. I also noticed that the university had installed call boxes at both ends of the trail. It was wonderful to feel my own strength and recovery, as well as to recognize the efforts that had been made to prevent sexual assaults.

I lean my bike along the railing of a new ultramodern footbridge that spans the Willamette River near downtown Eugene and reflect on the social changes that have occurred since *The Sexual Healing Journey* was first released in 1991. Back then, it felt daring to write about sex and sexual abuse. Today these topics are far more popularized and appear in magazine articles, books, television shows, and movies. People are no longer shocked when an actress, politician, or author publicly discloses past sexual abuse. In general, victims are more believed and less blamed. A large body of scientific studies has validated the phenomenon of repressed memories of sexual abuse. The relationship between past trauma and dissociation has been examined more closely. It has been great to witness the serious attention and shifts in public opinion concerning issues such as sexual harassment, sexual addiction, sexual health, acquaintance rape, victims' rights, and child advocacy.

While we still have a long way to go in terms of our culture, we have made great strides in acknowledging sexual abuse and its aftereffects. A lot of healing has happened in just a decade's time.

Looking back, I see the tremendous influence the book has had on my professional career. It catapulted me into a life of travel, lecturing, media appearances, and more writing. I coproduced two videotapes on sexual healing for survivors and their intimate partners. I designed and presented a day-long "Sexual Healing Journey" seminar to thousands of professionals throughout the United States, Canada, and New Zealand. This day-long training continues to be in demand. I have been interviewed about sexual recovery on many radio and TV talk shows. I speak at major conferences and deliver public lectures for survivors and partners wanting to learn more about sexual recovery. I feel privileged to be part of a community of committed and caring people who are dedicated to recovery from sexual abuse.

My work on sexual healing has led me in two new directions: studying sexual fantasy and developing resources that inspire healthy sexual intimacy. Some survivors who read *The Sexual Healing Journey* asked for more help understanding and healing problems with sexual fantasies. I saw that such problems are common, though extremely difficult to bring out in the open. Intrigued, I went on to do clinical and survey research on sexual fantasy. I discovered more about the origins, types, and functions of fantasy and gained a better sense of the difficulties people experience when their sexual fantasies stem from negative sexual experiences or unresolved psychological issues.

Eventually, I developed healing strategies for survivors to use with troublesome fantasies. These strategies are described in *Private Thoughts: Exploring the Power of Women's Sexual Fantasies*, coauthored with my journalist friend, Suzie Boss. While the book focuses on women's issues, it also provides a lot of information helpful to men with sexual fantasy concerns.

I also turned to literature for inspiring works which could help survivors create new, positive images of sex. Working in the sexual abuse field for so many years and hearing about the destructive ways humans act sexually, I wanted to explore the life-affirming qualities and beauty of sexual interactions based on caring, respect, and real intimacy. As a result, I compiled two poetry anthologies, *Passionate Hearts* and *Intimate Kisses*, celebrating the joys of healthy sexual love and pleasure. It was healing for me to be exposed to so many vivid descriptions of healthy sexual sharing.

I am delighted that in the last ten years *The Sexual Healing Journey* has been so positively received. My colleagues in the therapy field tell me they regard this as the seminal work on how to heal the sexual problems caused by abuse. The book has been lauded for providing a flexible approach to sexual recovery that combines mind, body, and relationship healing techniques. It is listed on many bibliographies—and now, web pages—for survivors, intimate partners, and therapists. Since it was first published, *The Sexual Healing Journey* has sold more than 100,000 copies.

Survivors around the world have sent letters of appreciation. An Australian woman recently wrote, "Thank you for your truth and honesty and your style of thinking, relating, and writing. The tone is gentle, yet firm, and covers all facets of the problems, appropriately and professionally." And a survivor from Connecticut sent a card saying, "*The Sexual Healing Journey* is an incredible resource. It's very healing to read other people's stories and quotes. I've worked on intimacy issues for many years now and can finally see, feel, and know that some powerful positive changes have occurred. Your book has been very healing for me and I just wanted to let you know that."

While I treasure these letters, I also understand that the book is, and always has been, an accumulation and sharing of information acquired from the life experiences of many people besides myself. My primary role has been that of a conduit for survivors, partners, and other therapists. I'm most proud of having helped bring the material to people who can benefit from it.

I hop back on my bike and head back home, thinking about how happy I am that *The Sexual Healing Journey* has remained in print and available for so long. In celebration of the book's ten-year anniversary, I've revised and updated sections where needed. I found myself altering the language a little, here and there, to reflect the stronger confidence I now have in the effectiveness of the approaches and healing techniques described in the book. As a more seasoned therapist, I am much more optimistic now about people's ability to heal fully and to create intensely rewarding and richly satisfying sexual lives after abuse. Experience has also taught me that when people solve their sexual problems, they often improve their self-esteem, assertiveness, and relationships. To flourish in life, we need to feel good about ourselves sexually.

This edition includes an improved and expanded Resources section to provide you with current information on books, articles, organizations, and residential treatment facilities. You'll also notice new listings for web sites that can be helpful to survivors, partners, and therapists involved in sexual recovery work.

In your hands you hold a safe, private way to begin sexual healing. This book outlines a model for healthy sex and describes the journey that can take you there. It offers you new insights into what happened, how it influenced you, and how you can change ingrained sexual attitudes and behaviors that hinder your enjoyment of life. I want to help you feel comfortable addressing and discussing sexual issues with others and to give you the tools you will need to accomplish your own sexual healing.

This book is based on my firm belief that *no one should have to suffer through life sexually damaged because of something that happened in the past. Healthy sex is something everyone deserves and can achieve.*

Wendy Maltz
Eugene, Oregon
May 2000

Most of the quotes and stories in this book come from questionnaires, interviews, counseling sessions, and workshops. Names and identifying details of the surviviors and partners mentioned have been changed. In some cases, composite accounts have been created based on the author's professional expertise.

Introduction

About the Sexual Healing Journey

Life is an adventure to be explored, not a problem to be solved.

—A Survivor

When I was in junior high I was captain of a girls' softball team. One cool, dewy morning we huddled on the pitcher's mound, trying not to feel self-conscious in our shorts and ironed shirts as packs of boys ran laps around the surrounding field. A starched and scrubbed physical education teacher began giving us tips on the upcoming game. After she finished citing a few rules, she paused and then quickly added in a whisper, "If the ball hits your crotch, grab your *knees* and scream. If the ball hits your breasts, grab your *head* and scream." We looked at each other in puzzled, embarrassed silence until a few girls giggled. Looking back, I realize that we were coached not to mention the real part of us that hurt. The message was clear: Sexual hurts were considered unmentionable.

Old cultural taboos against paying direct attention to sexual concerns can create a "knees and head" approach to sex. This attitude may obscure our ability to address our sexual concerns directly. We may ignore, sidestep or downplay sexual issues out of embarrassment, shame, and fear. It's almost as though we don't see the word *sex* in the phrase *sexual abuse*. But sexual abuse does cause *sexual* harm.

As a therapist who specializes in sexual abuse and sex therapy, I help survivors travel their own sexual healing journeys. One of their common goals is to have a healthy sex life, something each one of us has a right to enjoy. To get there survivors of sexual abuse have to overcome the damage of the past and to build their own, new models of sexuality based on a sense of choice, renewed self-respect, and a commitment to emotional intimacy.

Although each journey is personal, many survivors move through similar territories and challenges as they sexually heal. This book is designed to be your guide in navigating these sometimes turbulent waters. I will present a variety of techniques and exercises to help you evaluate and overcome the effects of past sexual abuse.

At the start of your healing process, it may help you to know that old, hurtful myths about abuse—myths that may have caused you to bottle up your own pain for many years—are being challenged and dismantled. That "knees and head" approach to talking about sex, which has for years inhibited frank discussions of sexual abuse, has finally grown as outdated as my old gym teacher's starched shirt. Talking honestly about the parts of us that hurt is no longer considered taboo.

As a society we have finally begun facing important facts about sexual abuse.*

This dissemination of new information and change in social attitudes about sexual abuse has helped some survivors to remember abuse they had long ago repressed. For other survivors—such as those, like me, who were victims of date rape—it may take time and a new awareness to accurately label past events as sexual abuse. With less shame and in increasing numbers, both men and women survivors are stepping forward and declaring, "Yes, this happened to me, too."

That's seldom enough to effect healing, however. For many survivors past abuse continues to interfere with their enjoyment of sex and intimacy. They may feel anxious about sex. They may feel anxious even talking about sex.

Indeed, a history of sexual abuse can disrupt many facets of our sexuality. Past abuse may continue to affect

- how we feel about being a man or a woman
- how we feel about our bodies, sex organs, and bodily functions
- how we think about sex
- how we express ourselves sexually
- how we experience physical pleasure and intimacy with others

By learning to face sexual issues directly, survivors can overcome the sexual harm that was done to them.

* See box, pg. 4–5.

SEXUAL SYMPTOMS OF SEXUAL ABUSE

Sexual abuse creates specific kinds of problems with sex. Here is a partial checklist of the most common problems I see in my clinical practice. These symptoms and others will be discussed in more detail later, but for now you may want to consider whether any of these statements apply to you.

TOP TEN SEXUAL SYMPTOMS OF SEXUAL ABUSE

_____   I avoid, fear, or lack interest in sex.
_____   I approach sex as an obligation.
_____   I experience negative feelings such as anger, disgust, or guilt with touch.
_____   I have difficulty becoming aroused or feeling sensation.
_____   I feel emotionally distant or not present during sex.
_____   I experience intrusive or disturbing sexual thoughts and images.
_____   I engage in compulsive or inappropriate sexual behaviors.
_____   I have difficulty establishing or maintaining an intimate relationship.
_____   I experience vaginal pain or orgasmic difficulties.
_____   I have erectile or ejaculatory difficulty.

These symptoms can show up immediately after sexual assault, emerge slowly over time, or come on suddenly, long after the abuse occurred. They can exist both before and after we've identified ourselves as survivors.

Sexual symptoms of sexual abuse don't often go away on their own. To overcome them, most survivors must actively work at healing. Although addressing sexual symptoms can be rough going at times, it is possible to heal. Recently a survivor shared, "I had almost all of these symptoms when I started sexual healing several years ago. Now many have gone, and the few that are left are manageable."

Don't be surprised if you feel anxious, or even afraid, about beginning your own sexual healing journey. Such feelings are common and will diminish as you proceed. It can help to remember that on this trip you are in the driver's seat, controlling how far and how fast you travel. To prepare for the journey and to give you an idea of what you can expect along the way, I'll address some concerns you may have.

INFORMATION ABOUT SEXUAL ABUSE

Sexual abuse is epidemic. Research estimates indicate that about one in three women and one in four to seven men have been victims of sexual abuse as children.* Adult forms of sexual abuse, such as date, acquaintance, and stranger rape, and other types of sexual exploitation are also extremely prevalent.

No one is immune to sexual abuse. Sexual abuse happens to women and men of all races, ages, cultures, religions, socioeconomic levels, and sexual orientations.

Victims of sexual abuse are not to blame. The responsibility for sexual abuse rests solely with the offender.

Sexual abuse is difficult to remember. It is estimated that about half of all survivors suffer from some form of memory loss. It is often not until survivors feel supported and secure that they begin to recall their sexual abuse.

Sexual abuse is difficult to disclose. Because of feelings of shame, embarrassment, or fear, many victims of sexual abuse do not report sexual abuse experiences. Many survivors have endured years of silent suffering.

Sexual abuse has serious long-lasting effects. The trauma of sexual abuse can be at the root of many psychological problems such as depression, anxiety, low self-esteem, self-abusive behaviors, social problems, sexual problems, and food, chemical, or sexual addictions. In addition, sexual abuse has been linked with such medical problems as headaches, asthma, heart palpitations, stomach pain, spastic colon, pelvic pain, fainting, dizziness, and a variety of chronic physical complaints.

Recovery is possible. Survivors can recover from the effects of sexual abuse using steps that involve recognizing effects, dealing with memories, overcoming guilt feelings, developing self-trust, grieving for loss, expressing anger, disclosing the abuse, resolving feelings toward the offender, improving health care, and learning that sex can be safe, healthy, and enjoyable.† A variety of resources for healing have become available to help survivors recover. These include books, tapes, newsletters, television discussions, counseling centers, support groups, sexual abuse organizations, and conferences.‡

*For sources on the prevalence of sexual abuse, see studies reported in *Child Sexual Abuse* by David Finkelhor, *The Secret Trauma* by Diana Russell, and *Abused Boys* by Mic Hunter. Figures on prevalence of sexual abuse are constantly changing, with increases primarily in the number of males estimated as victims. All four of these books are listed in the Resources section at the end of the book.

Complete publishing information for sources not appearing in the Resources section is given in the footnotes themselves.

†For a more detailed description of these stages, see Ellen Bass and Laura Davis's *The Courage to Heal* and Mike Lew's *Victims No Longer.*

‡See the Resources section for a listing of organizations and support groups.

WHO CAN GO ON THE SEXUAL HEALING JOURNEY?

Anyone. You don't have to first remember your abuse or identify yourself as a survivor of sexual abuse. Sexual healing can help you to determine whether you were ever sexually abused and to what extent. To take this sexual healing journey, all you need is a desire to learn about sexual healing or a feeling that this book may help you improve your sex and intimacy experiences.

While this book primarily speaks to survivors of sexual abuse, it also provides a resource book for intimate partners, therapists, friends, and family members of survivors who want to learn about sexual healing as well as to support survivors who are making changes. In addition, many of the ideas and exercises in this book can help people overcome sexual problems from other causes, such as antisex upbringings, psychological stress, relationship difficulties, medical illness or injury, sexual addiction, and other negative sexual experiences besides sexual abuse.

You can go on this journey alone or with an intimate partner. If you are single, you may wish to begin sexual healing without a partner. Nancy, a forty-year-old rape survivor, worked for months on sexual healing before considering becoming involved in an intimate relationship. Several months after her therapy ended, Nancy entered her most stable and satisfying relationship ever. By first healing alone sexually, she had laid the groundwork for new sexual intimacy.

If you have an intimate partner, he or she can help you by providing support and understanding. A man survivor told me his wife's ability to talk frankly with him about sex reduced his long-standing sexual anxiety. And a woman survivor found that her partner's interest in learning about sexual abuse and attending counseling sessions with her helped her feel she wasn't alone and abandoned. Sexual abuse and the recovery process affect both partners in a couple relationship. When couples learn how to work together in sexual recovery, they can heal individually and strengthen intimacy together.

HOW DOES SEXUAL HEALING WORK?

Sexual healing is a dynamic process. We gain understanding about how our sexuality has been affected by sexual abuse, make changes in our sexual attitudes and behaviors, and develop new skills for experiencing sex in a positive way. One type of change encourages another.

Lynn's experience as a twenty-seven-year-old married survivor illustrates this process. When Lynn was a child her older brother would often take her into the bathroom, fondle her, and attempt intercourse with her. Years later Lynn married her high school sweetheart, Hal. Throughout their marriage Lynn had difficulty becoming sexually aroused and enjoying sex. Sex became rare and was often an upsetting ordeal.

Before Lynn sought counseling she had no idea that her sexual problems with Hal might have resulted from the earlier sexual abuse. It wasn't until Lynn wept uncontrollably after sex one night that she realized a serious problem existed and that she needed help. While in counseling, Lynn made a connection between her ongoing sexual problems and the molestation by her brother. She discovered that she had learned to view sex as a duty, an act without choice, and an experience strongly associated with vaginal pain. Her sexual withdrawal from Hal was related to her old fears.

This new understanding prompted Lynn to begin changing her attitudes about sex. Lynn wondered if what she thought was sex was really sex *abuse*. She began to feel she had been cheated out of learning that sex could be something desirable, pleasurable, and fun. And she realized she could be a sexually healthy person after all.

With the help of counseling, Lynn learned new skills. She learned to create a temporary moratorium on sex, giving her needed time to heal and helping her realize she had a choice to say no to her husband's sexual advances. Lynn stopped associating sex with obligation, guilt, and pressure. She spent months learning to initiate and enjoy nonsexual touch. With Hal's cooperation she did special exercises to relax and stretch her vaginal muscles to make intercourse more comfortable. Lynn worked intensively for more than a year, and slowly she understood and resolved her feelings about the abuse.

As Lynn practiced new skills, she experienced her sexual feelings in a new way. Her responses changed. Eventually, Lynn's sexual experiences came to feel within her control and for her own pleasure.

> I didn't know what "sexual person" meant before. To allow myself to become sexually aroused has been a wonderful learning experience. I'm still learning to deal with sexual feelings . . . not to turn them off but to let them grow and become more sexual. I can just hug Hal if I want to do that, or make love, if that's what both of us feel like doing. If it's not right I can say so. I've never felt like I had these choices before.

You can also begin a sexual healing journey. You can identify your sexual concerns, learn how sexual abuse has affected your sexuality, get rid of old attitudes and behaviors that resulted from the abuse, and develop a new, healthier approach to sexual enjoyment.

Healing our sexual injuries allows us to heal in a basic way. We journey from intimate injury to sexual health. Through sexual healing we can overcome the harm and empower ourselves to experience sex anew.

HOW LONG DOES SEXUAL HEALING TAKE?

There are no easy answers or quick fixes. Sudden breakthroughs in healing occur rarely. In most cases changes come little by little, over months or years. Sexual healing usually takes a long time and involves real effort. New information and understanding are constantly being integrated as significant changes in attitudes and behavior are being made. It takes time to change established patterns of thinking and responding. Sexual healing is usually never as fast as survivors and intimate partners would wish. As one survivor said, "It takes as long as it takes." When you give yourself the time it takes, the rewards are well worth the experience.

HOW DOES SEXUAL HEALING RELATE TO GENERAL HEALING FROM THE ABUSE?

Healing can begin at many starting points. Different people heal in different ways. For many therapists and survivors alike, addressing sexual issues is seen as a final stage in sexual abuse recovery. Sexual concerns often emerge naturally after survivors have resolved feelings of anger and fear about the abuse and toward the offender, and after survivors have begun to feel better about, and take better care of, themselves. Many survivors seem more prepared to address the difficult topic of sex after having recovered generally from the abuse.

This traditional sequence makes a lot of sense in theory, but it's not always the way it works in practice. Sexual concerns come up at all points in sexual abuse recovery: beginning, middle, and later stages. Sometimes a specific sexual problem provides the impetus for a survivor to seek treatment in the first place. Mitch, a survivor of molestation by a woman neighbor, entered therapy to deal with a troublesome sexual problem. "I would ejaculate as soon as intercourse would start," he explained. "It was embarrassing. I knew something was wrong because I had no trouble lasting when I was by myself."

Looking for the cause of his sexual problem led Mitch to recall the abuse he had experienced as a teen. He needed to resolve his feelings of anger toward women, as well as a fear of humiliation that had resulted from the abuse. Mitch sought therapy as a way of helping him overcome the problem that concerned him most, his sexual functioning.

Sexual issues may emerge in the middle stages of general healing as we realize more about what happened to us and how it has affected our attitudes, our self-esteem, and important relationships in our lives. If sexual issues are not dealt with to some extent when they come up, we may inadvertently undermine our progress in general healing.

Mary, a lesbian survivor, lost all interest in sexual contact while she was in therapy with me working through her feelings from childhood sexual abuse. Although this is a common reaction for a survivor to have, it created havoc in her relationship with her partner, Joann. Joann was angry and depressed about the lack of sexual interaction. Joann's biggest fear was that Mary had stopped loving and trusting her. Mary had trouble keeping her mind on her general recovery because she was so disturbed by and concerned about Joann's reaction. Before Mary could resume work on general recovery, she and Joann had to work through their sexual issues and find new ways for intimate sharing and for expressing love. Sexual healing enabled Mary's general healing to continue.

Taking time to resolve specific sexual problems often assists other recovery work. George, a twenty-five-year-old male survivor of molestation by his uncle, found himself at an impasse in recovery from alcohol abuse. Often George would go home from his alcohol recovery group meetings and compulsively masturbate to degrading pornographic pictures. His compulsive sexual behavior was generating feelings of self-loathing and shame. He felt bad about himself and unable to share honestly and intimately with members in his recovery group. For George sexual healing became important in enabling him to break free from the hurtful cycle he was in. His sexual healing helped him gain understanding and control of his sexual impulses. As a result his self-respect and self-esteem were finally able to improve.

Sexual healing and general recovery need to work together in the same way that music and lyrics work together to make song: They alternate and blend together at different times. They are complementary, not isolated, experiences.

By incorporating sexual healing into a broader healing journey, survivors can flexibly shift back and forth from general to sexual healing when necessary. Sexual healing allows survivors to grow stronger.

WILL I NEED SPECIAL HELP ON THE PATH TO SEXUAL HEALING?

Sexual healing is profound personal growth work. During the process you will probably look closely at who you are, how you feel, what has happened to you in the past, and how you now take care of yourself and relate to others. The journey can be filled with many emotional highs and lows. While it can be uplifting to increase understanding, to make changes, and to gain new skills, you may also become depressed or upset at times. Your daily routines may be upset, or your day-to-day functioning may suffer. Having special help can be an important way to take care of yourself and to facilitate your healing.

You may want to work with a therapist who specializes in sexual abuse treatment.* Survivors can benefit from joining a therapy or support group and spending time with friends who are familiar with healing

---

* Sexual abuse and sex therapy specialists can be found in social work, psychology, psychiatry, and counseling professions. The academic degree is less important than whether the therapist is specially trained to heal the sexual repercussions of sexual abuse. See the list of organizations and programs in the Resources section.

For information on sexual abuse treatment and sex therapy, and for advice on how to find a therapist, you may want to read chapter 11, "Getting Professional Help," in *Incest and Sexuality* by Wendy Maltz and Beverly Holman.

from sexual abuse. If you are currently in therapy, talk with your therapist about your desire to focus on sexual concerns.

If you are a survivor of sexual abuse and find yourself caught up in self-destructive or extreme behaviors, seek qualified professional help. Your sexual healing won't be as productive, and may even be stymied, if other more critical issues aren't addressed. Any of the following problems should be resolved with the help of a professional: alcohol or other drug abuse, suicidal thinking, violent behavior, self-harm, criminal or offensive sexual activities or addictions, psychological problems such as severe depression or multiple personalities, or participation in an abusive relationship. Once you have begun to address these more crucial problems, sexual healing can be incorporated as part of your total recovery.

HOW CAN I BEST USE THIS BOOK?

This book can be used in a number of ways to help you sexually heal. If the idea of sexual healing brings up a lot of anxiety or fear, you may want to approach the material in this book with the understanding that you are primarily going to "read about" sexual healing. I have organized the book in progression, the information in the early chapters providing a foundation for the more active healing work discussed later. In this learning approach you may choose to read about the exercises, suggestions, and new skills, but not to do them yet. When you have read through the book once, you will have an idea of what sexual healing involves and where it can lead. This understanding can help you feel ready to do more active sexual healing in the future.

You can also take a pick-and-choose approach to the material in this book. Read about sexual healing, and do the exercises and suggestions that appeal to you now. Everyone heals differently, so it is important to be able to individualize the contents of this book to meet your needs at this time in your life.

Some survivors, especially those who have done a lot of work in sexual abuse and sexual healing already, may want to use this book more actively. You can use it, pencil in hand, as a workbook, marking the inventories and doing the exercises—jotting down ideas and reactions as you go.

It may be a good idea, whatever the degree of your active involvement, to keep a journal while you are reading the book. Sexual healing requires you to face your most personal feelings. Writing about them as you work through the book may help you resolve feelings now and may give you a record of personal growth that can help you in the future.

For survivors who are in counseling, you can use the book to augment your therapy. It can help you identify areas to focus on with your therapist. You might take an inventory or do an exercise and then discuss your responses and feelings in therapy. You may want to underline or highlight passages in the book that you find particularly significant and to share them with your therapist.

As you can see, there is no right way to use this book. It is designed to be a healing resource you can refer to at different times in your life.

HOW DO I BEGIN MY SEXUAL HEALING JOURNEY?

Begin your journey only when you feel ready for it. Go slowly. Pace yourself. Trust yourself. Remember: This is *your* journey.

So let's get started. You *can* repair the damage done to you in the past. You can look forward to a new surge of self-respect, personal contentment, and emotional intimacy. When you reclaim your sexuality, you reclaim yourself.

PART ONE

Starting Out

Becoming Aware

1

Realizing There's a Sexual Issue

Your pain is the breaking of the shell that encloses your understanding.

—KAHLIL GIBRAN, *The Prophet*

It was a cool November evening. Wrapped in big, fluffy towels, Sally and Jim crept onto their secluded backyard deck, took off the cover of their hot tub, slipped out of their towels, and eased into the hot water. Relaxing in their hot tub was one of their favorite things to do together. For Jim it was the only time Sally seemed comfortable letting him touch her anymore. Since their wedding day six years earlier, their sex life had been a problem. No matter what Jim tried, Sally never seemed aroused. Now they would let a month or two go by without having sex. Lately Sally would even pull away from him when he would start to give her a hug.

But something felt different tonight. Once in the tub Sally began touching Jim. He was surprised—even shocked—at first. Sally stroked him in ways she never had before. Jim laughed, telling her he felt attacked. He was delighted too. All of a sudden Sally broke down. She sobbed uncontrollably. Jim was shattered.

Jim leaned toward her. "What is it, honey?" he asked. Slowly and tearfully, Sally said, "I don't know why, but I find you a sexual bore. I'm not interested in having sex with you in the least. I'm real close to having an affair with another man."

Jim couldn't believe what he was hearing. He had no idea Sally felt this way. They'd always avoided talking about the sexual part of their relationship even though they both knew it was a problem. He felt like

15

his whole world had fallen apart. Is it me? Is it her? he wondered. I just don't know. I'm scared to death.

Sally was confused as well, later recalling that

> the biggest thing on my mind was that this other man, a virtual stranger, had aroused me sexually. That had never happened to me before. I didn't think I was capable of getting so aroused, and it scared me. I thought, why can someone else turn me on when my husband doesn't? That night in the hot tub, all these feelings and words just came pouring out from I'm not quite sure where. It was awful. I knew it was important at the time to finally get my sadness out. And it got us talking a lot and admitting that something was definitely wrong.

Neither of them will ever forget the moment they realized they had a serious sexual problem. But once the problem had surfaced, they could begin to do something about it. Sally and Jim's family physician referred them to me for therapy. Sally had previously told the physician that she was a survivor of sexual abuse.

In counseling, Sally and Jim were again surprised. I suggested that Sally's lack of sexual interest in Jim and her attraction to this other man might be repercussions of the molestation she had suffered years before by her brother. Sally explained her confusion:

> I couldn't figure it out. . . . When I talked to people before about having been sexually abused, they tended to downplay it. I thought it wasn't a big deal because I knew what had happened, who had done it, why it had happened. . . . I was led to believe that meant I had come to grips with it and it wasn't causing me any problems. That first day of counseling we began exploring the abuse in much more detail, and discovered that it was the crux of the problem.

Today, seven years and two children later, Sally and Jim look back with pride on their sexual recovery process. They have told me that they enjoy a deeper intimacy and a more satisfying sexual life than they ever thought possible.

I hear many stories like Sally and Jim's in my practice. No one comes to see me feeling excited or happy that they've recognized a sexual concern. Rather, they usually enter therapy feeling emotionally pained and desperate. Unresolved sexual issues may be straining their relationship, but even though they want help, it's not uncommon for survivors to resist looking at sexual issues. Many couples are unclear what role, if any, past sexual abuse could be playing in their current problems.

Sexual concerns *are* hard to face. They're personal and embarrassing. When we have a sexual problem, we may try to deny it or hope it will just go away by itself. Sometimes we worry that admitting our problems will cause others to reject us or think less of us. We may go through a lot of pain before we're willing to admit we have a substantial problem and want to do something about it.

How do we finally come to admit we have a sexual problem that needs attention? Often the admission comes at a key moment, like a flash of discovery. We're able to acknowledge a problem for the first time. Or if we've already been aware of a problem, we're suddenly able to see its significance more clearly. It's often not until we feel confused, hopeless, unfulfilled, or self-destructive that we can no longer ignore the real source of our trouble. Then our pain can open a door. Thus the sexual healing journey begins.

COMMON SITUATIONS OF SURVIVORS

Let's first take a look at four common situations survivors may find themselves in when they realize they are facing a significant sexual issue. Consider whether any of them apply to your own life.

_____ I'm acting in strange ways that don't make sense.
_____ My sexual problem isn't getting any better.
_____ My partner is hurting.
_____ New circumstances have made me more aware.

"I'm acting in strange ways that don't make sense"

Sexual issues can surface when *we begin acting in strange ways that we can't deny and don't understand.* We may have unusual reactions to routine situations.

After visiting her gynecologist for a routine Pap smear, Doris found herself sitting in her car for half an hour, crying. Michael became sick to his stomach when he entered a public restroom. Myra was shocked and disturbed that she became sexually aroused after reading a story about sexual abuse in the newspaper.

Normal social interactions can generate feelings of panic and fear. Receiving a friendly pat on the shoulder or a gentle hug can cause some survivors to stiffen. Thinking about asking someone out on a date can trigger feelings of overwhelming anxiety.

A gay psychology student found that his reactions to touch prevented him from learning a new therapy skill.

> I wanted to study bodywork. The training involved giving and receiving many types of massage. I became sickly afraid of having people touch me. Lots of fears came up in class. When I got home, I wasn't able to relate sexually with my boyfriend. It was then I realized that I had a problem with touch and sex.

Survivors may react strangely to the possibility of sex. They may end up feeling pulled in two directions, simultaneously wanting and not wanting sex. "There is a grip on me," one survivor said. "I don't even know that it is there until I try to be sexual. Then I feel like a victim, and locked in."

Some survivors realize they have a sexual problem when they find themselves giving their partners mixed messages about wanting sexual intimacy, such as one woman described:

> I want my husband to find me sexually attractive. I'll go to great lengths to improve my appearance so that he will. I wear sexy clothes and paint my nails. But if he gets sexually excited and interested in me, I'm annoyed. Why do I feel disappointed when I should be glad?

Some survivors are alarmed to find themselves having strong sexual feelings at times when sex is impossible. "I'll get filled with passion when I'm at work during the day," one man said. "Yet I retreat from the idea of sex at night or on the weekends, when sex is possible. I avoid it. Sometimes I'll watch television, fall asleep on the couch, stay up late, work, or wait until it's pretty late before I come home."

A woman survivor had a similar experience. "I'll start fights with my partner just to keep from having sex," she said. "On weekend mornings I'll plan an entire agenda to keep us busy so I don't have to be close. I don't understand why I'd rather clean the toilet than have sex!"

Survivors may be shocked at their unconscious reactions to touch and sex. They may find themselves suddenly doing odd or hurtful things to their intimate partners. In the middle of the night, while still asleep, a woman survivor hit her husband in the back. He was stunned. A gentle man by nature, he turned over, calmly woke her, and asked her to stop. It concerned her that she was expressing feelings toward him that he didn't deserve.

A partner's request for sex and sexual activities can trigger an abrupt response, as this woman described: "I got very angry with my husband if he wanted sex. Once I got so angry I *bit* him. I had no idea why I was that angry."

Survivors may realize their sexual behavior is inappropriate. After a kiss on a first date, a seventeen-year-old incest survivor shocked herself by unzipping her date's pants and performing oral sex on him. She had no conscious memory of ever engaging in oral sex in the past.

> I felt in a trance. It was as if a part of me had been waiting, trained and ready to go. The boy told me to stop. I felt embarrassed and stunned. I was shocked I had touched him in the first place.

Rachel felt frustrated by her sexual behavior, as well.

> I was involved in a relationship which I truly valued. I began to experience serious problems in intimacy. I found myself becoming irrational, and alternately spiteful or clinging. I began to crave sex and attention. But I would weep uncontrollably when my partner would try to make love, and if we did end up having sex, I was so anxious I couldn't climax.

Fran became concerned when she began squelching her own enjoyment during sex.

> In the middle of sex I became obsessed with a little bump on my partner's back. The obsession filled my mind to the point that I emotionally checked out. I shut down all feeling, and had to stop. I was unable to go any further.

Angie was also upset at how she denied herself sexual pleasure.

> I was having sex with my boyfriend when I suddenly became uptight and anxious. My thoughts scattered and dispersed like detergent in a pool of oil. I was totally unable to have an orgasm. I couldn't focus. I kept short-circuiting before I'd get there. I didn't know what was happening with me. It was scary.

Although such reactions can seem irrational and upsetting, they draw our attention to the fact that we have a problem. Awareness brings motivation to change, as this survivor's story illustrates.

> My husband and I were making love. Suddenly I was washed over by an overwhelming wave of anger. Inside my head I was screaming things like *"I hate men! I hate penises! I hate it that they enjoy this and I don't!"* I rolled over crying and screaming. After awhile the screaming was replaced by a voice of resolve inside me that said, *"I don't want it to be like this anymore!"* Soon after, I sought out counseling, and the memories of my abuse began to surface.

"My sexual problem isn't getting any better"

We may realize something's wrong when *we have a specific sexual problem that doesn't go away, has no medical cause, and is causing us more and more anxiety.*

Six months after being raped, Dawn was upset that she still didn't want sex with her husband. Jo, an incest survivor, couldn't reach orgasm with her lover even though she loved, trusted, and felt safe with him.

Some survivors may repeatedly sabotage their own best efforts to form close relationships. A twenty-five-year-old survivor wanted to start dating, but he froze when meeting women.

> I was very unhappy because I would become shy and clam up, saying little or nothing at all around women I liked and wanted to know better. If I did start talking with a woman, I would find myself feeling uncomfortable, very nervous, and somewhat scared.

It hurts to realize we've been denying ourselves pleasures other people enjoy. Some survivors feel caught in a web of negative sexual attitudes, inhibitions, and unfulfilling experiences. "The worst part of sex is foreplay," a woman survivor said. "Intercourse isn't so bad because I know it's almost over." Another survivor felt similarly:

> Sex is an ordeal, not an opportunity for closeness or pleasure. I'll tell myself, Okay, I'll do it this time—maybe it won't last too long—when it's over I'll be safe for a while. It bothers me that I think of sex like taking out the garbage—something that has to be done regularly, with small reprieves in between.

Self-denying or secretive behavior may finally cause survivors to admit something's wrong. They may fake enjoyment, focus solely on the partner's pleasure, or not communicate what they need to feel satisfied sexually. This behavior can create emotional distance, resentment, and self-loathing in relationships. The consequences can bring pain. A survivor described such a result:

> I have shut down my own sexual feelings and shifted my focus to satisfying my partner's sexual needs and desires. I often feel used and degraded as a result of not paying attention to my own feelings.

Survivors who routinely deny their feelings can become caught up in a charade. Candy faked orgasms for two years. As more time passed her behavior became unbearable for her. Although it was extremely hard to do, she decided to tell her boyfriend the truth.

> I needed to be special to men in some way—and the best way I knew was sexual. I'd get them sexually intoxicated with me. It didn't feel like I was denying myself for a long time, since I got a lot of mental satisfaction witnessing how much I could get them turned on. But lately since I've been valuing myself more and liking my boyfriend more as a friend, it just felt too phony not to tell him.

Although her boyfriend was shocked and hurt, he appreciated the new level of honesty and trust her disclosure made possible. As a couple they had begun their sexual healing journey.

Many survivors reach a point when they no longer want to engage in self-denying behaviors. They admit they have a problem that needs to be addressed.

Survivors may feel out of control with sex. That also can provide the impetus for a survivor to realize a problem exists. Survivors may find themselves consumed by their own compulsive drive for sex. They may be unable to stop themselves from being promiscuous, having secretive sexual affairs, or engaging in dangerous sexual activities. It's frightening. "I feel like I'm living in a house that's perched on a cliff," a survivor said.

Secrecy, shame, guilt, and fear are the by-products of being out of control with sex. These feelings can eat at our sense of self-worth. Our addictive and compulsive behaviors can prevent us from forming healthy intimate relationships. A twenty-three-year-old woman survivor explained:

I woke up one day and realized I was in the midst of "dating" three men at the same time. I had slept with all of them on the first date and was continuing to sleep with them all. I felt completely out of control, hated myself, enjoyed *none* of the sexual experiences, cared *nothing* for any of the men! My life was a mess and I was headed for disaster. I started to feel suicidal. Somehow it dawned on me that I needed to take control and take care of me. For the first time in my life I realized that I did not want nor have to be sexual. I just couldn't anymore. Within a month of cutting off these relationships and being celibate, I remembered the abuse experiences with my father.

Fear of sexually transmitted diseases such as AIDS has sparked many people with sexually addictive behaviors to recognize the seriousness of their out-of-control sex. Sexually promiscuous survivors may fail to use protection such as condoms or birth control. Then they become frightened to realize that the need to please a partner or get sexual attention could make them sick or lead to infertility, unwanted pregnancy, or even death.

Concern over solitary sexual behavior and thoughts can be yet another impetus for admitting that a problem exists. Some survivors compulsively masturbate, use pornography or need abusive fantasies for arousal, or habitually give sexual meaning to everyday experiences. A survivor who can't join in a game of volleyball, for example, without becoming sexually aroused by his teammates may be ready to admit he has a problem.

"My partner is hurting"

Survivors must pursue sexual healing because they want to, not because they feel they have to in order to save a dying relationship. Yet, we can realize we have a sexual issue when *we learn more about our partner's emotional pain and want things to improve.*

Often the partner of a survivor suffers most from a sexual problem. Survivors may not be concerned that they have sexual addictions, lack satisfaction in sex, or avoid sex. "I'd be just fine if we never had sex again," a survivor might say. What may be most disturbing is witnessing how much our partners hurt. A survivor explained her dilemma:

I was pushing my partner away because I would freeze during sex and I didn't know why. I never thought of the abuse when we had sex, but apparently my subconscious did. My partner felt as if there was something wrong with him and that I didn't want him. He felt as if he was a horrible person for wanting sex. He's been deeply affected, and it hurts me to see him this way.

Partners often suffer from anxiety, depression, and emotional stress that result from the sexual problems in their relationship. When survivors withdraw from physical intimacy or are not emotionally present during sex, partners can feel rejected, inadequate, and sexually unattractive.

Daniel sat next to his wife, a survivor, at their first counseling session and explained:

It hurts when my wife gives the message that sex is disgusting. She'll say, "All right, just get it over with. How can you want me, I'm so fat. You don't care about me, you're just using me." Why is she so defensive? She assumes I'm out to get her. Lately, even were she to initiate sex, I don't think I'd want it. For her there is no con-nection between expressing love and having sex. I have given up. Sexually, I'm withdrawn and I feel withered up. I have only general love and friendship feelings toward my wife. But my heart is closing up. I lack faith in her ability to change. I have no expectations for change anymore. I'm thinking of moving out. I'm tired of feeling anger and frustration all the time.

Survivors who are compulsively drawn to sexual activity may cause their partners pain. A survivor who sneaks around or lies to maintain secretive sexual behaviors can hurt a partner. Bev, a bisexual survivor, was shocked when her female partner became very upset and threatened to leave the relationship. Bev said, "I finally realized how much it hurt her when I'd complain that we weren't having sex enough or turn away from her to flirt with others."

It's not uncommon for partners to develop sexual problems of their own. They may lose interest in having sex, or they may start experiencing trouble climaxing or reaching orgasm too quickly. (In chapter 11 we will discuss how partners and survivors can address specific sexual problems.)

This was true for Meg, the wife of a survivor. She began experienc-ing sexual problems in response to the troubles her husband was having in lovemaking.

During sex my husband gets so nervous and uptight that he tells me not to move around a lot. I used to love moving around. It was a big part of my total enjoyment of sex. Now when he tells me not to move, I just start checking out of what is happening. I stop lubricating and my vagina hurts. Sex has become painful. I don't feel I can say anything though, because I fear I might discourage him from trying again. Sometimes at work or at a party a friend will come up to me and just give me a hug or a touch on the shoulder. When this happens I remember how much I like touch and how easy it used to be for me before this relationship.

In some relationships a partner may become dissatisfied and have an affair. While this action can shock a survivor into realizing a serious concern exists, the overall effect of the affair can harm the survivor's ability to trust the partner. Survivors may feel angry and betrayed and may have trouble focusing on the original sexual issue that led to the affair. Or survivors may jump desperately into sexual healing, fearing further abandonment by their partner. Either way, progress may be handicapped.

Many partners feel trapped. They want to remain in the relationship but are angry and sad because they've lost physical intimacy.

It can be difficult for a survivor to witness a partner's emotional pain. Many survivors have a tendency to feel ashamed, angry at themselves, or responsible for their partner's suffering. If this is true for you, remind yourself that the abuse creating stress in your relationship was not your fault. Your partner's reactions are normal for the situation, not a reflection of what you hoped or intended for the relationship. And remember that your sexual healing will improve the relationship for you both.

"New circumstances have made me more aware"

Like the last drop of water that makes a cup run over, we may acknowledge a sexual issue when *we have one final experience in a series that forces us to look at things differently.* We see our problem for the first time or in a new perspective.

Marsha suffered through seven unsuccessful relationships, one after another, until she realized she used sex like bait.

After the breakup of my last relationship, I started to look at the role sex played for me. I found that I used sex to hook a man into a relationship with me so I could get my need for affection and security satisfied. Often, once I felt sure of the man's commitment, the sexual relationship would sour.

Once she recognized the pattern, Marsha could no longer avoid facing the many sexual fears and discomforts that had been hidden from her conscious awareness.

The last drop fell into Howard's cup one evening at a community gathering. He was in a restaurant, seated at a table with a large group of friends.

> I looked around the room and realized that I had had sex with all of the women in our group, but I had an intimate relationship with none of them. Yikes! I knew something was wrong.

A moment of realization often comes when survivors are recovering from another problem, such as a chemical addiction, an eating disorder, physical ailments, criminal behavior, or psychological problems. The process of recovery gives them a new perspective. They get a chance to take an honest, sober look at themselves. Sexual problems that were well masked or denied before often come into focus.

An incest survivor found that her sexual problems surfaced when she stopped using drugs.

> For about four years prior to becoming aware of sexual abuse in my past, I had been using marijuana, and later combining it with cocaine, to be able to enjoy sex. As I worked on my healing, I decided to stop using drugs. When I did, my sexual relationship became very unsatisfactory. It felt shallow and lacking in any expression of intimacy or love.

The drugs, like a narcotic fog, had been masking the pain caused years before by abuse.

Matt, a thirty-two-year-old survivor of incest perpetrated by his mother, was involved in an Alcoholics Anonymous twelve-step recovery program* when he realized he had acted in sexually abusive ways himself. While making a rigorous inventory of hurtful things he had

---

* The Twelve Steps of Alcoholics Anonymous were originally developed to guide men and women in recovery from alcoholism. These steps have been adapted for many kinds of self-help programs that address addictive and codependent behavior. The steps include admitting powerlessness over a problem, recognizing the need for help from a Higher Power such as God, making an inventory of past behavior, openly admitting and making amends for past wrongs, surrendering to receive help from one's Higher Power, and eventually achieving spiritual awakening.

done when drinking, Matt admitted he once raped a woman he dated. He recalled the effect of this admission:

> When doing this step in my recovery, I realized I had intimacy problems and a lot of sexual anger towards women. I thought the alcoholism had caused it, but I was wrong. Being an offender has caused tremendous guilt and a desire to make amends. I want to know why and how not to do it again.

As a result of realizing he was an alcoholic and a sexual offender, another survivor, Cory, began addressing sexual issues. Afraid that he might be sexually abusive again, he resolved to deal with his own problems. Sexual healing became a major goal in his recovery program.

> I went into treatment because I had been drunk and tried to fondle my nephew in bed. I basically got caught and thrown out of my home. That was the last night I drank, and that's been two and a half years. My thought processes didn't change, though, and it was driving me insane to think of the sexual things I did. I knew that I had to find out more about me or I might get loaded again, and not feel, and hurt someone else. In treatment I saw that I drank for so many years to hide the confusion, guilt, and shame that I felt about my sexuality. By becoming sober and learning how to feel things, I was able to take a look at me, my actions, and what had really happened to me.

Marilyn, a survivor who suffered from multiple-personality problems, did not identify her sexual issues until she was well into recovery. For many years Marilyn had a separate personality that would surface during sexual activity. As Marilyn progressed in therapy, this once split-off personality began to merge with other parts, and eventually it disappeared. Marilyn started to feel anxious about sex and had problems with sexual functioning. Having these feelings about sex was actually a milestone in her overall healing. But Marilyn wasn't too happy about experiencing them.

> The split that handled sexuality for me had very few problems other than wanting to maintain control during sex. I have more trouble with sex now, with more of myself present.

For many survivors, healing from abuse can flush unrecognized sexual problems out into the open. Images of past sexual abuse may start to haunt us, and we may get in touch with how vulnerable we feel during sexual activity. Nattie described her reaction:

> Until I discovered the sexual abuse, I had no trouble with orgasm. In the past four years since remembering the abuse, I have had difficulty feeling sensation, becoming aroused, and reaching orgasm by myself in masturbation and with a partner as well. I can't ignore these problems now that they're here.

Becoming aware of sexual issues is seldom easy. As a male survivor confided to me:

> I see myself in all four situations where survivors realize they have a sexual issue. It hurts like hell—I have become keenly aware of how isolated I've been all my life.

Recognizing sexual issues may hurt. But with the pain comes an entry point into the sexual healing journey. When sexual problems do surface, they often tell us we have reached a core issue in overall recovery. Once we admit something is wrong, we can direct our energy toward understanding and healing. And healing our sexual concerns can lead us to profound insights about ourselves and to improved relationships with others. The journey has begun.

2

Acknowledging
the Abuse

. . . My despair was not the darkness, but the injuries hidden within it.

—LOUISE WISECHILD, *The Obsidian Mirror*

One evening several years ago, I tuned in "The Barbara Walters Special." She was interviewing one of my favorite television actors, Don Johnson of "Miami Vice." As he reclined on a couch in his lovely home, Don told Barbara about the joys and difficulties in his life. He talked of past struggles with drug and alcohol abuse and work addiction. Then he spoke of his relationships with women—how exciting and attractive he found them. I could see his energy rise and his breath quicken as he spoke. An air of intoxication seemed to fill the room.

Don said his problem was he liked women too much and found it hard to be with one special partner over a long period. He would develop a deep friendship and intimacy, but then his eyes would wander.

I thought to myself, this man has been sexually abused! His problems sounded identical to those of adult survivors I counsel in my practice. But then I reconsidered: Maybe I've been working too hard. Perhaps I'm imagining a sexual abuse history that isn't really there.

Then it happened. Barbara leaned forward and, with a smile, asked, "Don, is it true that you had your first sexual relationship when you were quite young, about twelve years old, with your seventeen-year-old babysitter?" My jaw dropped. Don grinned back at Barbara. He cocked his head to the side; a twinkle came into his blue eyes. "Yeah," he said, "and I still get excited just thinking about her today." Barbara showed no alarm.

The next day I wrote Barbara Walters a letter, hoping to enlighten her about the sexual abuse of boys. Had Don been a twelve-year-old girl and the baby-sitter a seventeen-year-old boy, we wouldn't hesitate to call what had happened rape. It would make no difference how cooperative or seemingly "willing" the victim had been. The sexual contact was exploitive and premature, and would have been whether the twelve-year-old was a boy or a girl. This past experience and perhaps others like it may very well be at the root of the troubles Don Johnson has had with long-term intimacy.

Don wasn't "lucky to get a piece of it early," as some people might think. He was sexually abused and hadn't yet realized it.

Acknowledging past sexual abuse is an important step in sexual healing. It helps us make a connection between our present sexual issues and their original source. Some survivors have little difficulty with this step: They already see themselves as survivors and their sexual issues as having stemmed directly from sexual abuse. A woman who is raped sees an obvious connection if she suddenly goes from having a pleasurable sex life to being terrified of sex.

For many survivors, however, acknowledging sexual abuse is a difficult step. We may recall events, but through lack of understanding about sexual abuse may never have labeled those experiences as sexual abuse. We may have dismissed experiences we had as insignificant. We may have little or no memory of past abuse. And we may have difficulty fully acknowledging to ourselves and to others that we were victims.

It took me years to realize and admit that I had been raped on a date, even though I knew what had happened and how I felt about it. I needed to understand this was in fact rape and that I had been a victim. I needed to remember more and to stop blaming myself before I was able to acknowledge my experience as sexual abuse.

By acknowledging sexual abuse we can save ourselves years of confusion, anguish, and even misguided therapy. Jean, a middle-aged survivor, explained her frustrating sexual history:

> I was married at age nineteen for a few years. I hated sex and tried to avoid it. Eventually my husband left me for another woman. I went through a series of short affairs, sleeping with many different men, looking for something, wanting to feel something. I went to therapists. One told me I should look for a man who was equally uninterested in sex. Another told me to get a book on masturba-

tion and a vibrator. I became orgasmic and learned about my body, but I still felt nothing when I was with another person. I tried rebirthing, meditation, and so on, but not until ten years later did someone ask me if I was an incest victim. Now I am on a new path.

Once she had identified the incest, Jean was able to get to the real source of her sexual difficulties. From then on her healing efforts proceeded more effectively.

In this chapter we'll survey ideas and work with tools that can help you fully acknowledge your sexual abuse. We'll cover four specific areas:

Understanding sexual abuse
Overcoming blocks to recognizing sexual abuse
Remembering sexual abuse
Telling others about the abuse

UNDERSTANDING SEXUAL ABUSE

Understanding the full meaning of sexual abuse can help you determine whether, and how, you were abused.

Although abuse can take many forms (see box, pg. 31–32), a consistent thread connects each type of abuse: *Sexual abuse occurs whenever one person dominates and exploits another by means of sexual activity or suggestion.* Sexual feelings and behavior are used to degrade, humiliate, control, hurt, or otherwise misuse another person. Coercion or betrayal often play into sexual abuse.

The abuse can take a direct, painful, and obvious course, such as in stranger rape. Or abuse can be indirect, perhaps even subtle, such as when a victim is gently fondled by an offender who professes love.

Touch plays a part in many episodes of sexual abuse. But abuse can occur—and cause sexual harm—even when no touching is involved. A person who has been forced to pose for pornographic pictures, or sexually harassed by telephone, has suffered sexual abuse, even though his or her body may never have been touched by the offender.

Expanding the definition of sexual abuse has helped many survivors identify their experiences more accurately for themselves and better convey the damage of their experience to others. "In the beginning of my marriage, nineteen years ago, I told my husband of a 'sexual relationship' I had had with my stepfather," a survivor wrote. "*Sexual abuse* was not a term in use in 1969, and *rape* and *incest* (no blood relation)

COMMON TYPES OF SEXUAL ABUSE

The clinical definition of sexual abuse continues to expand as our society recognizes a broader range of activities perpetrated by sexual offenders. A single episode of sexual abuse may fall into several categories.

Child Sexual Abuse: sexual abuse of children by adults or by older children or peers who dominate and control through sexual activity. Older boys who make girls undress and then fondle them, for example. It can be committed by strangers but most often is perpetrated by adults or older children in trusted caretaking roles.

Incest: the most common form of child sexual abuse. Sexual abuse of children by other family members, including mother or father, step-parents, siblings, aunts, uncles, cousins, and grandparents.

Molestation: sexual abuse involving sexual stimulation to body and genital areas, including penetration. It can happen at any age, by a perpetrator of any age.

Stranger Rape: violence, anger, and power expressed sexually in an attack on a victim. It may involve penetration of body openings (oral, anal, and vaginal) but does not have to.

Date or Acquaintance Rape: sexual abuse, not necessarily violent, perpetrated by someone known to the victim, often a peer in a trusted social relationship.

Marital Rape: sexual abuse perpetrated by one spouse on the other, or by a sexual partner in any long-term committed relationship.

Sexual Assault: physical attack to victim's sexual body parts, often involving force or violence. This term can cover a wide range of activities and often describes the rape of boys and men.

Exhibitionism or Exposure: displaying the naked body or parts of the naked body in an effort to shock, intimidate, or sexually arouse a victim.

Voyeurism: invasion of a victim's privacy either secretively or openly with the intent of gaining sexual gratification.

Obscene Phone Calls or E-mail Messages: invasion of a victim's privacy with sexually suggestive messages over the telephone or Internet in an effort to shock, intimidate, or sexually arouse a victim.

Sadistic Sexual Abuse: sexual abuse in which the offender incites or tries to incite reactions of dread, horror, or pain in the victim as a means of increasing the offender's sexual arousal during the abuse. May involve use of physical restraint, quasi-religious rituals, multiple simultaneous perpetrators, use of animals, insertion of foreign objects, mutilation, or torture.

Sexual Exploitation: objectification and use of victims, by means of sexual activity or photographic imagery, to gain money or sexual gratification.

Sexual Harassment: use of gender, status, and power differences to intimidate or control a victim, or to require sexual involvement. May be expressed as flirting and sexual suggestiveness.

Gender Attack: exposure to actions that demean the sexual gender of a victim, often with sexual overtones, such as cross-dressing a child or verbally denigrating a victim's gender.

Gay Bashing: verbal or physical attacks directed against a victim's perceived homosexual orientation.

Sexual Violence: acts of violence involving or harming sexual parts of the victim's body.

Note: Legal definitions of sexual abuse are much narrower and can't be relied on in determining if an experience was sexual abuse. Unfortunately, in many parts of our country, no laws protect victims from certain types of sexual abuse, such as spousal rape, sexual harassment, gender attack, gay bashing, unwanted Internet pornography, and abuse perpetrated in indirect and subtle forms.

didn't seem accurate enough to be honest." Sadly, for many years, this soft language prevented her husband both from realizing that she really had been sexually abused and from understanding the extent of the damage the abuse had caused her.

To help you understand the meaning of sexual abuse, and to identify whether you have been sexually abused, consider these four questions. A *yes* response to any of them can distinguish an experience as sexual abuse.

1. Were you unable to give your full consent to the sexual activity?
_____ YES   _____ NO

If you were harassed, intimidated, manipulated, or forced into the sexual activity, you were not able to give full consent. If you were under the influence of drugs, alcohol, or medication, you were not able to give full consent. If you were asleep, unconscious, or otherwise not mentally alert, you were not able to give full consent. As a result of age, size, and power differences, children are not informed or mature enough to give full consent to *adult types* of sexual activity.

2. Did the sexual activity involve the betrayal of a trusted relationship?
_____ YES _____ NO

If persons who were supposed to be taking care of you or who were in an authority role used their position to force or encourage you to engage in sexual activity, you were sexually exploited and thus sexually abused. This can occur in situations in which a parent, relative, teacher, religious leader, or therapist compounds the trusted caretaking relationship with sexual involvement. An employer who uses his status to gain sexual favors is abusing his power. (It makes no difference if you initiated the sexual interaction. Caretakers betray trust and responsibilities when they respond.)

3. Was the sexual activity characterized by violence or control over your person? _____ YES _____ NO

Any sexual situation in which you were restrained or bound against your will, physically forced, or harmed constitutes sexual abuse. Humans need to be in control of what is happening to them physically. When this is denied by someone else in a sexual situation, it constitutes abuse.

4. Did you feel abused? _____ YES _____ NO

Finally, for purposes of sexual healing, what matters most is whether *you* feel you were sexually abused. Your feelings are genuine. They can't be erased. You need to trust your own feelings about an experience. If it felt funny or exploitive to you, regardless of how others perceive it, it has had an impact on you. That is what counts.

When I treat sexual abuse survivors from the perspective of sexual healing, I keep in mind this working definition: *Sexual abuse is harm done to a person's sexuality through sexual domination, manipulation, and exploitation.* Sexual abuse is harm done that robs a person of any or all of his or her sexual rights. When these rights are infringed on in the course of sexual abuse, the victim's sexuality suffers harm.

During many years of working as a sex therapist, I have identified eight sexual rights that protect us and enable us to develop positive sexual attitudes and behaviors:

SEXUAL RIGHTS

- The right to develop healthy attitudes about sex
- The right to sexual privacy
- The right to protection from bodily invasion and harm
- The right to say no to sexual behavior
- The right to control touch and sexual contact
- The right to stop sexual arousal that feels inappropriate or uncomfortable
- The right to develop our sexuality according to our sexual preferences and orientation
- The right to enjoy healthy sexual pleasure and satisfaction

Perpetrators of sexual abuse can confuse their victims about many of these rights. Perpetrators often objectify and exploit victims to satisfy their own emotional and physical desires, ignoring victims' rights and often leaving victims feeling powerless. Perpetrators rationalize what they do, ignoring the needs and feelings of the people they abuse. Sexual abuse is a highly self-centered act. And although some offenders may try to convince themselves and their victims otherwise, sexual abuse does not occur by accident. Abusers either intentionally harm their victims or they take actions that they know could cause harm. Either way, victims are robbed of their sexual rights.

Acknowledging our own sexual abuse usually demands more of us than simply being familiar with the names and definitions for different types of abuse and knowing, in theory, that we have sexual rights. We may need to challenge specific blocks that have kept us from recognizing or fully acknowledging sexual abuse.

OVERCOMING BLOCKS TO RECOGNIZING SEXUAL ABUSE

It can be difficult to acknowledge our sexual abuse fully when we are blocked in any of these ways:

- Feeling unsure how to evaluate a particular experience
- Feeling confused by the special nature of the abuse
- Holding on to our own personal biases and discounts

By examining these three major blocks to recognizing sexual abuse, we can uncover new perspectives that can help us overcome them.

Block 1. Feeling unsure how to evaluate a particular experience

Survivors may be unsure how to distinguish sexual abuse from other experiences. We may not know where to draw the line or how to evaluate a particular experience.

Identifying sexual abuse can be a matter of degree and circumstance. We may need to look at the full context of an experience to determine whether it was sexual abuse. For instance, a father may take a bath with his three-year-old daughter, help her wash her vaginal area, and snuggle with her in her bed at night, never once sexually abusing her. But the same series of events *would* be sexual abuse if the father had forced the girl to come into the bath with him when she didn't want to, if he purposefully hurt her vagina or wouldn't stop touching it, or if he told her not to tell anyone, rubbed her with the intention of sexually arousing her, or got sexually excited himself.

Nudity, body touching, stroking, kissing, and hugging are natural human experiences. They become abusive when put into an abusive context, where appropriate boundaries aren't respected. In some situations we need to look at the dynamics of a relationship to judge whether sexual abuse occurred.

When I was about five years old, I used to play with a neighbor named Bobby who was also five. We played house and catch, and went on swings together. One day Bobby said, "Come with me. Let's go in my dad's car in the garage." Happy and excited, I followed. We opened the car door and climbed up on the shiny vinyl seat. Then Bobby said, "I'll show you mine, if you show me yours." He waited for my response. It was okay with me. For about ten seconds we knelt awkwardly on the seat of the car, pulling down our pants and showing each other our genitals. (I think we both were a bit surprised at what we saw.) Then we left the car and went out to play some more. I never told anyone about this episode because I knew it was a secret we shared, and I felt somewhat embarrassed. But I never felt bad about it either. I still don't. This was child's play. Perfectly normal.

Many of us can recall a similar experience from childhood. Such interactions are common, healthy expressions of sexual curiosity that are important to developing positive feelings about one's own sexuality. Bobby and I were similar in age and size. Neither of us felt intimidated or controlled by the other. Neither of us felt pressured or coerced. Neither of us felt we had been in any way tricked, harmed, humiliated, or betrayed. The experience in that car seat was not sexual abuse, neither for me nor for Bobby.

Sexual trauma, such as that caused by accidental injury or medical procedures, can be as upsetting as sexual abuse and can even have sexual repercussions similar to those of sexual abuse, but it may not fit the definition of sexual abuse. If you are riding a man's bike and someone intentionally shakes the handlebars, causing you to slip and hit your genitals on the crossbar, you may feel as if the person has hurt you sexually. You feel humiliated, your genitals hurt, and you know you were harmed on purpose. What you experienced *was* abuse, but it was not necessarily intended to harm or exploit you sexually.

In adulthood we may have negative sexual experiences. On occasion you may feel like a partner doesn't care about your sexual pleasure. You may experience pain or discomfort during sex. You may feel hurt if a partner gets up and leaves abruptly after having sex. But these situations aren't in and of themselves sexual abuse.

While you may not feel such sexual traumas or negative sexual encounters were sexually abusive, it is important to keep in mind that the path to healing from them can be quite similar to healing from real sexual abuse. You can still benefit from the sexual healing journey.

Block 2. Feeling confused by the special nature of the abuse

Survivors may have difficulty recognizing sexual abuse because circumstances that surrounded the abusive experience make recognition difficult. One or more of the following circumstances may be hampering your efforts to fully acknowledge an experience you had as sexual abuse.

Sexual abuse that was labeled something else.   Many perpetrators operate in a state of denial. When confronted they try to defend or explain away their actions. Their denial can confuse you.

Let's say you're out on a date and your date suddenly reaches inside your clothes and starts grabbing and pinching. You're uncomfortable and tell your date to stop. You might get a reply like "Hey, what's the big deal? Why are you so uptight? I was only kidding around!" You in turn question yourself, was it sexual abuse or was I uptight?

Perpetrators have been known to give victims amazing rationalizations for their behavior: "I'm teaching you about sex so you'll be a good lover." "We were just having fun." "You asked for it because of the way you dressed." Some survivors believe these falsehoods. As a result they have trouble identifying that they were abused.

Abused as a child by her mother, Liz did not understand for many years that she was an incest survivor. Her mother had given her a false explanation for what was happening.

My mother would come into my room at night with a flashlight and give me an enema. She'd come at night because during the day I fought her about it. She'd also stick her finger in my vagina explaining that she was checking to see if it was growing straight. She got pleasure from inflicting pain. I also remember her sticking suppositories in me, sometimes several at a time. She had lots of these rituals for hurting me. I'd tell her what she was doing wasn't necessary, and she'd just say she knew better than anyone else.

I did not perceive this as sexual abuse when I was a child. I accepted my mother's statements that what she did to me over and over again was a necessary medical procedure. Even when I grew older and discovered such sadistic torture was not medicine, I kept thinking she must mean well and is just making a mistake. Mentally, I filed it under *m* for medicine, instead of *s* for sexual abuse.

John, another survivor, was also given a false explanation for what happened to him. When he was two years old, John began wetting his bed. His mother's response was to diaper him. She continued to diaper him until he was *thirteen years old*. Sometimes she would miss with the pin and stick him in his bottom. The diapering was a humiliating, upsetting, and sexually loaded experience for him. Several years after his mother stopped diapering him, she sexually assaulted him.

In counseling, John realized that the diapering also constituted sexual abuse. He recalled that at school, one week after the assault by his mother, he disrobed and stuck a girl with safety pins.

Most victims of sexual abuse do not go on to sexually abuse others. Those who do, however, need to accurately identify the abuse that happened to them. Recalling his mother's abuse helped John to understand why he later abused the girl at school.

Some perpetrators confuse the victim by saying that what they are doing is a form of loving: "Come on, princess. Daddy is not hurting you. Daddy likes to make you feel good. This is how Daddy shows his love in a very special way." Believing what she is told, the little girl may fail to recognize that Daddy is doing something bad.

Many survivors of sexual abuse in early childhood report that they were unable to correctly label what was happening because they were too young to talk, lacked a knowledge of sex, or had no vocabulary to describe what was being done to them. Their innocence may have left them particularly susceptible to false explanations by the offender.

Sexual abuse that developed gradually and repeatedly over time. Sexual abuse can be difficult to identify when it evolves gradually over time. Perpetrators may "groom" their victims by engaging them over a long time in activities that progress from less threatening and nonsexual to overtly sexual. A mother may have her teenaged son massage her legs every night for months before she slowly encourages him to be more sexual with her.

Perpetrators may find their grooming tactics sexually exciting. Grooming can also give a perpetrator leverage over the victim to maintain the secret of the abuse. "If you tell, no one will believe you didn't want it. You've been doing things with me for a long time," a perpetrator may say.

Tom, a client, told me when he was five his father would lie with him on the couch watching TV. His father would lie on his back and spread his legs, and Tom would be on his back in the V of his father's legs, resting his head on his dad's genitals. After many months of doing this, his father began to get up during the commercials and slip into the next room, where he would masturbate, knowing that Tom was sometimes watching. Months later, his dad made Tom undress and raped him anally with his finger. Looking back, Tom could see his dad had been preparing him as a sexual partner for years before the sexual contact began. He began to understand that all the experiences had been sexual abuse.

Sexual abuse that was indirect, secondhand. Sexual abuse can happen in a secondhand manner. I became aware this could happen when Barbara, a client, told me she feared sex and sexual touch, and was angered by her husband's sexual demands. Barbara could recall no experiences of inappropriate sexual contact. Taking a closer look at her past, she explained that her stepfather did some things in the home that upset her as a child.

> Some mornings when my sister and I were seated at the kitchen table and my mom was making breakfast, my stepfather would come up unexpected from behind our mother, grab her breasts, and begin fondling them right in front of us. We'd get upset and want to leave, and Mom would tell him to stop, but it did no good. He'd keep touching and make us watch.

Even though Barbara herself was never sexually approached by her stepfather, she suffered the secondhand effects of sexual abuse by coming to associate fear, male dominance, and control with sexual activity. *Injury occurs whenever victims are exposed to other people who have a sexually abusive way of thinking and behaving.* One offender in the family can teach sexual abuse attitudes, contaminating even those who are not directly abused. (In chapter 5 I will discuss in more detail a way of viewing sex, learned from abuse, that I call the sexual abuse mind-set.)

Many types of indirect sexual abuse can occur in childhood. A child might be exposed to degrading pornography, secretive sexual activity, humiliating sexual remarks, and a variety of inappropriate and humiliating forms of sexual behavior. In some families sexual abuse becomes part of the daily atmosphere, lingering like stale cigarette smoke.

Sexual abuse that was masked by sex role expectations. Sexual abuse can be masked by social attitudes and roles that prescribe how men and women should behave. Our culture still defines women as sexually passive and men as sexually aggressive. This can cause us to overlook experiences that are sexually abusive.

Several months ago, Tina, a seventeen-year-old client, rushed into a therapy session, quite distressed, waving a newspaper clipping of a nationally syndicated advice column. A teenage girl had written to the columnist complaining that whenever she visited a friend's house, her friend's father insisted on greeting her with a hug and a kiss on the lips. She also wrote that while she and her other female friends assumed the father was just being friendly, his behavior made them very uncomfortable. The columnist responded to the young girl's concerns by advising that the next time she sees her friend's father, she should greet him with a smile, turn her head, and simply request a kiss on the cheek, rather than on the lips. My client Tina said, "I can't believe that kind of advice. Wasn't that sexual abuse? Don't those girls have a right to tell the guy to bug off completely?" Tina was right. This was sexual abuse.

The advice columnist failed to see sexual abuse because she was more focused on encouraging girls to show respect to elders and be polite. After all, this is what girls and women are expected to do. But this man was exercising sexual privilege. He was using his age, size, and position to force the girls to show him intimate physical attention. The columnist's response suggests the girls forget their true feelings and let him kiss them as a social courtesy. This attitude plays into abuse.

When we reverse the sexes of the people involved, we can see the experience from a new perspective. Imagine a letter to an advice columnist where it is the mother of a seventeen-year-old boy who approaches each of his friends, uninvited, with a hug and then a kiss on the lips. Wouldn't we automatically cringe, thinking she must want sex with them? Wouldn't she get to be known as the perverted older woman? If a boy told her to stop, or avoided physical contact with her altogether, would we blame him?

Sex role assumptions can also prevent us from seeing the sexual abuse of boys by girls and women. Like Don Johnson, boys may be sexually abused by women and not recognize that what happened to them was sexual abuse.

Fred, a survivor, was also sexually abused by his baby-sitter. In therapy Fred explained the circumstance:

> One night when I was seven years old, I went to bed early because I wasn't feeling well. My fifteen-year-old baby-sitter got in bed with me and told me I could suck her breasts. She showed me how to put my fingers in her vagina, too. I always thought of this as sexual experimentation. But when I think of a male sitter being sexual with a little girl, I have no trouble defining it as sexual abuse.

Block 3. Holding on to our own personal biases and discounts

Survivors may have trouble identifying experiences as sexual abuse because of personal beliefs that discount, minimize, or assume responsibility for the abuse. Even when we know something bad or inappropriate happened to us, we may have trouble identifying the significance of the experiences as sexual abuse.

Some survivors find it hard to let go of their established false beliefs even when, intellectually, they know better. These beliefs may serve a psychological function. We may wish to protect our image of the offender as a good person, like the survivor who said, "Grandpa was a wonderful grandpa. He took me fishing, read me stories, and watched me perform in school plays, when no one else did. He could never have done anything intentionally to hurt me." By denying what we know to be true, we may avoid the pain of feeling betrayed or not remember how upset we were by the experience. These strong needs can keep us from acknowledging abuse.

Our biases and discounts may include:

But I offered no resistance.   While shouting, screaming, talking, and fighting back can sometimes prevent or stop sexual abuse, the reality is that in many instances resistance is not effective. When I was date raped, my offender was so quick and crazed that I instinctively felt that resistance would be futile and harmful to me. Because I chose a tactic of not fighting back, it made it difficult to acknowledge I had been raped.

Children, and many adults, do not use force to deal with an overwhelming threat. When we see the offender is older, bigger, or more powerful, we may naturally decide our best option for survival is to play possum. When we have no place to run, and if no one hears our cry for help, we may have no choice but to submit. In addition, sexual abuse can happen so suddenly there is no time to struggle. Abuse is abuse even if you didn't fight back. Submission does not mean consent.

But I liked it at the time.   Some victims adjust to sexual abuse by using the experience to obtain attention, affection, favors, or rewards. During the abuse they may actively cooperate and may experience emotional or physical pleasure from it. The abuse may meet emotional needs that weren't being met for them any other way. But this creative way of coping does not lessen the abusive nature of what occurs. The activity still ignores the victim's long-range best interests, carries social stigma, and teaches exploitive sex. The tremendous secrecy and guilt that accompanies abuse can cause the victim to feel psychological strain and stress.

A gay survivor who had been abused by an older brother said his recovery work made him aware that teenage boys seldom, if ever, "seduce" older men. He told this story:

I hear gay men who are pedophiles justify their actions with comments like "I seduced this kid" or "This teenaged boy seduced me."

When I was a teenager I tried to seduce my uncle, who was molesting my sister. It didn't work, which I thought was unfortunate at the time. But looking back today, given how I think now, if he had sex with me I would classify it as sexual abuse. He was an adult and would have been responsible for his sexual relationships. It would have been up to him to know the difference between healthy and unhealthy sex. Just because I was gay and wanted to have sex with my uncle didn't make it okay.

But my body responded.   Our bodies are sensitive. Most sensitive are the nerves in our sexual parts. When these are stimulated, through thought or physical sensation, nerves respond. Sexual responses can be automatic. A male teenager might see an offender's erection and automatically become aroused himself, or a girl may suddenly find her nipples harden when stroked by a rapist. High stress and anxiety can themselves trigger sexual responses. Abuse is abuse whether or not you responded sexually.

But it was no big deal.   Survivors of repeated sexual assaults may become desensitized to sexual abuse. Abusive activities begin to seem "normal" and expected. A survivor of repeated childhood molestation described her reactions after a recent attempted rape:

> It was a gorgeous day. I went into a rest room at a park, and a guy grabbed and started fondling me. I told him I had a boyfriend outside with a big white dog. He let me go. Later my boyfriend said he was surprised at how I downplayed the experience. My thoughts were, but this happens all the time. Later I realized I had built up such a tolerance to sexual abuse that I couldn't see it when it happened to me.

Some survivors minimize the abuse because it did not involve overt sexual conduct, result in penetration, or culminate in orgasm for the offender. Many studies show that attempted intercourse and "incompleted rapes" have similar impact on the victim as when the assault is "complete." A little sexual abuse is sexual abuse.

Survivors may be operating a double standard when it comes to recognizing the seriousness of their abuse. They may feel more compassion for a close friend who has been abused than they do for themselves, even if they experienced similar abuse.

Once survivors learn to stop minimizing abuse, they may feel a weight lift. A survivor who had been molested by her grandpa as a child explained:

> Once I overcame my denial of the abuse I had to work through another barrier of minimizing it. I'd tell myself, "It wasn't that bad. He only touched my chest. I was the one who made it out to be sexual." But the denial made me feel crazy and depressed. I learned that fondling a girl's breasts under the shirt is sexual abuse. My depression went away when I put the responsibility on my grandpa, the offender. It's the only way.

But my abuse wasn't as bad as other people's. Your experience is valid for *you*. There is no benefit in comparing how badly you were hurt to the experiences of others. Individuals respond differently to sexual abuse. We all have different strengths, tolerances, and supports. One victim may be just as traumatized as another whose abuse lasted longer and was more painful. If you have been abused—no matter how bad compared to others—your sexuality has been tainted by the experience. The harm done to you is real and matters.

But it was my fault. No one is responsible for the abuse except the offender. Blaming yourself for the abuse may be an attempt to gain some sense of control or influence over what happened. Believing we caused the abuse counters our feelings of helplessness and powerlessness: If I think I caused it, it means I could have stopped it. No matter how you behaved, you had a right not to be sexually abused.

Survivors may feel they deserved what happened as punishment for being bad or misbehaving. If I had just stayed out of his way, my uncle wouldn't have touched me, a survivor might think. Tragically, the false view that victims can "cause" the abuse continues to be perpetuated in our society, confusing victims even more. In the media and in the courtroom, victims of rape, especially female victims, are further victimized by suggestions that they "asked for it" by their clothes or their life-styles. Releasing ourselves from these false and hurtful societal messages can help us identify experiences as abuse.

Victims of sexual abuse often doubt their own innocence in circumstances in which there has been seduction, manipulation, or no weapon, or if the abuse took place in their own home or a place they went to willingly. Jean, an incest survivor, entered therapy distraught over a sexual relationship she had had with a former female therapist.

Their sexual affair went on while Jean was still attending weekly sessions with the therapist. Even though the affair so confused and upset Jean that it led her to terminate the therapy, Jean felt uncertain she had been sexually exploited. To overcome this false belief, Jean had to learn that *every* therapist has an ethical and moral obligation not to have sex with a client. Even if she had actively seduced the therapist, Jean would not have been responsible for the affair. It was the therapist's responsibility to prevent the affair from taking place. By releasing herself from fault, Jean was finally able to acknowledge that the therapist's actions constituted sexual abuse.

Recognizing that an experience was sexual abuse can be hard to do, but denying it also takes great mental energy. When we are finally able to overcome our biases and discounts, we free up our mental energy to channel into healing.

REMEMBERING SEXUAL ABUSE

About half of all survivors experience some memory difficulty. Survivors may have absolutely no memories of sexual abuse or only incomplete memories. We may blank out details of events but can recall feelings such as anger or fear. "I don't know where I was or who I was with, but I remember feeling terrified that my genitals were going to be hurt and then feeling ashamed," a survivor said. Others may forget emotions and recall only the events that transpired. A client once told me about her incest so unemotionally that she sounded like a reporter on the evening news. It wasn't until she could recall emotions that she really *felt* she had been victimized and could acknowledge the abuse.

If you sense you were sexually abused and have no memories of it, it's possible that you were. Memories can remain dormant for many years. Suspicions about sexual abuse don't arise out of the blue, for no reason. Suspicions can be agonizing and painful. No one likes the idea that he or she might have been harmed in the past, perhaps by a loved one. When people have continuing suspicions of sexual abuse, it's often because something did happen to them.

Memory loss has a reason

Memory loss occurs for many reasons. We may have been so young when abused that we were unable to form thoughts or put our feelings into words. If we could talk, we may have lacked a vocabulary for the adult types of sexual activities that went on. It's harder to remember an event when we have no words available to describe it. Similarly, abuse can be hard to recall if it occurred when we were unconscious, asleep, or under the influence of alcohol or other drugs.

Memory loss can be an important way of coping with abuse. If dad is doing something we feel strange about, something that might change the way we think of him, we may unconsciously decide it's better to forget the abuse. Victims of extremely violent and bizarre abuse may suffer traumatic amnesia, in which the shocking, violent nature of the abuse causes absolute memory loss of the event.

Memory loss protects us from overwhelming or continuous psychological strain after the experience. Sexual abuse is often confusing, painful, upsetting, shame inducing, and humiliating. We may have no one with whom we can talk openly about it and no opportunity to resolve our emotional feelings. Some people we talk with may discount our experience or blame us for it. We may convince ourselves that if we forget about it, we can get on with life.

Memory loss also protects us from painful feelings that are indirectly related to the abuse. A survivor might fear that remembering would bring up other issues—Why didn't my mother protect me from what my father was doing? She must have known. *Didn't she care?*

Most of the survivors I talk with who suspect they were abused but have little recollection wish they could remember more about what happened to them. "Not remembering my past is like being dead and not being able to remember my life," a woman told me. Another survivor commented, "It's hard for me to accept there may be parts of me I've forgotten—things which happened to me that I don't know about." As we pursue healing we may want access to these locked-in memories.

Memories can't be forced

Recalling the specifics of sexual abuse is not essential for sexual healing. But if memories do return, that can help the healing process. Remembering sexual abuse may enable us to acknowledge abuse more fully and to direct our healing efforts more efficiently.

Survivors often remember abuse when they are ready to and no sooner. Robin, an incest survivor, began to recall her abuse when she felt stronger, more assertive, and secure in her life. Her memories emerged gradually. "I didn't let myself know more than I could handle. I feel grateful to the part of myself that kept this repressed until now," she said later.

Remembering takes time and energy. As one survivor said, "If I could put as much time into remembering the abuse as I did into forgetting it, I believe I could remember a lot more."

You're likely to find that memories will surface simply by your proceeding on this sexual healing journey. Sexual healing encourages thinking about sex and sexual abuse, which in turn can stimulate recollection.*

When we pay close attention to our sexual reactions and thoughts, we can often discover a link to past sexual abuse. One survivor's fear of getting anything gooey on her body led her to remember her grandfather ejaculating on her when she was a little girl. A male survivor traced his fear of men touching him on the shoulders to an early experience of being forced to orally copulate his uncle. As upsetting as these discoveries are, they do help to solve the mystery of why a strange reaction or thought existed in the first place and to bring the memory of the abuse to the surface.

For Bonnie, a thirty-three-year-old married client, clueing into her sexual reactions and behavior led to a profound memory. When Bonnie entered therapy she suffered from several sexual problems common to survivors: She was not orgasmic, hated touching her genitals, and avoided sex with her husband. Bonnie had no recollections of sexual abuse, but she did have a sense that something could have happened between her and her father. It now seemed curious to her that as a teenager she had insisted on having a deadbolt for her bedroom door.

One day in counseling, Bonnie shared that on a recent morning she had screamed uncontrollably after seeing a strand of pubic hair in the bathtub and that soon afterward she dreamed that she was six years old. In the dream, her father gave her some balloons, then he put her on the bed and began touching her sexually. Bonnie woke from the dream as her body convulsed in a sexual climax. She knew that the dream replayed the event that had really happened with her father years ago. Because her first orgasm occurred during the abuse, Bonnie had avoided having orgasms ever since. "A bug doesn't go back to the heat once it's felt the fire," she remarked. But once the specific memory of abuse was out, Bonnie was able to begin the slow process of learning to experience orgasm free from associations with abuse.

---

* See box, pg. 48–49.

Trusting our memories

When memories of events and feelings do start to surface, trust them. They may not make sense initially, but when many are added together you can get a better picture of what happened to you. As one survivor explained:

> The process was like finding pieces of a jigsaw puzzle, each in a separate drawer, and fitting them together to see a picture I had never seen before.

For another survivor, specific memories of incest came back in a sudden vision during a group therapy session. She recalled, "I had a vision of my father lying on top of me, kissing my face. I started crying in disbelief. After that, the vision kept coming and more was revealed."

Though most people are relieved to recall past abuse, be prepared that you might also feel upset, even extremely frightened or angry. You may temporarily experience sexual problems caused by the upsetting sexual nature of the memories.

Hank was surprised when, eighteen years later, he remembered the emotional feelings that accompanied being seduced by an older woman when he was sixteen years old and a virgin. An entry from his journal shows how the process of writing helped him to understand his feelings:

> I was surprised, almost shocked, to find myself feeling bitterness, regret, sadness, and a sort of crazy or helpless feeling of having been persuaded to do something I really was not sure I wanted to do. It's hard to believe that these feelings have been repressed all this time. She started hugging and kissing me, then she told me to take off my clothes. I felt like I had no choice, like I had to do it. I'm confused as to whether this was rape or something close to it. Something was wrong. I didn't feel I had a right to consider whether I was really ready to go all the way sexually. We had a two-week affair. Then it was over. I never felt close to her or able to be myself around her. This is so sad that in writing about this I start crying, something I never did before about this experience. She got pregnant by me. I said I couldn't be much of a father. She insisted on raising the child herself with her husband, which has had a deep effect on me over the years. I have always had trouble trusting and being intimate with women.

No matter how difficult the process of remembering is, remind yourself that you are stronger than the things that happened to you. You survived the abuse, and you can survive the memories. And the memories can help you heal.

SEXUAL HEALING APPROACHES TO REMEMBERING

Although memories of abuse often surface naturally when survivors are ready to handle them, some survivors feel stuck. They may want to make a more active effort to facilitate remembering. Survivors can attend ongoing therapy sessions to create a consistent setting where memories can unfold. Having professional and personal support can help survivors feel safe and understood, which is so important to remembering. Survivors can use a variety of methods to help them remember, such as hypnosis, investigating their past by talking with relatives, or looking at old picture albums, floor plans of old homes, memorabilia, and so on.*

If you feel ready to investigate your memories of sexual abuse, the following exercises may help you. These exercises consider sexual clues and activities directly. What you recall may cause you to feel unsettled, uncomfortable, perhaps even temporarily fearful. Go slowly. Seek support. Give yourself a safe opportunity for your memories to return. Don't try to force recall; memories will emerge when you are ready to handle them. Recording what you learn in a journal may help you.

1. Reflect on your childhood. Were there any periods in your childhood in which you displayed any of the common signs of sexual abuse, such as insomnia, nightmares, bedwetting, excessive masturbation, regression to more infantile behavior, explicit sexual knowledge, behavior or language unusual for your age, depression, withdrawal, frequent genital infections, severe headaches, unexplained gagging, self-cutting or mutilation, recurrent abdominal pains, eating problems, drug and alcohol abuse, suicide attempts, truancy, change in school performance, limited social life, running away, overtly seductive behavior, attention-getting or delinquent behavior?

Were there times in your life when you were particularly vulnerable to sexual abuse? Was there anyone in your past whom you feared or consistently avoided? Was there anyone in your past who had the opportunity, interest, and inclination to perpetrate sexual abuse?

2. Think about your earliest sexual experiences. Who did what, when, and how? Were these experiences, in reality, sexual abuse?

3. Pay attention to the feelings, images, and thoughts that come up for you during and after sex. Take seriously any strange or irrational reactions you may have. Are you strongly drawn to, or extremely afraid of, certain sexual activities? Are you upset with stimulation to certain body parts? Do you avoid certain types of touch? How long have you had these feelings? Under what circumstances did they originate? How might these activities relate to sexual abuse?

4. Pay attention to your sexual dreams and sexual fantasies. Are there repeated themes that pertain to power, control, humiliation, or violence? Do you have recurrent dreams or nightmares that involve sexual abuse?

As feelings and memories surface, keep in mind: You are the most important judge of your past. Unless they participated in or witnessed an experience, no one—no family member, friend, therapist, or doctor—can tell you for sure what did or didn't happen to you. Be patient. Keep an open mind. Trust your strong emotional, physical, and sexual reactions.

While remembering sexual abuse can facilitate sexual healing, recollection is not a requirement for recovery. Regardless of your level of recall, you can move forward and develop healthier sexuality.

* See the Resources section for books on general recovery from sexual abuse. In particular, Ellen Bass and Laura Davis, *The Courage to Heal;* Laura Davis, *The Courage to Heal Workbook;* and Mike Lew, *Victims No Longer.*

TELLING OTHERS ABOUT THE ABUSE

"Your secrets make you sick" is a popular phrase in Alcoholics Anonymous. It applies to sexual abuse recovery as well. Secrets usually maintain our shame and damage our important relationships. While we can know inside that past experiences were actually sexual abuse, our acknowledgment of sexual abuse is not complete until we share it with others. Sharing with others often liberates us from the past.

Even though it can be an important step in sexual healing, many survivors hesitate to share the secret of their abuse. They may have to overcome old injunctions to remain silent and not to tell. They may need to resolve worries and fears about what others might think of them. And they may need to come to grips with the reality of what happened to them on a new, deeper level.

If you know you were sexually abused, perhaps you have already shared your abuse with others or perhaps the idea of sharing is new for you. By exploring some of the reasons adult survivors hesitate to share, you can gain an understanding of what might block a deeper acknowledgment of your sexual abuse.

"I don't want to be seen as a victim"

Sharing that we were sexually abused means admitting to ourselves and others that we were once victims. This can be hard to do. Few people like to think of themselves as victims. Our society places a great emphasis on self-determination and independence. We don't like to see ourselves as having been in situations that went beyond our control, that we were powerless to change, and that led to our exploitation.

Regardless of what we would like to believe, we do not always have control over what's happening. Acknowledging we were once victims is an important acceptance of our human vulnerability.

Although survivors didn't have control over the abuse in the past, they do have control now over how they respond to it. Believing that we have to remain silent about something confusing and painful that happened to us can be another form of victimization. "I had to acknowledge I was a victim before I could see myself as a survivor," one man said.

"I'm embarrassed and ashamed of the abuse"

Sexual abuse is an intimate offense. It's hard to talk about our sexual encounters with others. We may not be used to sharing anything so personal. Most of us would rather admit that someone stole our car or punched us in the face than share that, against our will, someone touched us on a private body part.

Sexual abuse involves sexual feelings and often sexual parts of our bodies. Survivors who feel ashamed to discuss these intimate injuries need to remember that they did nothing shameful themselves. If we had faced breast or prostate surgery, we would have sought the support of our loved ones and discussed our experiences. We should not hesitate to ask for the same kind of support now.

"I'll be seen as less of a man"

Men survivors often have an especially difficult time revealing their abuse histories. One male survivor recounted his experience:

The very hardest part of recovery for me was coming out and saying that I am a sexually abused person. I didn't know until two years ago that men and boys could be raped. We're not supposed to be victims.

Our society gives boys the message that men should be able to stand up for themselves and fight off danger. They're also told that if a man gets hurt, he should go it alone instead of seeking help. A boy or man may worry that sharing the abuse would mean he had failed at being able to protect and take care of himself.

Males are also taught not to show their sensitivities and emotions. A man may fear that sharing the abuse would be like opening a flood-gate—dammed-up pain and emotions would come gushing out. He may fear he would be overwhelmed.

Men may also hesitate from disclosing they were abused because they worry about their sexual image. Our culture presents sex for males as an adventure, something they should feel excited about at any time. Male victims may doubt their masculinity because they didn't experience sex that way in the abuse. Because most abuse of males is perpetrated by other males, heterosexual male victims may worry they will be seen as homosexual if others hear the details of what occurred. Gay men may wonder if the abuse made them gay.

Men have to challenge some of these limiting social views of masculinity that restrict their humanness. Sharing that one was sexually abused is not a sign of weakness. On the contrary, being honest with yourself and others requires a tremendous amount of courage and strength.

In recent years a number of men, such as star hockey player Sheldon Kennedy, Olympic gold-medalist Greg Louganis, and Michael Reagan, adopted son of former president Ronald Reagan, have made their abuse histories public. Since one in five males are estimated to have been sexually abused as children, these disclosures are helping men overcome unnecessary shame and emotional isolation.

"I'll lose social status as a woman"

Women survivors have a different set of social injunctions to overcome. Women may worry that when they share the fact of their abuse, they will be seen as sexually loose or damaged. Our society has set up these fears. Rape laws, for instance, were written originally because husbands and fathers wanted a way to protect the value of their wives and daughters. Women were seen as property, vulnerable to damage by other men. But times are changing. This view of women as chattel is becoming outmoded. In recent years, many prominent women have been stepping forward and publicly saying they were sexually abused. Senator Paula Hawkins of Florida, talk show hostess Oprah Winfrey, former Miss America Marilyn Van Derbur, and actress Kelly McGillis have taken their stories public.

Since nearly half of all women are sexually abused in their lifetimes, a woman who openly acknowledges having been abused need not fear being alone. I have begun sharing that I was sexually abused when I give lectures and conference presentations. Although I used to fear that people would think less of me, my experience has been quite the contrary. Invariably, when my presentation is over, several people comment that they appreciated my ability to openly discuss that I am a survivor.

Sexual abuse does not lessen a woman's worth or a man's maleness. Like being robbed, *sexual abuse is a crime against you, not an indicator of who you are.*

"I was told not to tell"

If the perpetrator who abused you is still alive and around, it can be an additional burden. You may fear the offender would hurt you if he or she was to find out you had shared the story of the abuse with anyone. It may be difficult to trust even a highly confidential, private relationship.

Survivors may remain irrationally afraid of the offender for years. I call this the "Santa Claus is watching you" phenomenon. Given that many offenders were authority figures, some survivors may imagine the offender has special power to control their lives: He knows when you are sleeping, he knows when you're awake, he knows if you've been bad or good, so be good for goodness sake.

Survivors who have felt this way need to remind themselves that they are not powerless. They have support now that was probably lacking when the abuse occurred. It is offenders who have a lot to fear—

socially and legally—from survivors who are no longer willing to keep sexual abuse a secret.

"I'm afraid of other people's reactions"

Sharing about sexual abuse is risky. We can't predict how others will react. Although social awareness about sexual abuse has increased in recent years, many people may still respond in negative ways. They may not believe it really happened, say you were to blame, question why you didn't do anything about it sooner, or convey the impression that they believe you were somehow irrevocably damaged and made worthless.

A survivor told what it was like to share about her abuse with a partner whose response was upsetting:

> I began having memories of the sexual abuse while I was dating a man I didn't know well. I would tell him I had a new memory and what it was. He didn't understand why I wanted or needed to dig up the past (as if I had a choice). He was unsupportive about the actual memories and the emotional wreckage the memories brought up. He kept suggesting quick ways to fix the problems. I felt guilty, unsupported, and angry. I subsequently terminated the relationship. Since then my ex-partner has told me that his response was based on *his difficulty at seeing me in such pain.*

Another survivor admitted feeling terrified when, at age thirty-nine, she decided to tell her parents that she had been sexually abused by her mother's brother—thirty-three years earlier. She worried that they wouldn't think it had been sexual abuse, that they'd defend her uncle's actions, or that they wouldn't respond. Those fears and worries led her to confront her own doubts about what happened. Was this really sexual abuse? Did it really happen? Not until she felt clear in her own mind about what had happened, and about who was responsible, could she share the abuse with her parents.

> By the time I finally dialed my parents' phone number, I felt strong enough in myself that I knew, no matter what kind of response I got, that I wouldn't abandon myself. Naturally I hoped for a supportive response from them. But I knew that the benefit for me in my healing was in being able to say it—in hearing myself say it. For me, hearing myself say I had been abused meant I had overcome my shame and doubt.

Sharing is something we choose to do for ourselves, to help us heal. Because it is so risky, we need to be careful and share in ways that we believe will be beneficial to us.

When survivors decide they are ready and want to share that they were sexually abused, they can reduce risk and help themselves increase the likelihood of having a positive acknowledgment experience by planning their disclosure thoughtfully and carefully. Here is a slogan that can help: *Share in safety and in steps.*

Start talking about the abuse with close friends, with family members or lovers who have shown their emotional support for you in the past, with a counselor in a confidential session, or with other survivors of sexual abuse. These are people you believe will have a nonpunitive, caring interest in what happened to you. A survivor who shared her abuse with her therapist said, "I needed someone safe to tell. I needed a witness where there was none before, someone who would not shame me or intrude with their own reactions."

There is no formula to determine who the best "witness" will be for you. Consider who will be receptive, supportive, and caring about your needs. Sometimes the best listeners can be found in support groups.

> The survivor support group provided me with an opportunity to find out I wasn't alone, that there were others who had similar experiences. It also provided people who understood and didn't judge me. It was the beginning of being able to talk about sexual abuse and to trust others.

Not everyone is knowledgeable about sexual abuse. Before sharing your experience, ease your way into the topic, educating your listener as you go. You may even want to give them reading material about sexual abuse to clear away old myths before you proceed. (In chapter 9, we will talk more about how intimate partners can become better informed about abuse and thus more supportive.)

Talk in broad terms at first: "Something happened to me in the past that is difficult for me to discuss." Test their interest level: "I'd like to share more with you, but I want to know if you're interested in learning about it." Tell them what you need: "Since this is a sensitive subject for me, I'll need your understanding and support in hearing about it. Does that sound okay to you?" Reveal the details of the abuse gradually, as it seems safe: "I was molested by someone." "My uncle molested me." "My uncle had oral sex with me."

Be prepared for varied reactions. If people blame you in any way, you might remind yourself and them that the abuse was the offender's fault, not your own. If they wonder why you have kept silent about the sexual abuse for so long, tell them most survivors have trouble admitting and disclosing abuse. If they want to confront your perpetrator, remind them they must not do so without your approval, that you must control the resolution of issues related to your abuse.

Don't be surprised if you get some positive reactions too. When you *share in safety and in steps*, this is likely to happen. A survivor described her experience:

> When I first told my partner that my brother had sexually abused me, he was shocked, pretty speechless, but he seemed to me to be understanding and nonjudgmental. I felt relieved that at least that much was out in the open. It was a *big* weight off my shoulders.

And another survivor told of her situation:

> When my husband and I came home after a counseling session, he asked me what exactly had happened when I was sexually abused. I felt ready to reveal more. I told him it was hard to talk about. Then I shared with him that my brother had touched me on my breasts and vaginal area and that he ejaculated on me. I cried and was shaking the whole time that I talked. My husband held me. He cried with me. I felt closer to him in that moment than I ever had before.

Sharing the abuse allows you to be honest about yourself with others. It can release you from unnecessary feelings of guilt and shame. Sharing is a sign of your strength and your ability to recover. Although in the short term it may be painful and scary, in the long term it can feel good, an empowering relief. "I'm so glad the sexual abuse is out," said a survivor. "Most of the ugly little creatures I held in my darkness have hatched out and died in the light."

By acknowledging abuse, you can recognize the experience of sexual abuse as part of your life history and can learn to use it as a source of strength. By acknowledging sexual abuse, you take back power and can begin doing something about the past. When you share the story of the abuse with others, you can do it with your chin held high. You are no longer a victim. You are a survivor, becoming a thriver.

3

Identifying the Sexual Impact

It was painful to look at the damage yet also freeing. Once I
found out what I was robbed of, exactly how I was hurt, I was
able to start making changes. It was tear filled and
empowering.

—A Survivor

Adam, a thirty-five-year-old survivor, had come to couples counseling
with his wife, Marge, to work on difficulties in their sexual relationship.
In recent weeks Adam revealed to Marge that when he was thirteen he
was sexually abused by a male camp counselor. It had taken him twenty-
two years to admit he was once a victim. Marge reacted at first with surprise, then sympathy.

In the aftermath of his disclosure, Adam became depressed. He
found himself suddenly crying at work. He began having trouble sleeping at night. Marge began to worry what the awareness of the abuse
would mean to their relationship.

One day in counseling Marge listened quietly to Adam while he
described his turbulent emotions. Then she became agitated and said,
"It's hard to see you in such pain. Can't you just put the past behind you
and enjoy the life we have together?"

Adam straightened up in his seat, took a deep breath, and let loose
with a flood of feelings he had long held back:

God knows, I wish it were that easy, but it's not. The abuse left me
thinking I might be gay. It made living a heterosexual life-style
with you and the kids seem like a hoax and a sham. Remember how

I used to pester you to have sex all the time? I did that to try and get my thoughts of sex with men to disappear. Not only did the abuse make me question my sexuality, but it left me with a reduced sense of my value as a human being. What that guy did to me back then has made it difficult for me to be able to be intimate with you now.

Adam's eyes filled with tears. Marge looked him in the eyes and said, "I'm sorry. I didn't realize how harmful an event the abuse had been."

Sexual abuse is not simply an event that happened, ended, and now is over. It can have an impact on every aspect of a survivor's life—attitudes, self-image, relationships, and sexuality. These are not past issues but very real and current ones. It takes enormous strength to learn about, evaluate, and change them. In Adam's case, through hard work, he is realizing the many ways he's been affected by sexual abuse and is making important connections between past abuse and his present sexual issues. Marge is becoming more aware as well. Their journey is well underway.

Many survivors who work to gain an understanding of the general effects of their abuse remain unaware of the specific ways that sexual abuse has influenced their sexuality. The traces of past sexual abuse can reach into the present life of a survivor and cause continuing problems.

Some sexual effects go away within months after the sexual abuse, but many do not. Effects can be hidden in a survivor's sexual attitudes and life-style, and may not become apparent until many years after the abuse is over.

Your current behavior might not feel like an "effect" of anything. If you avoid sex, you might think, I am just a person who doesn't like sex. Why does everyone make such a big deal about it? I get along fine without it. This could be true. It could also be true that your current feelings were shaped by past sexual abuse.

In contrast, if you are a survivor who is constantly seeking sex, you might rationalize your sexual problems and tell yourself simply, I enjoy sex. It comes natural to me. I'm good at it. I'd like to do it anytime with anyone. I don't see why people get so uptight about sex. That could be true, but it's possible your high desire for sex may come directly from hidden emotional stress and what you learned about sex as a result of abuse. You may be unaware of the extent to which your sexual behavior is negatively affecting you.

As you learn to identify the many ways sexual abuse may be affecting your sexuality, the realization can be upsetting. It's unpleasant to question our sexual attitudes and behaviors, and it's sad to get a sense of how profoundly we have been affected by abuse. We may see for the first time that something is definitely wrong with how we approach sex. One survivor recalled this feeling:

> The part about my recovery from sexual abuse that made me especially angry was realizing that the sexual abuse was still affecting me in ways I wasn't aware. Those were subtle ways, operating subconsciously. They had to do with how I formed intimate relationships and what I was drawn to for sexual excitement. I had to identify all those effects before I could recover from them.

While knowing about the aftereffects of abuse can be painful, not knowing can be worse. If we remain unaware of the many ways the abuse has harmed us sexually, we may be locked in years of confusion and pain, denying ourselves the enjoyment of healthy sexuality.

Identifying the sexual impact of abuse can be a guide to your recovery. Once you realize exactly how sexual abuse has influenced your sexuality, you can direct your energy so you can heal in specific ways. You become aware of particular areas to focus on and make changes in during later parts of the sexual healing journey.

In this chapter we will work through the Sexual Effects Inventory to help you identify how sexual abuse may still be influencing you sexually. If you have little or no memory of sexual abuse or have not identified yourself as having been sexually abused, this inventory can help you explore the possibility of sexual abuse. Several times in later chapters you can refer back to your answers as you work to change your sexual attitudes and behavior.

This inventory is designed to help you evaluate your present sexuality: What is your sexual life like today? What might be troubling you sexually now? As you complete the inventory, you can identify specific issues that you would most like to focus on as you heal.

In later chapters we will be learning more about these effects, how they developed, and how you can work to change them. For now, let's focus on taking an honest, thorough inventory of your sexuality. Each survivor's experience is unique. There is no right or wrong set of answers.

SEXUAL EFFECTS INVENTORY*

1. Attitudes about Sex

Sexual abuse generates negative, false attitudes about sex. These become hidden from your consciousness. You may have difficulty separating abusive sex from healthy sex. Offenders contaminate victims, imprinting them with an abusive way of thinking about sex, a sexual abuse mind-set. This mind-set can affect every aspect of a victim's sexuality: sexual drive, sexual expression, sex roles, intimate relationships, knowledge of sexual functioning, and sense of morality. How have you been affected by this sexual abuse mind-set?

Put a check mark (√) in front of each statement you agree with and a question mark (?) in front of each statement you sometimes or partially agree with. (Statements that don't fit either category should be left blank.)

_____ I feel sex is a duty I must perform.

_____ I feel sex is something I do to get something else.

_____ In sex, one person wins and one person loses.

_____ Sex feels dirty to me.

_____ Sex feels bad to me.

_____ Sex feels secretive to me.

_____ I equate sex with sexual abuse.

_____ Sexual energy seems uncontrollable.

_____ Sex is hurtful to me.

_____ I believe sex is something you either give or you get.

_____ I feel sex is power to control another person.

_____ I believe having sex is all that matters.

_____ I think sex benefits men more than women.

_____ I think people have no responsibility to each other during sex.

_____ I think sexual desire makes people act crazy.

* I developed the Sexual Effects Inventory based on items identified in my clinical practice, research review, and questionnaire study. It is designed to give survivors a general picture of their sexual concerns at this time. The items in the inventory are ones survivors and therapists believe to be associated with past sexual abuse (some have been empirically tested, others haven't). Sexual problems have many causes besides sexual abuse, such as medical problems, religious and social upbringings, relationship difficulties, and stress, that could account for any particular response to an item.

_____ I think males have a right to demand sex from women.
_____ Sex means danger to me.
_____ I believe sex is a way to escape painful emotions.
_____ Sex is humiliating to me or others.
_____ I feel sex is addictive.
_____ I feel sex is a game.
_____ I believe sex is a condition for receiving love.

2. Sexual Self-Concept

Sexual abuse, and its consequences, can unconsciously influence how you feel about yourself and about sex. You may now see yourself as sexually damaged, suffering a poor sexual self-concept. Or you may have developed a self-concept that is inflated, where you believe you're more powerful as a result of sex. Knowing how you view yourself as a sexual person is fundamental to eventually making changes in your sexual behavior.

Put a check mark (√) in front of each statement you agree with and a question mark (?) in front of each statement you sometimes or partially agree with.

_____ I am an easy sexual target.
_____ My sexuality is disgusting.
_____ I hate my body.
_____ There is something wrong with me sexually.
_____ I am confused whether I'm gay or straight.*
_____ I feel I will lose control if I let myself go sexually.
_____ I have no sense of being sexual at all.
_____ I feel like a victim in sex.
_____ I am sexually inadequate.
_____ I don't like certain sexual parts of my body.
_____ I want sex for all the wrong reasons.
_____ I have to stay in control during sex.
_____ I don't have a right to deny my body to any partner who wants it.
_____ I can be loved only to the extent I can give sexually.
_____ I am oversexed.

---

* I do not believe a particular sexual preference in itself is a negative effect of sexual abuse to be overcome. It's the confusion about sexual preference and orientation that can be troublesome.

_____   I have no right to control sexual interaction.
_____   My primary value is in sexually serving a partner.
_____   If I want sex, I'm as sick as a sexual offender.
_____   I blame myself for past sexual abuse.
_____   I deserve whatever I get sexually.
_____   I wish I were the opposite sex.
_____   I am inferior to other people because of my sexual past.
_____   I am damaged goods.
_____   I can easily be sexually dominated.
_____   I'd be happiest in a world where sex didn't exist.
_____   I couldn't live in a world without sex.
_____   I am a sexual performer.
_____   There are some things I have done sexually that I can never forgive myself for.
_____   I am a sick person sexually.
_____   I'm not lovable for who I am, only for what I do sexually.
_____   I am a sexual object.
_____   I feel bad about my gender.

3. Automatic Reactions to Touch and Sex

Sexual abuse can create a conditioned way of reacting to touch and sex. Some survivors get panicky, avoid sexual possibilities, and want to run the other way when sexually approached. Others freeze and feel helpless and unable to protect themselves. Still others get overexcited and may recklessly seek dangerous sexual encounters. You may experience spontaneous reactions to sex that cause you to numb sexual feelings, to divorce your mind from what is happening physically, or to become sexually aroused in inappropriate ways. Sexual settings and contact can bring back negative feelings associated with abuse. Flashbacks to sexual abuse may arise and interfere with sexual relating and satisfaction.

Put a check mark (√) in front of each statement you agree with and a question mark (?) in front of each statement you sometimes or partially agree with.

_____   I am afraid of sex.
_____   I have little interest in being sexual.
_____   I am afraid of some sexual body parts.
_____   I am preoccupied with sex.

_____   I withdraw from sexual possibilities.

_____   I am bothered by sexual thoughts I can't control.

_____   When I get horny I feel extremely anxious.

_____   I feel especially powerful when I'm having sex.

_____   I get sexually excited at times when I shouldn't be.

_____   I constantly look for sexual opportunities.

_____   I believe that when a person touches me, he or she wants to have sex with me.

_____   I lose all power to protect myself when sexually approached.

_____   I have unhealthy sexual interests and desires.

_____   I often have flashbacks to past sexual abuse during sex.

_____   Unwanted fantasies intrude upon my sexual experiences.

_____   I am sexually aroused by thoughts of hurtful sex.

_____   I get panicky feelings when touched.

_____   I feel emotionally distant during sex.

_____   During sex my mind feels separate from my body.

_____   I feel like I'm another person when I have sex.

_____   I feel very nervous during sex.

_____   I experience negative feelings such as fear, anger, shame, guilt, or nausea with sexual touch.

_____   I get sexually aroused when I don't want to be.

_____   I often feel emotionally pained after sex.

_____   I am very sensitive to certain smells, sights, sounds, or sensations during sex.

4. Sexual Behavior

Sexual abuse can shatter our capacity for healthy sex. You may have been taught abusive patterns of sexual behavior and introduced to unhealthy, compulsive, abnormal sexual activities. Now as a reaction you may associate your sexual expression with secrecy and shame. Some survivors may withdraw from sex, preventing any fresh discovery of healthy sex. Other survivors may become preoccupied and driven by sex. Sometimes survivors reenact the abuse in an unconscious attempt to resolve deep-seated emotional conflict related to the original abuse. These reactions need to be identified so you can better understand your behavior and eventually work toward healthy changes.

Put a check mark (√) in front of each statement you agree with and a question mark (?) in front of each statement you sometimes or partially agree with.

_____ I isolate myself from other people socially.

_____ I am unable to initiate sex.

_____ I avoid situations that could lead to sex.

_____ I am unable to say no to sex.

_____ I feel I have no physical boundaries when it comes to sex.

_____ I need to be under the influence of alcohol or other drugs to really enjoy sex.

_____ I spend money to have sex.

_____ I feel confused about how and when to be sexual.

_____ I engage in medically risky sexual behavior (using no protection against disease or pregnancy).

_____ I engage in sex for economic gain.

_____ I have had more sexual partners than was good for me to have.

_____ I act out sexually in ways hurtful to others.

_____ I manipulate others into having sex with me.

_____ I engage in sadomasochistic sex.

_____ I have more than one sexual partner at a time.

_____ I become involved with sexual partners who are primarily involved with someone else.

_____ I use fantasies of sexual abuse to increase sexual arousal.

_____ I feel addictively drawn to certain sexual behaviors.

_____ I feel compelled to masturbate frequently.

_____ I engage in secretive sexual activities.

_____ I engage in sexual behaviors that could harm me.

_____ I engage in sexual behaviors that could have negative consequences for others.

_____ I have sex when I really don't want to.

_____ I am confused as to what is appropriate and inappropriate touch in dating.

_____ I often rely on abusive pornography to turn me on.

_____ I find it hard to say no to unwanted sexual touch.

_____ My sexual behaviors have caused problems with my primary relationship, my work, or my health.

_____ I use sex to help me feel better when I'm down.

5. Intimate Relationships

Sexual abuse influences a survivor's ability to establish and maintain healthy sexual relationships. Abuse can interfere with our ability to

make good choices. Some survivors may have difficulty selecting partners who are emotionally supportive. Other survivors may be unable to
trust and feel safe with intimate partners who *do* care. Survivors may
fear intimacy or have a limited capacity to experience closeness.

The sexual difficulties a survivor may have as a result of abuse often
create emotional and sexual problems for the partner. Knowing where
relationship difficulties lie, and how abuse has caused problems, can
help you work with your partner to solve individual concerns and to
build a more intimate relationship together.

Put a check mark (√) in front of each statement you agree with and
a question mark (?) in front of each statement you sometimes or partially agree with.

_____   I am drawn to partners who demand sex from me.
_____   I am afraid of being emotionally vulnerable in relationships.
_____   I am unable to attract the kind of partner that would be good
          for me to have.
_____   I feel obligated to please my partner in sex.
_____   My intimate relationships always fail.
_____   I have difficulty being intimate and sexual at the same time.
_____   I don't trust that a partner could really be faithful to me.
_____   I hide my real feelings in an intimate relationship.
_____   A partner would reject me if he or she knew all about my
          sexual past.
_____   I experience difficulty initiating sexual contact with a partner.
_____   My intimate partner is continually unhappy with our sex life.
_____   Our relationship would end if we stopped having sex.
_____   I want, but am unable, to remain faithful to one intimate
          partner.
_____   My intimate partner reminds me of a sexual offender.
_____   My intimate partner perceives me as sexually abusive.
_____   I want to get away from my partner immediately after sex.
_____   My partner feels sexually rejected by me.
_____   My partner feels sexually pressured by me.
_____   I have difficulty communicating my sexual wants and needs.
_____   I am afraid to be emotionally close with my partner.

6. Sexual Functioning Problems

Sexual abuse can create specific problems with sexual functioning. Abuse may have taught you unhealthy patterns of responding to sexual stimulation. Stress and anxiety that originated with abuse may continue to shadow your sexual activity. Over time these sexual problems interfere with intimacy and long-term sexual satisfaction. As you identify problem areas in how you function sexually now, you are also identifying specific sexual concerns to work on in the healing process.

Put a check mark (√) in front of each statement you agree with and a question mark (?) in front of each statement you sometimes or partially agree with.

_____ I find it difficult to become sexually aroused.
_____ I have trouble experiencing sexual sensations.
_____ I do not like to touch my genital area.
_____ I have difficulty achieving orgasm when I stimulate myself.
_____ I have difficulty having an orgasm with a partner.
_____ I lack desire for sex.
_____ I am hardly ever interested in sex.
_____ I overcontrol sexual interactions.
_____ My orgasms seem more related to relieving tension than to feeling pleasure.
_____ My orgasms are not very pleasurable.
_____ Sex in general is not very pleasurable.
_____ I am limited in the types of sexual activity I feel comfortable with.

Men
_____ I have difficulty getting or maintaining a firm erection.
_____ I have difficulty ejaculating.
_____ I ejaculate very fast.

Women
_____ I do not like touch to my breasts.
_____ I am unable to be vaginally penetrated.
_____ I experience pain or discomfort with vaginal penetration.
_____ I orgasm very fast.

WHAT YOU CAN LEARN FROM THE INVENTORY

Now that you have completed the Sexual Effects Inventory, go back and review your responses. Remember: There is no grading system, no correct set of answers. Rather you are looking to identify the effects of abuse on your current sexual self.

For many survivors, taking the inventory leads to self-discovery, self-awareness. It's another step in your journey. Although *your* inventory is unique, you may learn from, or feel support from, the following reactions from other survivors.

"I didn't realize how much my sexuality has been affected"

Many survivors feel upset after taking the inventory. You may be surprised and even distressed at the number of items you have checked. "I checked nearly half of all items in each category," a survivor said. You may be shocked that you checked items in so many different categories. Yet checking items forces survivors to overcome their denial. Real problems exist. By acknowledging them you can work on them.

"Different items are more important to me than others"

The impact of particular sexual effects can vary from person to person. A repercussion that is merely annoying to one survivor might be extremely upsetting to another. A lesbian survivor who feels fear when seeing an erect penis may find this sexual repercussion unimportant. But the same fear might be extremely upsetting to a heterosexual woman or a gay man.

Some items—such as "I engage in sexual behaviors that could harm me"—signal immediate danger. You will need to give these kinds of statements a higher priority in your sexual recovery.

"I see trends and patterns in my responses"

Many survivors see trends in one of two directions: feeling negative about and withdrawing from sexual activity, or becoming compulsive and engaging in a lot of sexual activity. "I can see that I tend to withdraw from sex, even though I crave getting touched," a survivor remarked.

Some survivors notice trends in both directions. "I feel compelled to masturbate a lot, yet I withdraw from having sex with my partner," another survivor commented.

Many of the items in the inventory overlap. Our attitudes about sex influence our sexual experiences and behavior, and vice versa. You may notice patterns and links in the types of items you checked and how they relate to each other.

In the following statement by a woman survivor, I have added words in brackets to indicate the different categories of sexual effects she reveals.

> When I reached high school and college I began to experience intense fear whenever I was asked out [AUTOMATIC REACTIONS]. I was sure I would end up in a struggle over intercourse, even on the first date. I thought that was all these boys and men wanted from me [SEXUAL ATTITUDES]. I feared the idea of having sex with anyone [AUTOMATIC REACTIONS]. I thought sex was banal, ridiculous, something for weak-minded folk [SEXUAL ATTITUDES]. I never once went out on a date [SEXUAL BEHAVIOR]. My fear created a complete lack of interest in sex, dating, and physical contact [RELATIONSHIPS, SEXUAL FUNCTIONING PROBLEMS]. I became a total bookworm [SELF-CONCEPT].

Because items relate to one another, when you do begin to make changes in one aspect of sexual healing, you will automatically be making improvements in others.

"My responses are different than they would have been in the past"

Survivors often comment that they would have marked the inventory differently had they taken it one, five, ten, or twenty years ago. Sexual repercussions can show up in different ways in different stages of your life. For instance, many survivors experience a period of high sexual activity in their dating years, then encounter problems with sexual interest and functioning only after they have become involved in a committed, long-term relationship. Retaking the inventory at different times can help you see how sexual repercussions of abuse may have changed over time and point to areas where you are making progress. A survivor gave an example of age-related change:

> As a child aged ten to fifteen, I engaged in what now would seem like excessive masturbation and stimulation of myself with objects.

Then, in my teens, I didn't like to touch myself. Now I prefer to masturbate only when I am feeling good about myself.

And another survivor said, "It's good to see that I've stopped using sex to try and fill an empty feeling in my heart."

You may want to take the Sexual Effects Inventory again in the future. It can be a powerful resource to refer to at different times in your sexual recovery, helping you identify areas for change. The inventory can also give you a way of evaluating the progress you make in your sexual healing journey.

In taking this inventory you may have gotten your first real awareness of how profoundly the abuse may have harmed you sexually. If you are feeling upset by what you've learned, remember that yours is a common reaction and a crucial one. You may need to grieve your losses and to feel the emotional pain and anger. As we proceed through this book, you will have a chance to address all the concerns you have checked. You will grow, and your current outrage at how much you were hurt will help fuel your will to heal.

4

Deciding to Reclaim Our Sexuality

Sexual healing is very profound work. It takes great courage to work through problems caused by the abuse. Your body may feel like a battleground over which you fight ghosts who have great power, reclaiming territory which is your birthright.

—MIRIAM SMOLOVER, *Therapist*

I'm sitting poolside at a hotel in Portland, Oregon, resting and watching the sunset. Earlier that day I had made a presentation on sexual healing to a large group of survivors. A young woman attending the conference sits down next to me. She's about twenty-five years old and is wearing a flowered dress. She tells me her name is Alice. She also tells me she was molested by her grandfather as a child. During my presentation that day, Alice says she became aware of just how significantly sexual abuse has affected her sexuality. For the first time she has begun making connections between the sexual problems she has now with her lover and what happened to her in the past with her grandfather.

I've been walking around feeling really upset and angry. I hate the idea that I'm still trapped in some way by my grandfather's influence. It's like I'm somehow still being abused. I feel like a marionette puppet dancing on a stage. The ghost of my grandfather is the puppeteer, hidden from sight, pulling my strings. It's as if my sexuality is outside my control—not mine. I know I've got to find a way out of this bind, because unless I do, I'll feel like I'm letting my grandpa rob me of my right to an enjoyable sex life.

Listening to Alice, I realize that she has reached an important turning point in her sexual healing journey. Now aware of the impact of the past, she is deciding to address the injustice she still feels. Alice is making a decision to reclaim her sexuality: to bring her sexuality under her own control, free of the influence of her offender. And she wants to accomplish this primarily for her own pleasure and satisfaction. She is turning the awareness of her sexual effects into a desire to get back her sexuality for herself.

After taking the Sexual Effects Inventory in the last chapter, you may be having feelings and thoughts similar to Alice's. You may want to make changes in one or more of the six categories listed in the inventory—attitudes about sex, sexual self-concept, automatic reactions, sexual behavior, intimate relationships, or sexual functioning problems. Other survivors, who have also come to this point in the sexual healing journey, have offered the following statements to describe how they feel. Check any that apply to you now.

REASONS TO RECLAIM SEXUALITY

_____ I want to develop a more positive view of sex.
_____ I want to feel good about myself as a sexual person.
_____ I want to improve my automatic reactions to touch and sex.
_____ I want to engage in healthier sexual practices.
_____ I want to have a good intimate relationship.
_____ I want to address a specific sexual problem.
_____ I want to overcome the effects of the past.

If you do not identify with any statements now, that's okay. Some survivors don't develop a desire to make changes until they are farther along in the sexual healing journey. Each journey is unique.

Justine, a date rape survivor, decided to make changes once she realized how past abuse was interfering with her enjoyment of touch. On becoming aware of the connection with past abuse, Justine became enraged.

Living well will be my best revenge. I had no control over what happened to me in the past, but I do have control over what I decide to do about it now. I don't want any aspect of life to be beyond my grasp. I want to experience the full beauty and expression of my sexuality.

Regardless of when we make it, the decision to reclaim our sexuality is life affirming. It reflects a natural urge to liberate ourselves from past constriction and to live life more fully. The decision to reclaim our sexuality is also serious, creating new demands on our time and energy. It requires effort to make important changes. We need to cushion this decision with self-respect and kindness, honoring our own pace and being honest about our present abilities.

Three activities can help you at this point in the sexual healing journey:

- Identify and tame your fears.
- Create realistic goals.
- Reclaim sexuality *for yourself*.

These activities can help you feel more comfortable with deciding to reclaim your sexuality and can help prepare you to make future changes in your sexual attitudes, behaviors, and experiences.

IDENTIFY AND TAME YOUR FEARS

Most of us are afraid to change our sexual habits. This fear is natural. Even if our current sex life is unsatisfying or unhealthy, we don't know what changing it will do. New learning often generates fear because it is a departure from what we already know.

Some survivors worry that change will be too great. Others worry that they won't change enough. We can become frozen by our fear of what's to come, but we don't have to be.

The following are some common fears survivors have expressed when they start to consider making changes and reclaiming their sexuality. Check any that apply to you, or add your own to the list.

FEARS ABOUT SEXUAL HEALING

_____   I'm afraid I will have to be more sexually active.
_____   I'm afraid I will have to give up pleasurable sexual behaviors.
_____   I'm afraid I will fail if I try.
_____   I'm afraid my social life will diminish.
_____   I'm afraid my present relationship will fall apart.
_____   I'm afraid of being sexually victimized again.
_____   I'm afraid further memories of abuse will surface.

_____   I'm afraid to recall how I felt in the abuse.
_____   I'm afraid of changes in my intimate partner.
_____   I'm afraid I'll become self-centered.
_____   I'm afraid it will only make things worse rather than better.

_____   _____

_____   _____

These fears are natural in sexual healing, but we don't have to let them stop us from moving forward. We can acknowledge, accept, and understand them.

Fears aren't necessarily bad. They can reflect the hidden excitement we have about making changes. They can signal that we are about to have a breakthrough in understanding.

You can divide up your concerns and face them one at a time. Look at the issues you identified in the last checklist. Then take each one and think about what you could do specifically to prevent it or cope with it. Separate each strand of your feelings as if you were unbraiding a rope. As you mentally prepare yourself to cope with each concern, you can lessen the overall power of fear.

We can talk ourselves through what frightens us. Here are some ways survivors have talked through, and disarmed, their fears.

I'm afraid I will have to be more sexually active.   Remember, we each have the right and power to control how sexually active we will be. We can learn specific skills for asserting our physical boundaries and saying no to sex.

I'm afraid I will fail if I try.   Failure is doing nothing about a problem that bothers us. If our efforts don't go as we hoped, we still learn and can take a new approach next time. Mistakes and setbacks happen in every endeavor.

I'm afraid my social life will diminish.   We are in charge of our social lives. If we have been socializing with those who encourage self-destruction by engaging in hurtful sex, we can let them go and form new, healthy friendships, partnerships, and sexual bonds.

I'm afraid my present relationship will fall apart.   This is possible. Some relationships end because people avoid problems, and some end because people face problems. If your relationship is healthy, and you and your partner work on sexual healing together, your ties are likely to become stronger and more satisfying.

I'm afraid further memories of abuse will surface. Further memo-ries often do surface with sexual healing work. You can learn specific skills to handle them when they do.

When we aren't afraid of our fears, we can use them to help us steer our sexual healing toward a satisfying outcome. Fears often help us to spotlight our deepest concerns. Seeing our fears illuminated, we can better focus on the healing changes we wish to make.

Vern, a forty-five-year-old survivor who compulsively masturbated, was afraid that changing his behavior would mean a serious loss of sex-ual pleasure. He learned to trust this fear—as a reminder not to over-look his interest in sexual pleasure while he developed a new, healthier pattern for sexual release.

The fears you identify are likely to resurface at different times throughout sexual healing. When they do, don't be alarmed. Instead, take time out to look at them more closely and to find a way through them.

CREATE REALISTIC GOALS

Deciding to reclaim your sexuality can happen much more easily when you identify realistic goals for making changes. Unless you do this, you may feel overwhelmed by stringent goals or too-high expectations.

In developing your goals, keep in mind how seriously the sexual abuse may have harmed your sexuality. You may not ever be able to *com-pletely* overcome the sexual effects of abuse. In one way or another, the effects may sometimes bother you. But you can learn to cope with the effects and to refuse to let them stop you from having a satisfying sex life. This too is successful sexual healing.

Avoid broad goals that carry high expectations, such as "I want a ter-rific sex life" or "I want to want sex a lot." These will probably generate anxiety and make sexual healing difficult. Goals will serve you best when they are specific and nonthreatening. A survivor explained, "My long-term goal is to reach a point where the idea of sex is not a negative experience but a positive one."

You can generate specific goals for sexual healing by considering how you would like to change. For example, if you would like to develop more positive sexual attitudes, which attitudes are currently causing you problems? If you would like to address a specific sexual problem, which do you want to work on first? Taking another look at the Sexual Effects Inventory in chapter 3 can help you identify what you want to change.

Once you have identified goals, you can develop realistic ideas about what it would mean to accomplish them. How could you tell that a goal had been reached? What would be different in your life?

Let's walk through this part of the journey with a survivor who wants to overcome the negative ways she reacts to touch and sex. That's a major goal, and it might seem insurmountable unless she breaks it into smaller pieces. She narrows the focus, asking herself, "Which reaction do I most want to change?" Her answer, "I want to stop having flashbacks disrupt my sexual experiences." She then asks herself, "How would I know I had accomplished this?" Her answer, "I'd have fewer flashbacks or I'd be able to continue with sex even if I had a flashback."

By becoming more precise she has come up with a measurable goal. A few months from now, after learning skills to address flashbacks, she notices that often she can continue with sex after having a flashback. She has not completely healed, but she has made significant progress. Her ability to respond differently now shows her that she has reached her original goal. Her life has changed in a real way.

Another survivor may decide he wants to feel good about himself as a sexual person. He first asks himself, "What specifically do I want to feel better about?" His answer, "I want to stop feeling ashamed about my sexual past." He then asks, "What would show me that I am no longer feeling ashamed about my sexual past?" His answer, "I'd be able to tell others, without embarrassment or fear, that my older brother molested me." If he can do this he will know he's met this goal and is making progress.

Our goals give us something concrete to aim for in our healing, a specific destination for our journey. Sexual healing becomes more tangible and less of a mystery.

Denise, a twenty-two-year-old incest survivor, initially identified her goal for making changes in her sexuality as "wanting to have a good sexual relationship." By becoming even more specific, she came up with concrete, measurable target goals that could help her focus her efforts more effectively as she healed. She defined her target goals this way:

I want to learn how to be comfortable with men as people. I want to develop a friendship with a man. I want to have a sexual relationship that develops gradually, over many months. I want to learn how to talk about my sexual likes and dislikes. I want to be able to talk through my feelings during sexual activities rather than shut them down.

To help you through this goal-setting process, first brainstorm general changes you want to make in your sexual healing. Then translate these general changes into smaller, target goals. Remember to keep your goals specific and nonthreatening. You may wish to use the space below.

General goal 1

_____

Target goals   a. _____

             b. _____

             c. _____

General goal 2

_____

Target goals   a. _____

             b. _____

             c. _____

General goal 3

_____

Target goals   a. _____

             b. _____

             c. _____

These goals can serve as guideposts in your recovery, helping you to move in a positive direction.

Be cautious of trying to reach your goals too quickly. A survivor said:

I'm in a hurry to heal. I know what happened. I'm frustrated that all my knowledge and reason, along with twenty-one years of a good marriage, can't _instantly_ blot out the abuse in childhood and make sex a natural, sensuous experience.

Feeling in a hurry to heal can lead you to make your goals rigid or to set unrealistic time limits for when goals have to be achieved. Don't start with "By next summer I will no longer compulsively masturbate," or "A year from now I want to be enjoying sexual relations with my partner several times a week." These goals may do you more harm than good.

Sexual healing is a dynamic process, involving many aspects of your sexuality and your relationship. Realistically, it requires a flexible approach. Rigid goals and unrealistic time limits don't allow you to shift your healing priorities over time. You may start by focusing on changing one area of your sexuality and then switch to another. It's not uncommon for survivors to find themselves putting more time and energy than they had expected into practicing new skills, building trust, or resolving feelings from the abuse.

While it can be important to motivate yourself to move forward at a comfortably challenging pace, you don't want to set yourself up to feel that you have failed. Trying to make changes too fast can lead to your feeling overwhelmed or frustrated. Instead, gently persist at a pace that fits you.

Sexual healing involves a great deal of unlearning. Along the way, we learn a new way to think, feel, and behave sexually. We need to create goals that respect the time it might take us to integrate smaller changes. After many months of healing work, a survivor said:

> Sometimes it feels like things will never change, but when I keep working at it, one step at a time, small things do change. I never thought I'd enjoy hugging so much. Recovery's been taking much longer than I wanted it to, but the changes I've already made have really been worth the effort.

RECLAIM SEXUALITY FOR YOURSELF

As you approach making changes in your sexual attitudes, behaviors, and experiences, keep in mind that the changes you'll be making are *for yourself*. As we have discussed already, this journey is not for any other person. "I started sexual healing because I wanted to save my relationship," a survivor said, "but nothing much happened until I started doing it for myself."

If we try to make changes in our sexuality for someone else's sake, we run the risk of recapitulating sexual abuse. In sexual abuse, a victim is forced or expected to behave in ways that satisfy the offender's emotional and sexual desires. The survivor's emotional and physical feelings are ignored. Victims get the message that their sexuality exists to benefit others. The sexual experiences we end up having may still remind us of sexual abuse, because we are engaging in them primarily for someone else.

Reclaiming sexuality for ourselves does not mean becoming sexually aggressive, insensitive, or abusive to a partner. If we are in a relationship, we can take ownership of our bodies, be in touch with our emotional feelings and sexual needs, control our role in sexual interactions, and still be sensitive to our partner. It's a matter of reversing the priority from "partner first, me second" to "me first, partner second." In sexual healing, the needs and feelings of both people are still respected, as we will discuss in more detail in chapter 9.

Though it may seem strange, the process of sexual healing itself can unconsciously become associated with past abuse. Survivors may force themselves to make changes when they aren't ready. They may attempt changes because they think they should or according to someone else's timetable. When they do this it's easy to feel oppressed by the process of sexual healing. If forced, even sexual healing can start to feel abusive.

You can tell if you have fallen into this trap by listening to yourself talk about sexual healing. If you hear yourself using terms such as "*I have to* do my exercises" or "*I should force* myself to do this," you are probably associating healing with the abuse experience. You can counteract this tendency by reminding yourself that you are pursuing sexual healing *for yourself*—you are reaching *your* goals, at *your* pace, for *your* benefit. The motivation to heal needs to come from within yourself. Only then will you be able to travel the ups and downs of the sexual healing journey.

Try asking yourself these questions: What can I *discover*? Shall I *explore* this? What can I *learn, create,* or *invent*? This low-pressure type of self-talk will help you to maintain a positive, healing attitude.

Frame your healing as an adventure you are taking yourself on. Learn and make changes for your own personal growth and enjoyment. "It's exciting to me to be part of a creative process," a survivor said. "Sometimes, when I know I'm making changes for myself, it feels like I'm being reborn."

Remember that your sexuality is yours alone, and only you can reclaim it. As a survivor said, "I'm the one who is in this body. I'm the one with these sensitive body parts and nerve endings. So I'm the one who is entitled to experience the sensations and pleasures that happen when I'm sexual."

As you progress on your journey, remind yourself to address your fears, to create realistic goals, and to make sure you are reclaiming your sexuality for yourself. These reminders will help you stick with your decision to become free of the sexual effects of sexual abuse.

Sexual healing may stir up painful realizations for you. At times you may feel saddened by the extent of damage sexual abuse has caused you. When this happens, express your sadness. Let go of your pain. Acknowledging our sadness can itself be cleansing and empowering as we journey on the way to reclaim ourselves and our bodies. I keep a card in my office with this message as a reminder, "The soul would have no rainbows had the eyes no tears."*

Eventually, we can see that we have choices about our sexuality and intimate expression, choices that aren't determined or shaped by abuse. Our sexuality can become an integral, healthy part of our lives. As Jill Kennedy, a therapist, explained,

> Sexual healing has more to do with recovered feelings of sensuality than with the sexual act itself. To be able to feel aroused in the fullest sense of the word—without fear of betrayal, retribution, or abandonment—moves beyond culturally defined views of appropriate behavior to a deeper level of self-acceptance.†

* A personal greeting card with illustration by Sally Struthers, Anaheim, Calif.: Strand Enterprises, 1979.

† Excerpted from the clinician questionnaire Jill Kennedy filled out in the summer of 1989.

PART TWO

Moving Forward

Making Changes

5

Creating a New Meaning for Sex

The greatest revolution of our generation is the discovery that human beings, by changing the inner attitudes of their minds, can change the outer aspects of their lives.

—WILLIAM JAMES

The other day I came into the living room and found my seven-year-old daughter, Cara, playing with her Barbie dolls. I noticed that Ken and Barbie were naked and seemed passionately involved under a pink lace blanket. Cautiously, I asked Cara if she had any questions about sex. She hesitated for a moment and then said, "Mommy, I don't understand why rape is so bad. Isn't it just like what mommies and daddies do when they have sex?"

After I got over my initial shock of her asking such a mature question, I ventured an answer: "It's true, some of the same body parts are involved. And some of the same behaviors occur. But," I continued, "rape and lovemaking are really very different. Rape is a form of violence where sex acts are used to hurt someone. Rape hurts a woman because her body is not ready or wanting sex. And it hurts because she feels bad she's being raped. Lovemaking is different; it's sharing. Lovemaking is happy and joyous. A woman's body goes through changes which make it pleasant. It's something that feels good."

Cara nodded her head and seemed content with this reply. Then she added, "I think, Mommy, you should tell people who have been sexually abused what you told me so they won't think sex is a bad thing anymore."

Many survivors think about sex in a way that associates sex with sexual abuse. This is understandable: Sexual abuse experiences are often a survivor's first exposure to sex. For many of us who were abused as children, abuse provided our primary sexual learning. Even for survivors who were sexually active before, sexual abuse can be so traumatic and upsetting that it mentally fuses sex with sexual abuse. Regardless of how or when we were abused, sexual abuse can seriously impair our thinking about sex.

When I ask survivors who are new to sexual healing to finish the phrase *Sex is . . .* , they often respond with answers such as *bad*, *dangerous*, *overwhelming*, *dirty*, *frightening*, *a tool*, *a duty*, *violent*, *secretive*, *humiliating*, or *a powerplay*. And when I ask them to finish the phrase, *Sex is like . . .* , these same survivors may tell me *a nightmare*, *a drug*, *a punishment*, *murder*, *being robbed*, or *being tortured*.

Survivors' responses to both questions rarely reflect a positive view of sex as an expression of love and caring, as a pleasurable and fun experience in itself, or as a special bond and sharing between two people. Instead, survivors' meanings for sex often reflect a view contaminated by the offenders' distorted thinking about sex and the traumatic qualities of the abuse. The abuse robs survivors of the right to develop a view of sex for themselves, free from the influence of abuse.

THE SEXUAL ABUSE MIND-SET

When survivors' attitudes about sex are contaminated and determined by the abuse, survivors develop what I refer to as a *sexual abuse mind-set*. In this mind-set, sex is seen as bad and dangerous, something to avoid or to pursue secretly and shamefully. The sexual abuse mind-set cripples a survivor's ability to change his or her sexual behaviors or improve a sexual relationship with a partner. It prevents healthy sexual enjoyment and intimacy. Here are two stories to illustrate.

Linda, a forty-five-year-old survivor of long-term sadistic abuse by her brother and mother, learned to view sex only as pain and torture. She hated sex and had recently withdrawn from it completely. In couples therapy, Linda and her husband, Mike, were surprised to discover that different meanings for sex were at the root of much of their suffering and miscommunication. After Mike shared how depressed he felt that they had stopped having sex, the couple conversed:

MIKE: Linda, I love you. I find you sexually attractive. I want to have sex with you sometime in the future. (*Linda tenses as Mike says the word sex. She grabs a pillow and hugs it to her chest.*)

LINDA: I hate it when you say *sex*. To me sex is violent, disgusting, ugly, and sick. I want nothing to do with it. I don't understand how you can want to do it without wanting to do something bad to me.

MIKE: When I say I want to have sex with you, I mean that I want to share a special, private part of myself with you. I want us both to feel pleasure. You're my wife. You're the person I love. You're the person I want to have sex with. (*Mike's eyes become filled with tears.*) What is so bad about wanting to be physically intimate?

LINDA: Intellectually, I know you don't want to hurt me. And there's a part of me that's even glad you find me attractive. But it's just that I've always thought of sex as something bad. I have a hard time believing it could be positive and that I might enjoy it. I don't know what sex really is. I feel like a child who needs someone to talk to me about sex and teach me healthy attitudes.

Another survivor, Jack, had recently been realizing in counseling that his view of sex kept him locked in behaviors that were destroying his fifteen-year marriage to his wife, Donna. Jack described sex as "a drug to blot out pain." He compulsively masturbated, cruised in his car to look at women, and sometimes engaged in secretive sexual affairs outside his marriage. Though Jack said he loved Donna and found her attractive, he didn't like to have sex with her. Their marriage was failing because Donna felt isolated and betrayed.

Jack's views on sex began forming years ago. When he was twelve and out on a family picnic, a woman neighbor cornered him in the bushes, stripped off his clothes, and performed oral sex on him. He found the sexual experience overwhelming but also very exciting and intensely pleasurable. For years Jack masturbated to thoughts of sexual contact with controlling older women.

In therapy, Jack realized that what happened to him was abuse. His meaning for sex fostered his compulsive sexual activities.

My penis and my heart are disconnected. Sex is a way I reward myself when I've done well at work or console myself when I'm feeling depressed. It's not a way I show my love. In fact, I feel like I cheapen Donna when I do it with her. I dislike the rituals that go with making love with Donna, like kissing and hugging. I feel controlled by them.

For Jack, and for Linda in the previous story, sex was learned in an abusive situation, devoid of intimate caring, safety, or relaxed fun. They came to see sex not as a sharing of pleasure but as something bad that is done to you or that you do to someone else. To resolve their present-day sexual problems, Jack and Linda need to learn new definitions and ways of thinking about sex that can foster sexual recovery and healthy sexual enjoyment.

As we move forward in this chapter, my goal is to help you explore how the sexual abuse mind-set may have distorted your own view of sex, and to help you acquire an intellectual understanding that sex can be something good, healthy, and positive. I will show you tools that can help you create your own meaning of sex, free from the influence of abuse.

To begin, let's look at the sexual abuse mind-set more closely. In the mind-set, sex is seen in narrow terms and is confined to ideas that relate to sexual abuse. Survivors in this mind-set are unable to associate sex with healthy experiences of love and caring.

This is a damaging way of thinking. When survivors believe in the mind-set, they may be more susceptible to being revictimized or to acting in ways that could hurt themselves and others. This mind-set can be hard to detect, hidden from our own conscious awareness. It can be such a strong, ingrained belief that we fail to see it as wrong. Our deeply held beliefs can appear as truths when they're not.

To complicate matters, the sexual abuse mind-set is reinforced by our culture. Sex is often portrayed in the media as one person sexually dominating, manipulating, or exploiting another. Our society promotes the message that boys should be sexually aggressive and girls should be sexually accommodating. We are culturally exposed to the sexual abuse mind-set much more often than we are exposed to healthy ways of thinking about sex. The five conditions for healthy sexuality—consent, equality, respect, trust, and safety (CERTS)*—are seldom taught at home or in school, or reinforced in our culture.

To create this new, healthy meaning for sex we need to first cast aside our old, damaging ways of thinking about sex. This involves learning to identify, challenge, and overcome the ways we associate sex with sexual abuse. We must come to see ways that our thinking has been contaminated by the offender's unhealthy view of sex and by the traumatic repercussions of the sexual abuse experience itself.

---

* These five CERTS conditions were first presented in Wendy Maltz and Beverly Holman's *Incest and Sexuality*; see the Resources section.

FALSE IDEAS ABOUT SEX

The sexual abuse mind-set is made up of five false ideas about sex:

1. Sex is uncontrollable.
2. Sex is hurtful.
3. Sex is a commodity.
4. Sex is secretive.
5. Sex has no moral boundaries.

Survivors are usually affected by some of these more than by others. As we examine and challenge these falsehoods, pay attention to any ideas that apply to your current thinking about sex. It may be helpful to ask yourself, What meaning do I give to sex now? Reviewing your responses to the Sexual Effects Inventory in chapter 3 may help you to evaluate your current perspective.

False idea 1: Sex is uncontrollable

As a result of sexual abuse, survivors may believe that sexual energy is a wild force that cannot be contained or controlled. Once unleashed, they fear it can't be stopped. Angie, a thirty-five-year-old survivor of childhood incest, recently realized that her father, the offender, is still giving her the message that sex cannot be controlled.

> Several months ago my father stopped by to visit me on his way back from the Philippines. He entered my home and said, "I haven't seen a white woman in three months. You'd better watch out, I just might rape you. I might not be able to help myself." Not only were his remarks threatening and blatantly racist and sexist, but they showed me how sick my father is in his thinking about sex.

Some offenders don't admit they feel out of control themselves, but rather they project their feelings onto their victims. As an adult, Betty asked her father why he had molested her and her three sisters in the past. Her father replied, "I wanted to keep you from having to get your sexual needs met outside the family." The implication was that the girls had uncontrollable sexual needs that he should control. The girls were three, four, and five years old when he began abusing them. Betty's father had projected his own feelings of being out of control onto his innocent children and then had used his distorted thinking to defend his behavior. Victims like Betty who receive such a message may inaccurately conclude that their own sexual energy is uncontrollable.

Sexual abuse can leave survivors with the impression that sexual energy is impulsive. An offender may say, "I want sex and I have to have it *now*." Many offenders act in sudden, unpredictable ways, pressuring victims and communicating the false idea that sexual needs require immediate fulfillment.

Because sexual offenders often become unreasonable, unreachable, and emotionally distant the more sexually aroused they appear, survivors may conclude that sex causes all people to divorce themselves from everyday reality and responsible concern for others.

Sexual abuse gives survivors the message that sex is insatiable. An offender may say, "This will be the last time," and then come back to sexually molest the same victim again. Survivors may feel that sex is like an addiction: The more sex the offender gets, the more he or she craves.

Victims may also come to believe sex is uncontrollable because of the sexual feelings they experienced during abuse. A male victim may be shocked to get an erection, or a female victim may be shocked to vaginally lubricate during the abuse. Victims may feel that their own sexuality has turned against them. They may have difficulty understanding that their sexual reactions are natural physiological responses to sexual stimulation. Sexual responses indicate the body is functioning as it is designed to. The *abuse* is what's out of control, not the sexuality of the victim.

When survivors believe that sex is uncontrollable, their sexuality suffers. Some survivors withdraw from sex, fearing that if they let themselves experience it a little, they might become "addicted" like the offender. They may become sexually anorectic, starving themselves from any touch that might arouse their own sexual appetites.

Similarly, survivors may pull back from sex with a partner, fearing that their partners will want more sex if they get a little. The thinking goes that it is better not to have any sex than to be overwhelmed by the insatiable, uncontrollable sexual needs of a partner.

Survivors may feel that sex will lead them to a state of helplessness and absolute lack of control. Confusing sex with sexual abuse, they may believe they will always be powerless in sexual relationships. A survivor expressed this belief:

Sex is dangerous. It feels like invasion and ownership of myself and
my body by someone else. If I stay away from sex, I can stay intact;
if I give in to it, I lose myself.

In contrast, the idea that sex is uncontrollable can lead some survivors to act in sexually self-destructive ways. They may figure since
they can't control it they might as well give in to it. Survivors may compulsively and aggressively seek sexual activities. Believing sex is uncontrollable, survivors may become sexually demanding or may give in to
the sexual demands of their partners. They may ignore the need to use
birth control or safe sex practices, increasing their chances of having an
unwanted pregnancy or contracting AIDS and other sexually transmitted diseases.

Sexual abuse—not sex—can be seen as an uncontrollable force. The
offender's actions were not due to a driving force to *have sex* but rather
to a driving force to *sexually abuse*. The offender was addictively compelled to sexually abuse. Healthy sex is nonaddictive. In healthy sex, sex
has limits. It is controllable and fulfilling. It doesn't lead to feelings of
shame, self-loathing, or regret. It enhances your self-esteem and
increases feelings of safety and mutual enjoyment with a partner.

False idea 2: Sex is hurtful

As a result of sexual abuse, survivors may come to believe that sex is
always physically and emotionally hurtful. Sexual abuse can be painful
if it is violent and sadistic. But even when it's gentle, abuse leaves survivors with the pain of feeling betrayed and used by the offender.

The sex in sexual abuse can hurt physically for many reasons. In violent sexual abuse, offenders use sex as a way to express feelings of anger,
rage, and hostility. They may see sexual organs as weapons or targets of
injury and pain.

Some sexual abuse involves sadistic practices such as physical
restraint, force, torture, and bodily mutilation that are intended to
cause the victim pain. Many offenders are sexual sadists who psychologically enjoy making their victims suffer. They may have hurt their victims as a way to become sexually aroused.

Forced sex and abusive intercourse and penetration inhibit muscle
relaxation and lubrication in females. If we were children when the
abuse occurred, our bodies were too small and underdeveloped for sex-

ual intercourse and other forms of penetration. Abuse by a peer or sibling can also cause physical pain because child and adolescent sex offenders are often clumsy and have little understanding or regard for how hurtful their actions can be to their victims.

Survivors of physically painful abuse may assume that *sex* caused the pain they felt. They may have trouble seeing that it was the violent, sadistic, premature, or forced acts in *sexual abuse* that hurt them.

Sex in sexual abuse also hurts because it involves psychological betrayal and loss. Survivors may come to believe that it was sex that caused the loss of trust. "If it weren't for sex," a survivor of acquaintance rape said, "we could have stayed friends." An incest survivor expressed a similar feeling: "If it weren't for sex, Daddy would have been able to be a good daddy to me." In both cases it really was *sexual abuse* that damaged their relationships.

Angie, a thirty-five-year-old survivor, was a teen when her father, an avid hunter, ordered her to undress in front of him one afternoon while she was working on a quilt in her bedroom. Angie noticed that her father looked at her with the same excited stare he showed when he was duck hunting. "His breathing became faster, his mouth opened slightly, he started salivating, and the tip of his tongue protruded between his lips," she said. Turning around for him as he examined her naked body, Angie suddenly knew what it felt like to be prey.

> I felt like the duck looked as it tumbled to the ground. After he left I didn't want to look at or touch any of the things in my bedroom. I felt like I no longer had power over anything. I had lost the power of protection over my own body. My cut fabrics, my sewing machine, my stuffed animals, my books, everything I loved seemed humiliated and defiled too. Sex came to represent domination, emotional pain, and a feeling of spiritual death.

Sexual abuse hurts and destroys human closeness and trust. Healthy sex is quite the opposite. It doesn't hurt; it is nurturing and fun. Healthy sex expresses and encourages safety and caring.

False idea 3: Sex is a commodity

When people are sexually victimized, they often learn to see sex as a commodity, something to give, get, or withhold. A victim of childhood sexual abuse may learn that if she "gives" sex she will be treated more kindly and shown more affection. Sex may have become, in her mind, a "ticket for love." As an adult this same person may use sex as a reward to a partner for being nice or as a bribe to get a partner to be nice. Abusive sex teaches survivors that sex is a commodity that can be exchanged for attention, love, power, and security.

This commodity view of sex is also reinforced by our culture with phrases such as "*losing* your virginity," "*getting* laid," and "*giving* sex." In this frame of mind people are reduced to sexual objects, and sex becomes no more than acts of physical stimulation and release. Sex becomes something to obtain, a skill to possess, or a commodity to "sell" to others. Prostitution and pornography thrive on this way of thinking about sex.

Many survivors were bribed with the promise of jewelry, gifts, money, or job promotions as a method of coercing them into sexual activity. They learned that sex could be exchanged for wealth or status. Offenders may have portrayed sex as an economically powerful commodity. A teenaged survivor of father-daughter incest recounted her experience:

> When I was a girl my father would take me shopping. He'd point out a dress or a pair of shoes and ask me if I wanted them. When I'd say yes, he'd tell me if I did this and this and this with him sexually, he'd get me the things. Or he'd tell me if I did one sex act he'd give me such and such an amount of money, and if I did another sex act or let him take pictures of me, he'd give me more.

Another teen recalled a variation on this scenario:

> When I was younger, my dad would always show me pictures of naked girls in *Playboy* magazines. He told me about the girls—who they were and how they lived. He told me he'd be my manager when I got older and wanted to get into *Playboy*. I didn't know what a prostitute was then, but my dad would tell me that there were girls who would stand on street corners and sell their bodies and there were guys who managed them. The girls would get to live in fancy apartments and wear fancy clothes and buy fancy cars. He said all I'd have to do was what I was doing to him. He said he was showing me how to do it so I would be able to get ahead in life.

When sex is learned as a commodity, the pull to continue thinking of sex this way can be strong. Survivors may fear that without this view, they would suffer economically, feel bankrupt, or be deprived. A survivor who has thought of sex as a payoff for financial support from a partner may worry that she will be destitute if she begins to change her view of sex.

In the commodity view sex can also be seen as a payoff for love and faithfulness. I have to give it to him or he'll want to get it elsewhere, a survivor might think. Survivors who believe sex is a commodity fear their partners will leave them if they stop being sexual. Jason, a twenty-year-old survivor who attends college, exclaimed, "I think every woman I date expects sex of me and will be angry if I don't make a pass for it." When sex is seen as a commodity, it can feel like a job to be performed.

In sexual abuse, sex is often learned as an obligation. When Eva was twelve, her mother went into the hospital for a hysterectomy. Her father informed her that now she was the oldest female of the house and in that capacity had to be his sexual partner.

Some victims learned sex was something they had to do to protect their own lives or the lives of others. One survivor said she had sex with her stepfather to keep him satisfied so he wouldn't physically abuse her mother and herself, or sexually molest her younger sisters. A male survivor who was abused in satanic rituals was taught that if he didn't participate in certain sexual acts, he would be thrown into a fire. Survivors who have survived these kinds of life-threatening experiences may unconsciously continue to believe that they will be beaten or killed if they don't have sex.

Though it may be difficult for survivors to realize and to believe deep down, healthy sex is *not* a commodity. The kind of sex that is a commodity is abusive, unhealthy, and often degrading. Healthy sex is an expression of self-love and shared intimacy. Developing a new meaning for sex means moving away from the damaging view of sex as a commodity and toward seeing your sexuality not as an entity separate from yourself but rather as a part of who you are.

False idea 4: Sex is secretive

The sex in sexual abuse is secretive. Offenders often say to their victims, "Don't tell anyone about this" or "Let this be our little secret." An offender may threaten to do something hurtful to a survivor if the secret of the sexual activity is revealed. Some survivors may think they have to remain silent about sexual matters to survive.

Sexual abuse, especially in childhood, may teach that sex is exciting when forbidden and dangerous. Later, survivors may feel that if sex is open and approved by others, it isn't as satisfying. Sexual arousal may have been learned in circumstances in which sex was secretive. Sneakiness may have become associated with heightened arousal or "better sex." In abusive sex, sneakiness is routine.

Many survivors say secretive, compulsive sexual activity is the most intense and satisfying experience they know. Fear of getting caught may increase the adrenaline rush, fueling a chemical high in the secret sex. But like taking drugs, this high is a trap. To maintain the affair, the compulsive masturbation, the illegal sexual activity, the survivor has to lie over and over. Viewing sex as secretive can make it feel shameful. "This must really be bad if I can't talk about it," a survivor may think. This kind of sex becomes self-destructive.

A secretive view of sex makes communication about sex impossible. You can't speak about your real sexual feelings and needs. Because of the lack of open communication, survivors may feel the same as they did in the abuse—all alone during sex.

Seeing sex as secretive can have another negative consequence. Survivors may fail to get accurate information and education about sexual concerns. They may go through life with misunderstandings about their own sexuality, generating anxiety for themselves unnecessarily. "For years I worried that I had damaged my clitoris by masturbating as a child," a survivor revealed. "It wasn't until college when I talked to a sex education nurse that I found out I hadn't. What a relief."

Survivors who believe that sex is secretive may have difficulty understanding that sex can be private and personal but also a topic to be openly discussed at times when it is appropriate, such as with a partner or a medical care professional. Healthy sex does not promote secrecy and engender fear or shame. It is a good and natural human behavior of which you can feel proud.

False idea 5: Sex has no moral boundaries

In sexual abuse, sex is learned as having no limits. There is no right or wrong when it comes to abusive sexual expression. For the offender anything goes. A feel-good ethic pervades. An offender might think, If it makes me feel good, I'll go ahead and do it, or, I'll enjoy now and worry about consequences later.

In this view of sex, sexual fantasies are to be acted out, regardless of how hurtful their content. Pornographic material is to be acquired, devoured, and shared with victims no matter how abusive and humanly degrading its contents. Sexual offenders may ridicule people who want to put restrictions on sexual behavior as being uptight or sexually inhibited.

In sexual abuse, sex is like a game. Having sex means winning, even if it means someone else loses. That certain behaviors might be inappropriate, hurtful, and exploitive is seen as insignificant when compared to the overpowering importance of fulfilling sexual urges and desires.

Offenders do not consider the moral implications of what they do. They don't think about how their actions could affect their families, their communities, and the whole of humanity for years to come. They don't care if their victims are their own children, siblings, students, clients, or friends. They don't worry about the disruptions they are causing to established relationships. Offenders don't analyze what effect their behavior is having on their victims or what the long-term psychological or medical consequences might be—even if devastating. In all these ways, offenders teach a mentally, physically, and spiritually unhealthy approach to sex. Their actions threaten the whole human system that is based on mutual respect and trust.

Sexual abuse teaches that sex is something where anything goes and where anything can be gotten away with. Many offenders break laws and never get reported, caught, or punished for the sexual crimes they commit.

Associating moral neglect with sex can create many problems for survivors. Survivors may withdraw from sex, fearing it will lead them into moral decay. Survivors may act out sexually in inappropriate and hurtful ways without seeing the potential damage of their actions at the time. And, sadly, survivors may continually create abusive sexual fantasies and expose themselves to degrading pornography, thinking that these activities are *sex* when they are really extensions and replays of *sexual abuse.**

Unlike abusive sex, healthy sex involves a strong regard for fairness in human relationships. The potential consequences of one's behavior are kept in mind. Healthy sex encompasses a concern for the betterment of all individuals and humanity. Healthy sex is moral and just.

---

* For an excellent essay on pornography and its effects, see David Mura's *A Male Grief*, which can be found in the Resources section.

HEALTHY IDEAS ABOUT SEX*

"I grew up having absolutely no idea of what normal, healthy sexuality would be," said one survivor. "I didn't have a clue. I didn't know there was such a thing as a trusting sexual relationship between two people."

Another survivor, after realizing her beliefs about sex were really about sexual abuse, expressed a sense of bewilderment many survivors feel: "If sex isn't sexual abuse, then what is it?"

Many survivors have trouble conceiving of sex as something that encourages health and intimacy. This is understandable since little time is spent in our culture teaching people about healthy sex and its values. We may receive many messages about abusive sex on a daily basis—in television shows, movies, magazines, and jokes—and few if any messages about healthy sex.

To help you create a new concept of sex, let's take time to consider six healthy ideas about sex:

1. Sex is a natural biological drive.
2. Sex is powerful healing energy.
3. Sex is part of life itself.
4. Sex is conscious and responsible.
5. Sex is an expression of love.
6. Sexual experiences are mutually desired.

Healthy idea 1: Sex is a natural biological drive

All animals have an inherent sex drive. Even among humans, this is a natural and normal part of being alive. Our sex drive encourages us to reproduce as a species.

The human sex drive is strongly influenced by chemicals in our bodies that respond to messages in our brains. In healthy sex this drive involves more than procreation. Sex becomes a means to experience self-love and pleasure, as well as physical closeness and emotional intimacy with a partner.

We are not at the mercy of our hormones, however. We can regulate our sexual urges and responses by how we think about sex. If we feel sex-

---

* I would like to thank C. Leon Hopper, Jr., and Barbara Wells, ministers of the East Shore Unitarian Church in Bellevue, Washington, for contributing material on healthy sexuality from a spiritual perspective.

ual desire, we can choose whether we want to act on it. In healthy sex we exercise control and choice over our sexual drives.

Sex can enhance our self-esteem and physical well-being. A healthy, happy sex life—by giving us warmth, closeness, excitement, pleasure, and release—can put us in touch with a range of positive feelings. But sex is not a need like food, shelter, or clothing. Our individual survival does not depend on it. Though it may be a little uncomfortable at times, nothing bad happens to us physically if we have sexual urges and don't act on them. "Sex is a bonus in life," a survivor said. "Sex is one possible way of expressing love. It's an extra."

Sex is not something we can expect someone else to give us on demand, whenever we feel sexual urges. Nor do we owe anyone sex. In healthy sex, each person assumes responsibility for responding to his or her own sex drives and for deciding when and with whom to share intimacy.

Healthy idea 2: Sex is powerful healing energy

Sex tied to abuse is experienced as a bad kind of power—a power over others, a power to restrict and control, to own and hurt. But sex in a healthy setting is experienced as a good kind of power—a power to create, a power to give birth to life and love. Theologian Frederick Buechner suggests that sexuality, in its tremendous power, is much like nitroglycerin: When used in one way it can blow up bridges; used in another way it can heal the human heart.*

Sex is an energy that feels good. It can be relaxed, fun, and pleasurable. In sexual arousal we experience warming, soothing, exciting, and nurturing sensations in our bodies. Sexual climax can release muscular tension and can enable us to feel alive and warm inside.

Being sexual can enhance and strengthen our self-esteem. It involves feeling attractive and likable. The comfort and closeness of intimacy with a caring, respectful partner can help us feel good about ourselves. One survivor explained healthy sex this way:

> I now believe sex is a furthering of communication. It helps our relationship grow and be strong. For us sex is clean, innocent, pleasurable, and fun.

* Frederick Buechner, *Now and Then* (New York: Harper & Row, 1983), 87.

When lovemaking is mutually desired and joyous, it brings peace. Partners feel spiritually connected to each other and to the good energy in the universe. Rebecca Parker, a theologian, writes

> Sexual intimacy can serve as a resource for healing and transformation in our lives. Through it we can experience a restored sense of intrinsic joy in being, elemental goodness, personal power to affect and be affected, intimate connection with all of life, and creative potency. . . . When it functions this way in our lives, making love is a means of grace.*

From a healthy sex perspective, sexual energy has the power to bring individuals together, to express love and caring, to create life, and to fulfill our longing for unity and wholeness.

Healthy idea 3: Sex is part of life itself

Sexual experiences, whether they are alone or shared with a partner, can connect us with broader life energy. "Sex is the vital life force," say John Travis and Regina Ryan, authors of the *Wellness Workbook*:

> [Sex] is the energy of our aliveness. Sex is also the preservation of life—a type of communication in which the entire organism attempts to unify itself with another. . . . "Well-sex" is freely chosen, conscious of consequences, respectful, erotic, playful, expansive and unifying.†

Sex is one of the natural rhythms of the universe. Orgasm is like a wave: building strength, reaching a peak, spilling onto the shore, and then receding in calmness. Or sex can be viewed as a flower: starting as a bud, opening up, reaching a state of fullness, releasing beautiful scent, its petals falling off, the flower fading away. Building tension and releasing it in the pleasure of sex can nurture one's body and spirit.

And sex can be seen as sharing one's essence with a beloved, trusted

* Rebecca Parker, "Making Love as a Means of Grace." *Open Hands*, Affirmation: United Methodists for Lesbian/Gay Concerns, 3, no. 3 (Winter 1988): 8–12.

† John Travis and Regina Sara Ryan, *Wellness Workbook*, 2d ed. (Berkeley: Ten Speed Press, 1988), 185.

partner, feeling the momentary pleasure of union, like the pleasure of dancing together as one. A survivor described her thoughts:

> I used to view sex as a thing separate from myself that arrived like a package when two persons' genitalia joined. Now I see it as an experience I can design and create myself.

Sex is more than stimulation, sensation, or sexual acts. Sometimes it's expressed as a warm stirring inside—the pleasure of being happy and safe with someone for whom you feel an attraction. Especially in the context of sexual healing, we need to remember that sex is much more than intercourse or orgasm.

Our sexuality is a significant part of who we are. It exists within life, rather than outside or apart or secret from other experiences. Like the feeling of a breeze on our faces, the warmth of the sun on our skin, or the touch of a hand in ours, sex is part of a whole, large continuum of human touch. Sex is a way to tune into our aliveness.

Healthy idea 4: Sex is conscious and responsible

Sexual urges and attractions are normal and healthy. Whether and when we act on them is another story altogether. Sexual activity needs to be entered into with an awareness of possible outcomes and effects. We need to be sure that we ourselves, our sexual partners, and other people in our communities will not be hurt as a result of what we do. Sex involves ethical responsibilities.

Sex means being aware of what is happening in a sexual encounter. It means sharing feelings, thoughts, and needs with a partner, and listening and being listened to. The focus of sex is on the relationship, the emotional intimacy, rather than on any specific sexual act.

Healthy idea 5: Sex is an expression of love

Sex is not a way to *get* love. It is an expression *of* love that emerges out of relationship. We don't do it *to* someone or even *for* someone, we experience sex *with* someone. Sex is a way of showing caring and respect for another person. It is a physical expression of something that already exists in a relationship. It is not essential to a relationship, but it's one possible outgrowth of a relationship. When partners care about each other, are friends as well as lovers, the sexual experience can be a varied, continual renewal of their sense of unity. A survivor said:

> I now view sex as a very loving, caring act. Sex is one result of love, instead of the other way around. As long as I have sex in a healthy way, there is nothing wrong with it. I prefer to love someone first before having sex.

When sex is an expression of love, sexual arousal and pleasure can become personally associated with one's partner. The love we feel for another in our hearts is translated into warm, tingling sensations in our genitals. Sex becomes a way to express how happy we are to be with a partner. The editors of the *New Age Journal* write:

> Sex is our most intimate form of communication. At its most intense, communication becomes communion—a mutual opening and meeting beyond words and concepts from our deepest and most vulnerable parts. Such communication is only possible when there is openness, honesty, and regard for your partner as an equal. This may seem obvious, but it is the most fundamental aspect of sex, and one that is too often forgotten. Sex reminds us of our interdependence and oneness.*

Author Anaïs Nin said, "Only the united beat of sex and heart together can create ecstasy."

Healthy idea 6: Sexual experiences are mutually desired

Sexual relations require full informed consent and equality between partners. If a relationship is lopsided, undermining, controlling, or dishonest, the sexual relationship will also be.

In healthy sex, partners don't impose their sexual needs on each other. Rather, each person in the relationship takes responsibility for his or her own sexual urges and release. "If either one of us doesn't want to make love, the other person doesn't pressure or complain. We just accept that's the reality for now," a partner of a survivor said. Healthy, positive sex needs a healthy, positive context for it to exist within.

---

* Rich Fields et al., eds., *Chop Wood, Carry Water: A Guide to Finding Spiritual Fulfillment in Everyday Life* (Los Angeles: Jeremy Tarcher Publishers, 1984), 63–64.

CHANGING YOUR ATTITUDES ABOUT SEX

Once you learn about the difference between abusive sex and healthy sex, you may be amazed at how deeply you have believed in an abusive view of sexuality. For some survivors, the prospect of letting go of the sexual abuse mind-set and replacing it with healthy sexual attitudes may seem extremely difficult.

Changing our sexual attitudes makes us challenge our old assumptions about people and relationships. "I have always assumed that all men were just like the offender—wanting to hurt me, cause me pain, and make me have sex with them," a woman survivor said. "To change my views about sex and stop thinking of it as abuse, means I have to stop thinking men are uncaring, insensitive, and just interested in sex."

Survivors who were victimized by female offenders may have difficulty letting go of similar misconceptions about women. "It's hard for me to consider that a woman would really enjoy sex and not merely use it for her own purposes and gain," explained one survivor.

Survivors may also find it difficult to imagine that sexual relationships can ever be equal. As a result of abuse, they may believe that sexual relationships are inherently imbalanced, with one person dominating and the other submitting.

For some survivors the thought of changing their sexual attitudes can be frightening. They may worry that with new attitudes they will pressure themselves to give up certain harmful sexual behaviors they like to some extent. Making changes can involve facing some harsh realities and stepping away from what is harmful even if it is familiar. The fear comes from making a change, not from losing something that could be hurting you.

Changing our sexual attitudes takes time. We first develop a new intellectual understanding of sex and then need to translate and integrate this new understanding into our sexual behaviors. For awhile, even once we realize they are wrong, our old beliefs may still control our reactions at a gut level. One survivor recounted the slowness of the process:

> Once I saw how much sexual abuse was influencing my attitudes
> about sex, I couldn't just switch to a healthy perspective on sex
> right away. It took me months and years to stop acting based on my
> old attitudes. I needed lots of time to test out my new ideas and put
> the new meaning I've created for sex into practice.

As you work to change your sexual attitudes, you may need to constantly remind yourself that there is a difference between abusive sex and healthy sex. You may need to challenge one by one your old, negative beliefs about sex. Two lists that compare abusive and healthy outlooks on sex follow. You may want to refer to this summary table as you progress on your sexual healing journey, to measure how your sexual attitudes are changing.

SEXUAL ATTITUDES

Sexual Abuse Mind-set *(Sex = Sexual Abuse)*	*Healthy Sexual Attitudes* *(Sex = Positive Sexual Energy)*
Sex is uncontrollable energy.	Sex is controllable energy.
Sex is an obligation.	Sex is a choice.
Sex is additive.	Sex is a natural drive.
Sex is hurtful.	Sex is nurturing, healing.
Sex is a condition for receiving love.	Sex is an expression of love.
Sex is "doing to" someone.	Sex is sharing with someone.
Sex is a commodity.	Sex is part of who I am.
Sex is void of communication.	Sex requires communication.
Sex is secretive.	Sex is private.
Sex is exploitive.	Sex is respectful.
Sex is deceitful.	Sex is honest.
Sex benefits one person.	Sex is mutual.
Sex is emotionally distant.	Sex is intimate.
Sex is irresponsible.	Sex is responsible.
Sex is unsafe.	Sex is safe.
Sex has no limits.	Sex has boundaries.
Sex is power over someone.	Sex is empowering.

Unfortunately, you can't magically erase your old thinking and replace it with a healthier mind-set. You must learn to integrate changes in your thinking with changes in your sexual reactions and behaviors. You're involved in a process of relearning how you think about sex. Give yourself time to reinforce what you are now learning, gradually molding new ideas with new behaviors.

Here are some suggestions for ways you can facilitate making changes in your sexual attitudes.

1. *Avoid exposure to things that reinforce the sexual abuse mind-set.*
Avoid television shows, movies, books, magazines, web sites,* and other
influences that portray sex as sexual abuse.

Pornography is harmful to sexual healing. It conveys the idea of
unlimited sexual access to women, children, and men. Pornography
exploits the people who act in it as well as the public who buys it. It uses
sexual stimulation to make money, reinforcing the commodity view of
sex. Pornography evokes strong emotions, such as fear and excitement,
and encourages sexual arousal to abusive ideas and images. Pornography
depicts sex from the perspective of someone who has compulsive and
unhealthy sexual interests. Pornography gives us destructive and false
impressions about sex. It makes sexual aggression appear pleasurable,
increasing our tolerance of coercion in sexual relations. Pornography
teaches that one can never have enough sex; one never reaches a state
of satisfaction or satiety with sex.

Though they can be hard to find, some movies, books, and magazines use sexual stories and imagery without being abusive.† I call these
positive erotica. The sexual relationships they describe exist in a healthy
sex context, with consent, mutuality, respect, safety, relaxed fun, and so
on. Unlike abusive pornography, these erotic materials can increase
awareness of our sensuality and pleasurable connectedness with a partner.

In sexual healing, we can replace "hard-core" sex with "*heart*-core" sex.

2. *Use new language when referring to sex.* The way you talk about
sex influences how you think about it. Change your language so you
refer to sex as a positive, healthy experience you have control over and

---

* Due to the availability and anonymity of pornography and sex chatroom activities on
the Internet, many people are now at increased risk of developing sexual compulsions and
addictions. Internet-caused sexual addictions tend to develop quickly and intensely.
When left untreated, they can seriously harm a person's emotional health and interpersonal relationships.

† Because of the different abuse histories and sexual orientations of survivors, it's difficult
to suggest specific resources for "nonabusive" erotica. In my practice as a sex therapist, I
sometimes suggest clients read select contemporary romance novels (by Mary Jo Putney,
Nora Roberts, Susan Johnson, Jayne Ann Krentz, and others) which often portray sex as
consensual, mutually pleasurable, safe, and intensely rewarding. I also recommend my *Passionate Hearts* and *Intimate Kisses* poetry anthologies (see Resources section), as well as
videos on sensual massage and tantric sex. Some sensitively produced erotic videos are
available through New Leaf Distributors (call 800-326-2665 for a catalogue). I suggest you
have a nonsurvivor friend or support person screen materials to provide you with recom-
mendations.

can make choices about. Avoid slang terms for sexual contact, such as *fucking, screwing, banging,* and *getting a piece.* For many survivors these terms reinforce the sexual abuse mind-set. Instead, use terms such as *making love* or *being physically intimate.* Stop using words for sex parts such as *prick, dick, boobs, tits, cunt,* and *asshole.* In general, these terms are degrading and reinforce the idea of people as sex objects. Instead, use unloaded, accurate terms such as *penis, breasts, vagina,* or *anus.* After changing her sexual language, one survivor remarked, "I no longer think of sex as a four-letter word."

3. *Discover more about your sexual attitudes.* Spend time in activities that can help you change your present sexual attitudes to healthier beliefs.

- Imagine how your views about sex would differ if you hadn't been abused.
- Write about what you believe sex is or want it to be.
- Draw a picture or make a collage using pictures cut from magazines to show how you have viewed sex in the past and how you would like to think of sex from now on. You may want to use symbols to represent abusive sex, such as a knife, a hammer, fire, a dollar bill, or a teardrop, and other symbols to represent healthy sex, such as a heart, a happy face, a flower, a peace sign, or sunshine.

4. *Discuss ideas about healthy sexuality with others.* Talk about sex with your friends, partner, therapist, or support group members. Discuss the difference between healthy sex and abusive sex.

Bob, a thirty-year-old gay survivor of multiple forms of child sexual abuse, gained a new perspective on sex by talking with his partner.

> My partner told me that sex is a way he shows me that he loves me. Kissing and hugging are just as important to him as a specific sexual activity. For him to enjoy sex, it needs to be tender and caring, an extension of loving touch. Talking with him about sex has helped me trust him more emotionally. When we have sex, I feel it more centered in my chest rather than centered in my genitals.

Another survivor found discussions with her therapist helpful.

> I used to feel I had to earn love by being sexual. I learned that loving is something that just is.

5. *Learn more about healthy sex.* Because our society tends to expose us to an abundance of abusive ways of thinking about sex, to make changes in your sexual attitudes you will need to actively work at exposing yourself to ideas and images that portray sex as healthy and positive. Read books and articles* that can help you educate yourself more about healthy sex (see Resources section). You may also want to attend classes, lectures, or workshops at which healthy models for sex are being presented. These educational events can jog your thinking and encourage your progress, as one survivor explained:

> In a talk on spirituality and sex, my minister referred to sex as "beautiful." For days I couldn't stop thinking about what he had said. The words *sex* and *beauty* felt like opposites to me. I made myself a sign saying "Sex is beautiful" and posted it in my bedroom. I thought about the phrase daily. It took many months, but eventually I began to feel deep inside that this could be true.

Remember, it takes time to create a new meaning for sex separate from the influence of sexual abuse. Perhaps the most you can accomplish at first is to become more conscious of your previously held sexual attitudes and beliefs. You will not acquire a new meaning for sex overnight.

Once you do acquire an intellectual understanding of healthy sexuality, do not expect your behavior to change suddenly either. Expect to make changes gradually, one at a time, reinforcing your new attitudes about sex. These new attitudes will form the foundation for future growth.

Now that you have begun separating sex from sexual abuse, you are ready to redefine your sense of who you are apart from the influence of past sexual abuse.

---

* You may want to read my article, "The Maltz Hierarchy of Sexual Interaction," which describes how healthy sexuality differs from abusive and destructive sex (see Resources section). The full text of the article can be found on my web site at: www.HealthySex.com.

6

Finding Our
Real Sexual Selves

Abuse is something that is done to us. It is not who we are.
—EUAN BEAR AND PETER DIMOCK, *Adults Molested as Children*

When I was ten years old, I would walk to school with my arm stiff against my thigh, holding my skirt down. I can remember thinking that if people saw my underclothes, they would know—as I thought back then—that there was something wrong with me. This unwavering belief in my sexual strangeness persisted throughout most of my childhood. Boys would not like me, or ever want to marry me, I would tell myself, because there was something wrong with me. I was afraid to tell anyone about my thoughts for fear they would make fun of me or confirm my worst suspicions about myself.

Where did these false and damaging ideas about my sexuality come from? Why did I believe them for so many years? As an adult looking back on my own history, I can trace these thoughts to when I was six years old, around the time when an older male relative first made sexually suggestive remarks and advances toward me. Though now fairly vague, my memories of the abuse still fill me with a sense of revulsion and an urge to kick or push away. I can remember feeling fear mixed with sexual excitement when I was a child. I also remember that I felt guilty and strange that I enjoyed these sensations so much.

The abuse shaped the way I came to think about myself sexually. Because I had experienced strong sexual feelings prematurely, in a situation clouded by fear, and without anyone to help me make sense of the experience, I concluded as a child that there must be something terribly wrong with *me*.

103

How sexual abuse influences a survivor's sexual self-concept differs from person to person. For survivors who have developed a positive sense of themselves sexually prior to the abuse, and who received emotional acceptance and support after the abuse, the influence may be fairly limited. But for other survivors, perhaps most survivors, the damage can be profound.

Sexual abuse can harm how we feel about our sexual attractiveness and our sexual energy, leaving us feeling negative about our gender (being a man or a woman) or causing us confusion about our sexual orientation (being lesbian, gay, straight, or bisexual).

Our sexual identity is profoundly connected with our self-identity. When abuse hurts our sexual self-image, it hurts all of the ways we perceive ourselves. We may falsely conclude we are bad, worthless, undeserving, or damaged. This poor self-concept can trap us in a cycle of loneliness, shame, isolation, and despair. The more unworthy we feel, the more we cut ourselves off from others. And the more isolated we become, the more we may feel damaged, ashamed, and weak.

Sexual abuse may have overridden positive self-beliefs that were only beginning to form. A teenaged girl may feel attractive and sexually curious, only to lose this feeling after a date rape.

Similarly, sexual abuse may solidify negative beliefs that might otherwise have gone away. A teenaged boy may fear he is sexually inadequate, only to have this belief firmly established after a sexual seduction by an older woman in which he is unable to get an erection.

These negative feelings can wear us out, hurt us, and keep us locked in self-denying and self-destructive behaviors. When we feel poorly about ourselves sexually, we may neglect to care for ourselves, or we may engage in sexual behaviors that carry a high risk for sexual disease or revictimization. And, tragically, we may suffer years of unhappiness troubled by sexual difficulties we incorrectly believe are innate and irreparable.

This negative thinking can be so ingrained and long-standing that we may not realize it is a consequence of sexual abuse. Crippling and erroneous attitudes may appear as truths, as if we have seen ourselves only in a distorted mirror.

In this chapter you will have an opportunity to increase your understanding of how sexual abuse may have damaged your sexual self-concept. You have already begun to learn new, healthier attitudes about sex. Now you can learn to create a new sexual self-concept and to see yourself in a mirror that hasn't been warped by the abuse.

The insights you gain and the changes you consider at this time can mark a turning point in your sexual healing journey. When you develop a positive sexual self-concept, you create a foundation for making changes in your sexual behavior, overcoming sexual problems, and finding healthy enjoyment in sexual experiences.

BELIEFS ABOUT PERSONAL VALUE

From my work counseling survivors, I have identified three common conclusions that survivors reach about themselves. These are expressed in specific ways in the Sexual Effects Inventory in chapter 3. All of these conclusions are damaging and false. Believing in any of them makes us devalue and demean ourselves sexually, fueling a poor sexual self-concept. These mistaken conclusions, or false labels, are as follows:

1. I'm basically bad.
2. I'm a sexual object.
3. I'm damaged goods.

Let's begin by examining these false labels to see how each one may apply to your thinking.

False label 1: I'm basically bad

As a result of sexual abuse, many survivors feel that they are intrinsically bad. They may harbor great feelings of shame related to their sexuality and consequently may believe they are worthless, unlovable, or even evil. The belief of being intrinsically bad can develop because of events that happened before, during, or after the abuse.

I was bad before the abuse.   Jack, a thirty-five-year-old survivor, was fifteen when his parents entered his bedroom one Sunday morning and found semen stains on his bedsheets. His parents should have realized that nocturnal emissions, commonly called *wet dreams,* and masturbation are normal sexual outlets for a teenager. Jack's parents, however, humiliated and reprimanded him for these normal sexual expressions. "You are disgracing this family with your behavior," they said. From then on, whenever he ejaculated, Jack felt wrong and bad.

A year later, Jack was molested by a neighbor. The abuse solidified Jack's previous belief that he was bad and sexually out of control. His shame fueled years of acting out relief through compulsive masturbation, followed by more shame and more masturbation. In counseling, Jack has been realizing that his sexual feelings were normal: It was the *abuse* that was bad and sexually out of control, *not him*.

Nicky, a twenty-six-year-old bisexual survivor, remembered that when she was six her mother scolded her harshly for playing doctor with a little boy her own age. When Nicky was raped by an older boy from the neighborhood several months later, she concluded—on her own—that *she* had been bad again. Nicky's false conclusion about herself was due to the influence of her mother's scolding before the abuse combined with the abuse itself. The error she made was both understandable and tragic. Only years later did she begin to learn that her normal childhood sexual curiosity was healthy and good, and that it had nothing to do with the abuse.

Many parents give bad information, setting the stage for their children to reach the wrong conclusions about themselves. To sexually heal, Nicky and Jack need to learn now that their sexuality has always been fundamentally good.

Survivors may also falsely conclude that they are bad because of their need for intimacy and affection. Rochelle, a forty-year-old survivor, was three years old when she was molested by her father. One day, when she couldn't sleep on her own at nap time, she came into her father's bed to nap with him. As a child she concluded that it was her need for closeness that caused the abuse. Only now, more than thirty-seven years later, is she realizing that her desires for comfort were healthy and good, and didn't cause the abuse. Her father was bad by exploiting her desire for closeness as an opportunity to sexually molest her.

I *was bad because the offender said so.* Some survivors believe that they are bad because the offender said things like "You're a naughty boy," "You're a tease," "You seduced me and made me do this," or "You like to be bad, don't you?"

As adults these old, false messages may haunt us. The abuser's words may echo, becoming part of how we think about ourselves. Eventually we may forget where these deeply held ideas first came from.

Offenders make these kinds of statements to increase their sexual arousal. They may say these things to shield themselves from the responsibility for perpetrating abuse. Victims may sense that the offenders' actions are wrong, yet the offenders continue to project the guilt onto their victims. It can be difficult for a victim not to be influenced by an offender's projections of guilt. After all, offenders are generally older, stronger, more powerful, and possibly even a member of the family or in another position that normally demands respect.

"I feel guilty for all the things he did to me," a survivor said. It doesn't make sense rationally for the victim to feel guilt, but this sense of being bad and guilty may stick to the survivor anyway. It's hard for survivors, especially those who were young victims, to realize the offender was speaking from his or her own distorted thinking and fantasies, not describing who the victim intrinsically is.

Abusers sometimes use a child's normal curiosity about sex as a lure into sexual abuse. By shading curiosity with guilt, the offender might try to make the child feel responsible for abuse. "You wanted to know what mommies and daddies do when they're alone, didn't you?" a survivor recalled her molester saying. In reality children are by nature curious about new things and experiences—including potential dangers like razor blades, matches, and drugs. Their curiosity is not bad. What's bad is exploiting this curiosity then falsely labeling the curiosity as an excuse for abuse. Regardless of the circumstances, victims are *never* responsible for sexual abuse.

Unless sexual messages from the offender are thrown away, they can continue to block your sexual enjoyment. "If I enjoy sex, it will make me everything he said I was," a survivor said.

I was bad because I got something out of it.　Many survivors come to believe they were bad because they took gifts in exchange for sex, enjoyed special attention that came with the abuse, or felt pleasure during abuse. A woman who was molested by her father related her story:

> He liked to make me have orgasms. It made him think he was a
> great lover, satisfying his consenting daughter. I suffered from
> intense guilt for not having made him stop.

Another survivor, abused by her brother, described a similar experience. Eventually, she was able to see how her feeling bad because of her sexual responses contributed to problems with her husband.

> I remember times when I became sexually excited during the abuse.
> Afterwards, I'd feel so upset, ashamed, and disgusted with myself. I
> felt like such a bad girl. Now when I become sexually excited with
> my husband, I'll freeze as if to stop myself from having any pleasure
> during sex.

A male survivor liked his sexual feelings when his mother was seductive with him. He hated himself for fantasizing about having sex with her. "I felt very confused," he said. "Good boys don't want to have sex with their mothers."

If you feel you got something out of the abuse, it's important now to realize you are not bad. Your physical responses were normal given the circumstances. Your needs were understandable. The offender exploited those needs. Victim reward is a common ploy used by offenders. Abuse that satisfies some need in the victim is something many offenders strive for. Offenders know that victims who are getting something like money, attention, or sexual release are less likely to inform on the offender and more likely to remain available for future abuse. In addition, an offender might satisfy a victim sexually to pretend that his actions aren't really abuse.

In some abuse situations, having an orgasm was one way a victim could gain a degree of control over what was happening. Penny, a survivor of father-daughter incest, said, "The sooner I climaxed, the sooner he finished, and the quicker he'd let me go. Looking back on it, I see how my sexual response was how I took care of myself in a bad situation."

Regardless of the circumstances surrounding the abuse and the feelings you experienced during the abuse, you were innocent. You are good, and your sexuality is good, too.

I was bad because of actions after the abuse. Some survivors feel they are intrinsically bad because of things they did after the abuse. One survivor of childhood incest felt bad about herself because of how often she began lying after the abuse.

> As a child, I felt like a caged animal. I had to be on guard constantly. I had to plan ahead to avoid further abuse, which meant I had to learn how to lie and make excuses.

This was not a moral failure or an indication of being bad; lying helped her survive.

Many survivors act out sexually after abuse. They may develop new, unusual sexual behavior such as compulsive masturbation, sado-masochism, or frantic sexual activity. This makes them feel worse and may fuel more extreme behavior yet. Survivors may go through periods of being sexually self-destructive. They may socialize with people they know could abuse them, participate in degrading and unsafe sexual practices, prostitute themselves, or use alcohol and other drugs that impair their judgment. Some survivors may even sexually abuse others or engage in deceptive sexual practices such as having secretive affairs.

These acting-out sexual behaviors can become part of a negative cycle: Survivors feel so bad after acting out sexually that they come to believe these behaviors "prove" they were bad to start with and thus deserved the original abuse. Sexual acting out is a repercussion of sexual abuse, not an accurate reflection of a survivor's natural sexual self. Acting out may be a replay of the abuse, an attempt to blot out the pain caused by the abuse, or a cry for help.

Reactive sexual practices can generate intense feelings of guilt and shame. A gay male survivor of multiple forms of sexual abuse discussed his experience:

> My sexual experiences as an adult put me in a role of being domi-nated and humiliated, just as I was in the abuse. I'd go through periods of casual sex with many anonymous partners, which are very dangerous in this time of AIDS. I sought sex with strangers to ease my loneliness. My guilt feelings over having so many partners, and the humiliation, kept me in a constant state of feeling that I was a bad and worthless person.

By understanding that any sexual acting out after abuse was a reper-cussion of the abuse, you can begin to free yourself of continually feeling bad. A twenty-five-year-old bisexual survivor who was molested by her father when she was a toddler shared her story.

> During my childhood, from ages seven to fifteen, I had sex with many other children—boys and girls, many men, even one priest. I masturbated several times a day. I tried a lot of different sexual activities on myself. I even made sexual advances toward my sister and touched her in bed on several occasions. I knew it wasn't right. I believed there was something basically wrong with me. I knew I was out of the ordinary sexually. I knew I had sexual problems, but basically I thought I myself was the problem—that I was bad to begin with.
>
> It wasn't until several years ago that I began to stop blaming myself. I saw how the priest and other men took advantage of me. I hurt other children because of what my father did to me, not because of who I am underneath.

Considering these cases, it's good to remember that feeling bad may serve a purpose, even today. Often it may be an attempt to protect yourself from feeling powerless and betrayed. It can give you an illusion of control in a situation that was out of control. You can fool yourself into believing that you could have prevented or altered the abuse by making changes in your own behavior. If you focus on feeling bad about yourself, you don't have to admit that you felt vulnerable, powerless, unloved, exploited, or let down by others.

Finding out why you may feel bad about yourself can put you in touch with a lot of buried feelings. Tom, a thirty-year-old survivor, cried as he told me his story.

> I felt like a bad kid when my dad molested me. Dad always said we were sharing and loving in the sexual contact. I believed him, even though it hurt and felt humiliating. I thought I was to blame and that there was something wrong with me. I felt ugly and bad inside.
>
> Now, as I reject the idea that I was bad, I'm left with feeling that I had no control over what happened, and that *my father used me for his own sexual gratification.* I was merely an object to him. I get this awful feeling of a void inside, a big empty hole at my core. It feels like I don't really exist. No one's there, or is the real me in hiding?

While letting go of feeling bad can be painful, it brings relief. Another survivor told of the change it made in her life:

> I used to think that if I was to want to be sexual, I'd be bad, since the abuse was sexual and bad. Now I can see that my being sexual has nothing to do with abuse. I can enjoy it for myself and still feel good about who I am.

False label 2: I'm a sexual object

In sexual abuse, offenders treat victims as sexual objects. "You sexy little thing," a rapist might say. Offenders physically touch victims with no respect or regard for the victim's humanity or rights. Offenders treat victims as if they were mannequins come to life—living representations of their sexual fantasy objects.

As a result, survivors may also come to view themselves as sexual objects. They may feel they have lost their individual identity, believe that they must sexually please others, or view themselves as easily controlled by others. Survivors who conclude they are sexual objects keep themselves tied to the exploitive and hurtful thinking of the offender. When survivors continue to view themselves as objects, it permits the offender and the abuse to contaminate sexual relationships today. By understanding how the sense of being a sexual object is related to the abuse, survivors can start to free themselves from this harmful way of thinking.

Let's examine some common ways survivors feel they have become sexual objects.

I have lost my individual identity.   Sexual abuse forces victims into roles in which they are robbed of a sense of themselves as individuals with feelings, needs, and rights. "I felt like a pawn used to ensure my brother's heterosexuality," said a woman survivor who had been molested by her brother after he had been molested by an older man.

Sexual abuse can make some survivors feel they are sexual objects without gender. Andy, a twenty-nine-year-old survivor struggling to overcome the view of himself as a genderless object, explained:

> When I was ten I served as the lookout while my older brother had sex with my sister. After a time my sister started refusing my older brother, and my older brother turned to me for sex. I came to feel I was merely a sexual substitute for my sister, a creature without an identity of my own.

Shawna, a twenty-five-year-old survivor, felt that she lost a sense of her identity because she had to deny her own feelings and needs during the abuse. When Shawna was eleven, a fifteen-year-old male cousin cornered her in a barn and forced her to have oral sex. The experience left her feeling that being sexual means ignoring her own existence and rights. In group therapy Shawna explained this feeling:

> I can now see that my whole sense of who I am sexually started in the abuse. The experience with my cousin made me feel unattractive and dirty. I felt like an *object*, a plain, unimportant object. I was unworthy of affection and so unable to have *needs*, especially in connection with sexual activity. How dare I even think of asking for *anything!*

The sense of having no identity can be extreme in some survivors, like Tess, who was a victim of repeated sexual molestation and torture in sadistic rituals.

I see myself as not quite human—like an android with certain functions, like providing sex to anyone who requests it. I don't feel entitled to some very human things like love, a relationship, or marriage.

Even if you were treated inhumanely in the past, you are not without your own feelings, needs and rights. You can reclaim these now, as you sexually heal.

I am a sexual pleaser.   As a result of being treated like an object, some survivors build a sexual identity around pleasing a partner sexually. Survivors may literally live to please. "I am nothing without somebody," said a survivor who had worked as a prostitute. "I'm a commodity. My most attractive feature is my ability to distract and please males."

For some survivors this role of pleasing others is passive. A woman might make herself available to have sex with her partner whenever the partner wants it. For other survivors the role of pleasing is active. Looking back on how he saw himself as a sexual pleaser, a male survivor recalled his feelings:

I carried a tape in my head that said I'm bad and unworthy. I gained a false sense of self-esteem by being a sexual performer and mechanic. I would fix the sexual problems of my partners, help them have orgasms and feel satisfied. I often sabotaged my own enjoyment of sex by playing these roles. Inside I played victim a lot.

Survivors who are sexual pleasers believe sex is a condition for receiving love. They may look to sexual partners for approval and acceptance. "I used to think that if I did what my date wanted, it meant I was okay," a survivor said.

Pleasing a partner can take on a desperate quality. Some survivors hunt for the love they need by offering themselves sexually to partners. "The only way I feel I can be loved is if I am sexual," a survivor said. "If I can give someone really good sex, they will love me."

These survivors may believe their worth is determined by how many people want them sexually. Feeling this way can lead survivors to dress and behave seductively. They make their bodies into lures to catch partners. Sexual objectification is something others do to them and also something these survivors do to themselves.

Unfortunately, survivors who focus on sexually pleasing others may have difficulty feeling loved themselves. In seeing themselves as sexual objects for someone else's pleasure, they may interpret genuine caring love as just another bid for sex.

If you feel that your worth is determined by what you do sexually, you stay locked in a view of yourself as a sexual object. You deny the value of your whole personhood. By freeing yourself from acting like a robotic sexual pleaser, you give yourself the opportunity to feel loved for yourself, separate from sex.

I can be easily controlled by others. In sexual abuse, offenders force or lead victims into submissive roles. Victims must behave sexually without a sense of personal control or power. Victims may begin to view themselves as sexual slaves. A woman who had been abused by her brother recounted her experience:

> My brother would say, "You do what I want you to, when I want you to, and how I want you to." My feelings and reactions didn't count, so I learned to shut them off, ignore them completely. I was a tool for him to use, whenever he wanted to use me.

As a result of their past abuse survivors may come to see themselves as having no ability to influence the course of a present-day sexual experience. "I feel like a rag doll, with no mind of my own," a survivor said. The feeling of being controlled by someone else can creep into social relationships as well. A survivor who was abused by her father said:

> Men can control me. Whenever I get around a male I turn into a bubble-headed victim. It doesn't matter if the guy is thinking of me sexually or not. I don't feel I am in charge of myself. I feel automatically his.

To overcome this feeling of having no control, you need to remind yourself that you now have a choice. Being submissive may have been useful, and even imperative, during the abuse. But continuing to act submissive now will only hinder your ability to have a positive self-concept and satisfying intimate relationship.

If you see yourself as a sexual object, you can change this illusion. *You are not a sexual object; you are a sacred soul.*

False label 3: I'm damaged goods

Sexual abuse hurts. It causes mental and physical injuries. Survivors may conclude that they are damaged goods, that the abuse has rendered them sexually disabled, inadequate, or inferior. A survivor said:

> I feel like an amputee, without phantom nerve impulses. It's as though the connection between my heart place and my pelvic place has been severed. When I get in touch with this, I feel tremendous loss. My body feels like an empty, lifeless husk that houses my brain.

Survivors may feel they are unwanted—"No one would want me if they knew what happened to me"—or unworthy—"I'm not as good as others because I did not have normal experiences." Survivors may believe that what they have to offer is not good enough. Developing a new approach to sex and intimacy can be difficult if, deep down, you cling to pessimistic, limiting thoughts.

To break free from feeling damaged and inferior, you must first understand more specifically how you reached this conclusion. Here are some primary beliefs that keep survivors believing they are damaged goods.

I am the names the offender called me.   Survivors may come to believe that they are damaged goods because of messages they received from the offender. Sexual abuse is exploitation and subjugation. Many offenders enjoy calling victims vile, lewd, offensive names designed to humiliate and control. Offenders call victims names such as cunt, prick, asshole, slut, whore, bitch, shit, fag, homo, wimp, sleaze, or describe them as dirty, stupid, and frigid. Survivors often accept these labels, making them part of their sexual self-concept.

If you have internalized a name given you by an offender, it can help to realize that the name has to do with the offender's distorted, cruel, and sexually abusive thinking; it has nothing to do with who you are. You are not the labels given you.

I am what was done to me.   Survivors may have confused the abuse that was done to them with *who* they really are sexually. A survivor may think: A disgusting and bad thing happened to me, therefore I am disgusting and bad. This reasoning is unfair and untrue. Consider applying it to other situations when disgusting and bad things might happen to you: Say a car splashed mud on you as you walked down a road. Say you accidentally stepped in dog doo. Would those experiences make you disgusting and bad? The abuse is not you. It is an upsetting incident that hurt you psychologically, but you yourself—your feelings, thoughts, caring, and love—are separate from it.

I am less of a man or woman because of abuse. Survivors may believe false, hurtful cultural messages that imply a girl's worth is lessened by sex or a boy's masculinity is destroyed if he is sexually dominated. These old ideas blame and punish the victim, perpetuating the notion that women are property or that a boy's masculinity depends on his sexual prowess. Anyone can be sexually dominated and abused. Victims aren't responsible for abuse and do not deserve to be punished by society for what the offender did to them.

If you are a survivor who feels you have been culturally branded by the abuse, remind yourself that these cultural views are inhumane and cruel. You hurt yourself, and keep the abuse alive, when you believe in them.

I suffered permanent physical damage. Sexual abuse can cause lasting physical injuries and marks. Survivors may have visible scars or suffer repercussions of sexually transmitted diseases acquired in the abuse. Some women may have become pregnant by the abuser or may have been made infertile as a result of disease or damage suffered in the abuse.

Much suffering and loss can result when sexual abuse causes irreversible sexual damage. Scars and injuries are painful, continuing reminders of past abuse. Such survivors are like accident victims who need to find ways to go on with normal activities. They must grieve and cope with losses, and then learn to enjoy their lives, as much as possible, given the reality of their physical conditions.

Years back I worked in the local hospital, leading discussions on sexuality for people with spinal cord injuries, multiple sclerosis, cancer, herpes, and other problems that caused sexual impairment. Sexuality was a major issue for these patients. Yet some of them had very positive sexual self-concepts and enjoyed satisfying sexual lives. I was impressed with their attitudes and curious as to how they could feel so good about their sexuality, given the problems caused by their illnesses and injuries. What I found was that patients with positive sexual self-concepts defined sex and sexual behavior very broadly, as intimate, private touching and sharing. These patients made the best of intimate activities they were still physically able to participate in. They found creative ways for sexual expression, made intimate connections with their partners, and enjoyed themselves fully.

If you are a survivor who has suffered permanent damage, it may be helpful to remind yourself that your sexuality has more to do with your feelings of love and sensuality than with the look or functioning of a particular part of your body. You can still be a creative, loving, and sensual person, regardless of the extent of your injury.

Our sexual worth is not something we carry around with us like a balloon, which others can stick pins in, and destroy. Our sexual worth runs so deep no one can take it away, no matter what they say or do.

BELIEFS ABOUT GENDER AND SEXUAL ORIENTATION

To feel good about ourselves sexually, we need to feel good about being the man or woman we are, and comfortable with our sexual orientation, whether we are lesbian, gay, straight, or bisexual. Yet these two areas are often especially sensitive, confusing, and controversial for survivors.

Gender identity and sexual orientation are complex matters even without sexual abuse in the picture. They can be strongly influenced by a number of factors, including biology, upbringing, sexual experiences, cultural influences, and personal choice.

In this section we'll explore some of the ways that sexual abuse can negatively influence the feelings survivors have about their gender and sexual orientation. By understanding the impact of abuse, you can begin to free yourself from damaging beliefs and confusions that may have developed from the abuse.

I don't like my gender.   Because of abuse, survivors may detest their maleness or femaleness. A boy who was abused by his father might think, I don't want to be a man if men are like Dad. And a girl who was abused by her father might conclude, I don't want to be a woman if women have to be submissive and get treated like this.

Some survivors may believe their gender was the cause of the abuse. A girl might hate herself for being female because the abuse happened once she grew breasts. And a boy may hate himself for being male because his offender was sexually attracted to boys but left girls alone.

As a result of abuse you may have turned against yourself, putting down qualities that you believe are associated with your gender. A male survivor might always avoid initiating activities and expressing himself assertively. And a female survivor might refrain from allowing herself to reveal her natural beauty or express her emotional sensitivity. The rejection of your own sexual gender can lead to feelings of isolation, alienation, and self-loathing. A male survivor spoke of how he was affected by abuse:

> For many years I spoke in a high-pitched voice. I acted with female mannerisms. People thought I was gay, though I am not. I felt ambivalent about being a man and had not accepted my maleness. Over the last couple of years I have broadened my idea of what it means to be a man, and my voice has lowered significantly.

If you are a survivor who dislikes your gender, you need to remind yourself that sexual abuse is perpetrated by, and happens to, both males and females. The qualities that perpetrators and victims display during abuse, such as domination and submission, or control and helplessness, reflect the dynamics of sexual abuse. These are *not* qualities that belong to a particular gender.

Feeling good about your gender means realizing your strengths as a man or as a woman. You need to permit yourself access to a full range of human expression including positive qualities commonly associated with your gender: directness, receptivity, courage, caring, dignity, strength, and emotional vulnerability. To turn from your gender is to deny the beauty and power that go with being the person you are.

I'm different from others of my gender.   Sexual abuse can lead survivors to feel there is something that makes them different from other members of their sex.

Sometimes sexual abuse is a direct affront to gender identity. Zack, a fifty-five-year-old survivor, spent many years feeling he wasn't as masculine as his peers. When Zack was a toddler, he was frequently dressed in girl's clothing by his aunt and grandmother. They painted his nails and permed his hair. The dressing involved touching and stroking his body. This abuse taught Zack to be sexually stimulated by images of being feminized. Dressing as a female became a way for Zack to feel excited, accepted, and loved. The abuse robbed Zack of knowing what it would feel like to be a little boy who didn't want to dress like a little girl. Now, as an adult, Zack feels different from other men due to his desire to cross-dress and masturbate to thoughts of wearing women's clothing.

Sexual abuse can force survivors into roles that contradict accepted gender norms. Rick, a heterosexual survivor, learned a sexually submissive role when he was abused as a child by an older male neighbor. Now Rick finds it difficult to initiate intimate relationships and physical contact.

> I'm twenty-four years old, and I'm still a virgin. My fears about sex get in the way of being able to initiate contact. Many women I have dated have left me because they were uncomfortable that I wasn't sexually assertive the way guys are supposed to be. I'm a romantic at heart, but I think I've locked the sexual part of myself away. Recently I had a dream of a cage with its door opening up. A tiger was in there. I knew that tiger represents my maleness. This was a beautiful image for me.

Being forced into a submissive role can bring another set of consequences for males. In an attempt to compensate for feelings of sexual inadequacy and powerlessness, a boy survivor may express a caricature of what he thinks men do by acting tough, macho, and invulnerable. He may fight or destroy property in a vain attempt to prove he's not weak or feminine. Unfortunately, this strategy makes it difficult for him to identify in positive ways with other men. And it also leads many male survivors to act in sexually aggressive and demanding ways, which inhibit healthy sexual intimacy in adulthood.

Some women survivors feel different from other women because the sexual abuse taught them to be sexually active and aggressive. Acting in ways that contradict traditional female roles, these women survivors may suffer much confusion and rejection, making it difficult for them to form intimate relationships. A woman who had been molested as a child by her stepfather described her situation:

> I always felt different from other women. When I was a teen I liked sex more than the men I dated, and when I was married I liked it more than my husband did. I felt *too masculine*.

Girls and women can also act tough to cover up feelings of sexual vulnerability that resulted from sexual abuse. These compensatory behaviors can lead to feelings of being different from other females.

Alice, a twenty-four-year-old lesbian survivor, was physically abused by her father and was raped by her brother and his friends when she was ten years old. She became a star athlete in college on the women's volleyball team. She was known as the kamikaze player because she would dive for balls so hard that she sometimes hurled her body into the bleachers. Alice broke her fingers and bruised her knees, but she never cried, never showed pain.

In her adult sexual relationships, Alice wondered why she could give pleasure to her partner during sex but not receive pleasure for herself. She felt different from other women. Now, as she recovers from her early sexual abuse, Alice is realizing that she can overcome her sexual problems by accepting traits of softness and receptivity, which she has viewed as traditionally feminine.

If you are a survivor who feels different from others of your gender, you may need to take a close look at how sexual abuse has colored your view of yourself. You are a member of your sex as a result of your biology; the abuse didn't change whether you are male or female. Your gender is nothing you must prove or deny; it's a given.

While it's important to feel comfortable and affiliated with your gender, it's also important to keep in mind that healthy sexual relationships involve two individuals sharing intimacies. Both of you, regardless of gender, should be able to initiate sexual activities and receive pleasurable sensations.

I'm confused about my sexual orientation.   Sexual abuse can cause many survivors to question their sexual orientation. They may wonder whether the sexual abuse determined their present orientation or whether the abuse was the primary reason they are gay, straight, or bisexual.

The issue of sexual orientation is confusing for many people who have no history of sexual abuse. Even after conducting many studies, researchers discuss factors such as genetics, biology, upbringing, and social influences, but still do not point to any absolute "cause" of homosexuality or heterosexuality. Sexual orientation categories seem to blend together along a continuum rather than conforming to clear-cut distinctions. Very few people in the population at large feel completely gay or straight. Sexual orientation can be confusing for some people because their orientation has changed over time. For instance, a woman may live a married heterosexual life-style for many years, divorce, and later become involved in a lesbian relationship.

The issue of sexual orientation can also be a loaded one for survivors because of cultural biases against homosexuality, or, less often, against heterosexuality. While some survivors may simply be curious about sexual orientation issues, others may have extreme fear about the subject. A male survivor who succumbs to cultural prejudices and homophobia may worry that he might be gay. Some survivors experience similar biases against heterosexuality. A female survivor who is living a women-oriented life-style, for example, may become extremely upset when she considers whether she might be straight.

Although sexual abuse does not seem to exactly "cause" a particular orientation, the research on survivors does seem to indicate that, for at least some survivors, it can have a profound influence. Interestingly enough, the influence of sexual abuse on orientation can be in two different directions: Abuse seems to be able both to encourage and to impede the development of a particular orientation. Survivors may move toward or against the orientation they had in the abuse.

Some survivors *adopt the sexual orientation role they had in the abuse.* A girl abused by a girl cousin, for instance, may assume she is a lesbian, whereas a girl abused by a boy cousin may assume she is heterosexual. These assumptions are understandable, since sexual abuse is often a young person's first exposure to sexual roles.

This taking on of the sexual orientation role from the abuse will not present a problem if it is a role with which the survivor feels comfortable. If the girl who is abused by her girl cousin already *feels* herself to be a lesbian, this "adopting the role" influence becomes inconsequential. But if a survivor identified with a different sexual orientation before the abuse, or had not yet identified an orientation, this influence can be disturbing and confusing, and even lead to years of unhappiness. A lesbian survivor told of her experience:

> After the abuse by my stepfather, I assumed I must be heterosexual. I went through a horrendous period of having sex with male partners. It was painful physically and felt like an assault. This is perhaps because I'm not into men. I was with them to prove I was okay because I thought I was heterosexual at the time.

Similarly, some males who were sexually abused by other males may adopt the sexual orientation role they were made to assume in the abuse. Researcher David Finkelhor reported that adult male survivors who were victimized before age thirteen by an older male were four times more likely to be currently homosexually active than were those who did not experience any abusive male-to-male sexual contact.*

One reason that survivors may adopt the orientation role of the abuse is because of a self-labeling process. Researchers Robert Johnson and Diane Shrier, who studied boy victims, explain:

> The boy who has been molested by a man may label the experience as homosexual and misperceive himself as homosexual on the basis of his having been found sexually attractive by an older man, particularly if he has had no opportunity to be reassured and relieved of his guilt and anxiety about his role in the molestation experience. Once self-labeled as a homosexual, the boy may then place himself in situations that leave him open to homosexual activity.†

Similarly, heterosexual abuse experiences can cause a person who is homosexual to mislabel his or her orientation. The lesbian survivor who had been molested by her stepfather and assumed she was straight did just this.

In going through this self-labeling process, survivors may fail to see the distinction between healthy sex and sexual abuse. The sex that occurs in sexual abuse is not a homosexual act or a heterosexual act, but an act of *sexual abuse*. Most sexual abuse of boys is perpetrated by males who are heterosexual. Most perpetrators of sexual abuse of children are pedophiles (people who are sexually attracted to children, not necessarily to a particular gender). It's important to remember that the sex in abuse has more to do with cruelty, exploitation, and harm than with sexual activities on which to base a long-standing orientation.

Some survivors may adopt the orientation role of the abuse because they experienced sexual arousal during the abuse, and they may think that this arousal proves the orientation role they had in the abuse. You may have responded sexually during the abuse, but that does not mean that you are gay if it was homosexual abuse or straight if it was heterosexual abuse. Our bodies respond to sexual stimulation regardless of the sex of the person doing the stimulation.

Sexual abuse can teach us arousal patterns that affect how we define

---

* David Finkelhor, "The Sexual Abuse of Boys," *Victimology: An International Journal* 6 (1981): 81.

† Robert Johnson and Diane Shrier, "Past Sexual Victimization by Females of Males in an Adolescent Medicine Clinic Population," *American Journal of Psychiatry* 144, no. 5 (May 1987): 652.

our sexual orientation. Sexual abuse by a male offender, for example, can create mental images of men's bodies, sexual organs, and sexual release associated with sexual stimulation. A man who was molested by his male cousin expressed dismay about his sexual thoughts:

> I'm very confused about my sexuality—whether I'm gay or straight.
> I think I'm straight, but I don't like the obsession I have for the
> male penis.

These kinds of mental images and associations may be more of a repercussion of the abuse trauma than any real indication of sexual orientation.

Rather than feeling that the abuse led them toward the role they had in the abuse, many survivors feel that their current orientation evolved *as a reaction against the abuse.* A girl abused by her father, for instance, might turn away from heterosexuality because she associates relations with men with abuse. To her, male bodies may seem repulsive, triggering images of pain and fear. As she matures, she may seek women partners because they feel safer and more comfortable. Similarly, out of fear and negative associations with women's bodies, a lesbian girl who is abused by her mother might migrate toward relationships with men. The sexual abuse may have caused this survivor to have an antifemale reaction, making it hard for her to realize her desire for women partners.

Some male survivors also react against the orientation role of the abuse. A homosexual male, abused by a male, may later feel more comfortable relating with women. Likewise, a heterosexual male, abused by a woman, may be drawn to sexual activities with males.

One man who was abused by his mother when he was young, then abused again by a teenaged boy, suffered much confusion about his sexual orientation. He was both adopting and reacting against the orientation role of his two abuse experiences. Even with these conflicting influences, a basic heterosexual orientation seemed to persist for him.

> Growing up, my sexual concept was that of a little boy looking for
> the love his mother never gave him. I was very passive sexually and
> very afraid of women. I felt toward women the way I sometimes felt
> toward my mom—like I wasn't an adult male.
>   After I was abused by the older neighborhood boy, I decided
> temporarily that I was gay because I liked it, and I later sought out
> gay experiences even though I didn't feel attracted to men. Looking
> back now I think this gay time was easier than having to go

through my fears and mixed feelings about the women I really was attracted to. I'm now married and sometimes use gay fantasies to help me perform with my wife. I see this as a defense against intimacy with her. As I've come to understand and accept the origin of these fantasies, I seem to need them less and less.

Because of influences caused by abuse and negative cultural influences, many survivors struggle for years against a sexual orientation with which they would feel more comfortable. It is often not until they feel more secure, mature, and assertive that they can resolve their confusion.

If you are a survivor who questions your sexual orientation, remember that *all sexual orientations are valid*. In determining your sexual orientation, you may want to consider these questions:

- What was your sense of your sexual orientation before the abuse?
- Do you think you may have reacted toward or against the orientation role in the abuse, or do you think the abuse had no effect?
- Now when you do have romantic feelings, desires for deeper intimacy, consistent physical attraction, or fantasies of loving sexual contact, what is the gender of the person for whom you feel attraction?

Developing a healthy concept of yourself sexually involves feeling comfortable with your sexual orientation now. You may not be able to answer conclusively the questions you have about your sexual orientation. You will probably only cause yourself anguish if you strive for a particular orientation that you don't believe fits you at this time. What matters in sexual healing is accepting yourself and being able to express love and share intimacy with someone else.

GUIDELINES FOR IMPROVING YOUR SEXUAL SELF-CONCEPT

It takes time and effort to develop a positive sexual self-concept. Not only do we have to watch for the false conclusions and negative beliefs about ourselves that resulted from the abuse, we also need to replace old ways of thinking with new, healthy ones. Here are some suggestions for activities you can do—when you feel ready—to overcome the effects of abuse and to start developing a positive concept of yourself as a sexual person.

Befriend your inner child

Inside each of us is an innocent, creative, sexually curious child. This childlike vulnerability is a crucial part of our personality that was affected by the abuse. Many therapists and survivors call this child-self the "inner child."* Many survivors feel that their inner child is still hurting. Getting in touch with your inner child can help you overcome old hurts, heal old pain, and realize your intrinsic goodness.

One way to befriend your inner child is to give yourself the kind of emotional support and care you needed after the abuse but that you may not have received. Ask yourself: What did I need from a parent, care-taker, friend, or lover at the time of the abuse? Perhaps you needed to be held and comforted, to be assured that you were safe from further harm, to be validated for your emotional reactions, or to be given information to help you understand what happened. Even though many years may have passed, you now can start giving your inner child the validation and support it needs. A survivor of father-daughter incest expressed her needs:

> The little girl inside of me needs protection. She needs to hear it wasn't my fault, that I was in an impossible situation, that there was no way I could have avoided the humiliation.

Using your adult wisdom and what you now know about sexual abuse, you can connect with your inner child and tell yourself all the things you still need to hear. The use of meditation and affirmations (see box) may help your inner child heal from the abuse.

As you get in touch with your inner child you can also learn to respond to the child's unmet needs, as this survivor explained:

> I don't feel I ever had a real childhood. I didn't feel innocent and carefree like children should be. I missed out on a lot of relaxed fun that children have, like flying kites and being creative. I didn't get to explore my sexuality as my own or enjoy the discovery of sex as something good and natural.

---

* For more information you may want to read *Healing the Child Within* by Charles Whit-field (see the Resources section).

As an adult you can give yourself permission to do some things that you didn't get to enjoy as a child. What did you miss doing that you can do now? Fly a kite, dress up, dance, sing, paint, repair bikes? Freeing up the child energy puts you in touch with your natural curiosity and play-fulness—two important ingredients for a healthy sex life.

Adopt a clean-slate philosophy of life

Let the past be past, and give yourself a future. It's not fair to you to cling to the past image you have of yourself. You don't have to feel dam-aged forever. If you have felt like a sexual object in the past, you don't have to anymore. These ideas are not empty platitudes like "Let bygones be bygones." Rather, you can use your new awareness and acknowledg-ment of the past in an active way, to work toward change step by step.

AFFIRMATIONS TO HEAL MY INNER CHILD

In a safe, quiet, and relaxed setting, imagine that the adult you are now is sitting down and talking to the child or person you were at the time of the abuse. Say each statement aloud.

The sexual abuse was not your fault.
You are a valuable and good person.
You did not deserve what happened.
You are not bad because of what happened.
Your feelings and responses during the abuse were normal.
Your sexual energy is good and separate from the abuse.
You are a strong [boy/man] [girl/woman].
You can share your pain with others, and it will go away.
You are not alone anymore.

Be aware of your response to each statement. Are there some statements that are easier to take in than others? You may want to repeat each statement several times in one sitting.

This exercise can be adapted so that your inner child can repeat each statement as well. Thus, after you say, "The abuse was not *your* fault," your inner child can respond with, "The abuse was not *my* fault," and so on for each statement. You may also want to do the exercise while looking into a mirror. This exercise makes an excellent daily meditation.

I believe in what I call a *clean-slate* philosophy of life. This means that each day brings us a brand-new opportunity to create ourselves again, without being pulled back into our past. You can imagine that every night the blackboards of your life are wiped clean, leaving them fresh and open for the next day's events.

Who you are is who you decide you are. You are not strapped to the negative labels that the offender called you in the abuse or to the way you saw yourself later as a result of the abuse. These labels will disappear as you stop believing them and stop acting in ways that reinforce them. Keep asserting new, healthy concepts of yourself; they eventually will take hold.

Find your voice

An important way to stop feeling like an object is to speak up and assert your needs and feelings to others. By asserting yourself, you validate your existence. You affirm to yourself and to others that you deserve respect. To express yourself is to find your voice.

Linda, a thirty-six-year-old survivor of ritual abuse, found her voice in a group therapy session. It was the week before Halloween, and members of her group were planning a celebration with candles on a table. Linda felt panicky. She flashed back to her abuse, which sometimes involved candles on tables. As usual, Linda kept silent at first and started coming down on herself for reacting strongly against the event. She kept telling herself that the group would not hurt her and that she had nothing to fear. She felt silly for being afraid. But her panicky feelings wouldn't go away. Her inner child was screaming, "If you ever listen to me, listen to me now, and don't go!" Linda thought maybe she should avoid conflict and skip the next meeting.

Something else happened instead. Linda decided to tell the group members how she was feeling. To her surprise, they were responsive and agreed not to do a ritual. Each member praised her for her assertiveness. Linda felt apologetic, thinking she had spoiled everyone else's plans. She felt critical of herself for being so sensitive. But above these feelings she also realized that her reactions made sense. She became proud of herself for speaking up. Later in couples therapy, Linda told her husband, Mike, of her accomplishment:

> I see what I did in group as a major step in my sexual recovery. To
> be able to feel comfortable with having sex with you, I need to tell

you what I need and not feel bad when you make changes that consider my feelings.

I am finally feeling that I deserve to enjoy sex. It is something I want for me. It seems so elementary. I need to take time to know what I want. When I was young, I was never allowed to feel and make decisions. Now I can. I can decide I want it. I deserve to enjoy my sexuality, and we deserve an intimate life together.

After listening to Linda, Mike for the first time expressed hope for their sexual relationship. Changes did not happen overnight for them. Throughout the next several years, Linda slowly became more able to assert her feelings and needs in her relationship with Mike. This new ability allowed Linda and Mike to reach a new level of intimacy.

Finding your voice helps you to overcome the feelings of submissiveness you learned in the abuse. A survivor of father-son incest said

In difficult situations I used to sit back, withdraw, and shrug my shoulders. Or I would do things to distract attention from my true feelings. Now when I speak up, I feel that I exist, I am powerful, and I have an effect on other people. I feel good about myself and strong as a man.

Asserting himself helped Todd, another male survivor, overcome a tendency to withdraw socially. In therapy Todd realized that underneath all of his hiding he was a passionate and sensual man. At a party shortly thereafter, for the first time in his life he asked women he didn't know if they would like to dance.

I felt an incredible feeling of confidence as I asked these women to dance. Some friends later told me that they could sense a lot of sensual energy exuding from me. The experience feels like a coming of age for me. I was being acknowledged as a sexual being. I feel alive and thankful. I feel life is a wondrous, mysterious thing—and I'm part of it. I belong.

Learn to be in your body

We are our bodies. Taking good care of our bodies is taking good care of ourselves. Developing a positive sexual self-concept means keeping ourselves physically healthy and strong.

Because of abuse, many survivors fail to get the message that *your body belongs to you.* Internalizing this concept is essential to sexual heal-ing because it is a way of undoing the false, learned self-concept that you are a sexual object. Taking care of your body encourages you to keep in touch with what is happening to you on a physical level.

During and after abuse, many victims do not want or cannot stand to "be in their body." Many victims cope with physical and emotional pain by "leaving" their bodies to some extent. A young rape victim, for example, may block out sensation and awareness of her body, mentally distancing her consciousness from her genital area during the attack. For many survivors, tuning out body needs and disowning body parts may have been a way of surviving the abuse. Continuing to withdraw physically now, however, harms sexual recovery and enjoyment.

Learning to live in one's body after abuse is often a slow and gradual process. At the start of their healing some survivors may find it very dif-ficult to even look at themselves naked in a mirror. One woman had been abducted, raped, and tattooed by a motorcycle gang and could not financially afford to have the tattoos removed. She kept no mirrors in her apartment and avoided walking by windows and mirrors in public. To overcome her fear of looking at herself, her therapist asked her to think of something she enjoyed looking at that made her feel safe and happy. The woman thought of a little brown teddy bear she kept in her room. Next the therapist suggested that the woman hold the teddy bear next to a part of her body when looking at that part in a small mirror. Using this process, the woman eventually was able to look at all parts of her body and, finally, to view her whole body in a full-length mirror without fear.

Looking at yourself in a mirror can also help remind you how you have aged since the abuse. When it comes to sex, some survivors con-tinue to think of themselves as being the same size, age, and shape they were when the abuse took place. When you look at yourself in a mirror now, you can affirm the differences. (Many of the Relearning Touch exercises in chapter 10, such as Cleansing and Reclaiming Your Body, can be extremely helpful in improving body awareness and body image.)

Taking an inventory of the parts of your body that were hurt in the abuse can also help you. Janice, a survivor I counseled, drew an outline of her body on a big piece of paper. At first, it looked like a gingerbread woman, with only eyes, nose, mouth, and ears drawn in; the rest of her body she left blank. I asked her to think about what had happened to her in the sexual assault, then mark an X on her drawing to indicate each place on her body that had suffered pain or injury, or that she associated with emotional harm. Next to each X, Janice described the type of hurt she had experienced. For example, she wrote "bruise from being kicked" next to an X on her thigh and "teasing about the size of my breast" next to an X on her breast. When Janice was done, her drawing had many marks and words on it. Slowly, she stretched out her arm and touched her drawing. She began to cry. Seeing everything together at once, Janice realized how profoundly she had suffered from the abuse. Although painful for her, this awareness finally opened doors for her to reconnect with her body.

In a similar exercise, other survivors can identify how they feel about different parts of their bodies. Using a drawing or simply thinking to yourself, you may want to scan your body from head to toe, stopping at each body part. Repeatedly ask yourself these questions:

How do I feel about this part of my body?
How well have I been taking care of this part of my body?

You may want to record your answers in a journal so that you can refer to them later and evaluate your progress in changing how you feel about your body.

A woman survivor who had difficulty achieving orgasms realized through this exercise that she harbored many negative feelings toward her clitoris. She thought of her clitoris as her "recalcitrant member—disobedient and resistant to authority." Disturbing as this realization was, it was the key that would allow her to overcome her negative feelings and experience sexual pleasure. She began doing affirmations to remind herself that her clitoris was an innocent part of her body and that it belonged to her.

Some survivors learn to reconnect with "lost" body parts by having imaginary conversations with their anatomy. Strange though it may sound, giving your sexual body parts a voice can help you discover how you feel about them.

Jill, for example, got very upset when her husband would stimulate her breasts during sex. In therapy she said, "I hate my breasts. I'd just as soon cut them off and throw them away!" Jill's therapist suggested she "talk" to her breasts. Jill used her imagination and discovered that she had been blaming her breasts for her father's abuse because he had begun abusing her after her breasts developed. When in the imaginary conversation her breasts "spoke" back to her, they were able to clarify her confusion. It was her father, not her breasts, who had caused the abuse. Her breasts "told" her they had pleasure to offer, if only she would accept them. This dialogue helped her feel better about her breasts and herself.

Many survivors who do this exercise find they have a victim-perpetrator scenario playing between their mind and their sexual parts. For example, an imaginary conversation between a man and his penis might sound like this:

MAN: I don't like you. You are not much of anything. Regardless of how you feel, you are a thing I will use over and over again.
MAN'S PENIS: You treat me awful. You handle me without any love or affection, hurt me, and expose me to diseases. You don't care about me—you just want me to perform.

Sounds like the penis is a victim and the man a perpetrator, doesn't it? Even if the dialogue sounds silly, this type of exploring can open your self-awareness. You may be able to start taking better care of yourself once you understand how you view your own body.

MAN'S PENIS: I'm tired of being the receptacle for your anger and shame. I'm an important part of your body. I deserve your respect.
MAN: It's hard for me to see you as mine and think of you as deserving my respect. But I guess you are very important.

Reclaiming your body as your own also involves maintaining good physical health. The old adage that your body is a temple is a helpful one to remember. Basic care involves eating well, avoiding alcohol and other drug abuse, and exercising regularly. You can also empower yourself by learning more about sex, sexual reproduction, sexual diseases, and health care.*

By making yourself physically strong, you can change your image of yourself as weak and vulnerable. Exercise makes you stronger and releases anger and tension. Many survivors have taken up self-defense training and body building to gain confidence in their strength and ability to protect themselves from harm.

Living in our bodies is essential to developing a healthy sexual self-concept. A survivor said:

---

* For more infomation, I recommend reading *Our Sexuality*, an excellent text book on sexual issues, roles, and functioning by Robert Crooks and Karla Baur (see the Resources section).

To keep in touch with my body, I do bodywork therapy and am a dancer now. Living in my body has shown me a deeper safety and ability to function than ever before. This is where my sexual healing work is, in learning to live in me.

Develop a sense of boundaries

If you do not already feel you have them, physical boundaries can be important tools to use in improving your sexual self-concept. Most Americans begin to feel uncomfortable when another person comes within eighteen inches of their body. Those who don't want the intrusion can protect themselves by moving away or pushing others back. Survivors may lack awareness of this invisible cultural barrier. Because of violations of their bodies, many survivors have never learned they have a boundary. By keeping in mind the concept of an invisible bubble around your body, you can start to recognize and protect your own personal space. You can imagine the bubble to be as many inches as you want from your body in all directions.

Assert your right to privacy. If you want to undress alone, be in a bathroom alone, or be free of fondling by your partner while you sleep, you have a right to your wish. As you strengthen your boundaries, you gain a stronger sense of yourself. Then, when you choose to have contact with another person, you can feel more present, more in control, and more able to enjoy what you are doing together.

Find good role models

In developing a more positive image of yourself as a sexual person, it can help you to become acquainted with people who already feel comfortable with themselves sexually and who enjoy healthy sexual relationships. These people can serve as your role models. Think of persons of your sex whom you admire and respect as having a healthy sexual presence.

Recently I asked a group of survivors to think of someone of their own gender whom they saw as sexually healthy and positive. Only half were able to think of such a role model. The women who were mentioned were described as self-protective, assertive, and able to enjoy sex. The men mentioned were described as emotionally sensitive, assertive, and able to enjoy sex. When asked to name a television couple who represented a healthy couple, a number of the survivors mentioned Claire and Cliff Huxtable on "The Cosby Show." This couple is portrayed as sexually interested in each other, nonpressuring about having sex, and playful in their physical intimacy. It may be helpful to imagine yourself as such a woman or man.

Sexual abuse belongs to your past. If you have been blaming or punishing yourself because of the abuse, it's now up to you to break the pattern. You need to forgive yourself for having been sexually abused, to separate yourself from what happened to you, and to take active steps to become the sexually healthy person you have a right to be. After two years of sexual healing, a woman who had been raped by her father expressed her feelings:

> It feels strange to me to feel pleasure and pride in my sexuality, but it's wonderful too. I now know that my sexual song is pure and beautiful.

7

Gaining Control over Automatic Reactions

At any time, some signal in the present can rubberband a survivor back to old trauma and pain. One of the biggest challenges survivors face in sexual healing is overcoming automatic reactions which block clear access to present situations.

—GREGORY MULRY, *Therapist*

Judy, a rape survivor, reacts with fear every morning when her husband turns to kiss her goodbye. This instantaneous reaction confuses Judy—she loves her husband. When Tony, a survivor who is single, sits next to an attractive woman in a coffee shop, he immediately enters a sexual fantasy of dominating and controlling her. He feels trapped by his own sexual thoughts. Simple conversation with her is impossible.

Tony and Judy are experiencing "automatic reactions"—feelings, thoughts, and sensations that echo past abuse and inhibit healthy sexuality. These reactions represent ingrained reactions to sex, touch, and intimacy learned during the sexual abuse.

Automatic reactions are an extremely common and insidious repercussion of sexual abuse. They persist even when we have been changing our attitudes about sex and are feeling better about ourselves sexually. They reflect an interwoven pattern of physical and emotional responses. Automatic reactions often operate below our conscious awareness, making us feel confused, upset, and out of control.

As we sexually heal, we become more aware of our automatic reactions. We learn to pay more attention to our responses as we challenge ourselves to change long-standing patterns of sexual behavior. We may run into our automatic reactions as we attempt new ways of experiencing touch and sex. "It seems like the abuse is following me everywhere," a survivor told me.

Automatic reactions that were learned in the abuse can harm us sexually. They can inhibit and disrupt our present-day sexual experiences, keeping us trapped in patterns of self-denying and damaging sexual behavior for many years. And they can make us feel bad about ourselves and keep us from joyful sexual intimacy with a partner.

In this chapter information is presented to help you learn how to recognize, understand, and cope with your automatic reactions. You will find that the knowledge and skills you acquire here will aid you immensely in being able to change how you behave sexually and in learning new approaches to touch and sex.

RECOGNIZING AUTOMATIC REACTIONS

We react automatically in many situations in our lives. Keeping our hands from a hot burner on the stove, looking both ways before crossing the street, or hugging our children when they have been hurt are automatic reactions that are healthy and good. Problems occur when the automatic reactions we developed in traumatic and confusing situations, such as sexual abuse, interfere with our present ability to enjoy our sexuality. These automatic reactions cause us to react in strange or inappropriate ways that inhibit our ability to feel good about ourselves and close to people we care about.

Often operating subconsciously, automatic reactions may be difficult to recognize. We may not even realize when we are experiencing automatic reactions learned from the abuse. Consequently, we may inaccurately attribute our response to something else, a bad habit, or a failing in ourselves: "I am afraid of sex because I'm not a loving person," "I feel like masturbating when I see underclothes because I'm perverted," or "I move away when my partner touches me because I don't really want to be touched." We may suffer years of self-loathing and isolation simply because we are not aware of our automatic reactions and how they affect us.

To help you recognize your automatic reactions, we will begin by examining three main types: emotional responses, physical sensations, and intrusive thoughts. To aid in identifying your automatic reactions, first review your responses to section 3 of the Sexual Effects Inventory in chapter 3.

Automatic reactions that are emotional responses. One evening, Mandy, a thirty-year-old lesbian survivor, curled up on the couch with her lover, Chris, to watch a romantic movie on TV. During the movie Chris became amorous and began stroking Mandy's shoulders. Mandy immediately became scared. Her fear didn't make sense to her. She knew Chris would stop stroking her if asked. Mandy's feeling of fear was automatic, triggered by Chris's stroking her shoulder, which in some way reminded her of past sexual abuse.

Survivors can experience many different types of emotional automatic reactions related to sexual abuse. A list of some common ones follows. Check any you experience in situations involving touch, sex, and intimacy.

_____ I feel fear.

_____ I feel panic.

_____ I feel terror.

_____ I feel anger.

_____ I feel sadness.

_____ I feel shame.

_____ I feel disgust.

_____ I feel paranoia.

_____ I feel anxiety.

_____ I feel confusion.

_____ I feel suspicion.

_____ I feel emotionally numb or distant.

Automatic reactions that are physical sensations. Nancy, a forty-year-old survivor, is fine when she's on a date unless she starts to feel attracted to the man she's with—then her whole body tightens and shuts down. She gets short of breath, her body becomes hard and cold, and she starts to shake from deep in her guts. Talking becomes difficult. She spends the rest of the date anxious to get home where she can relax and be alone. For Nancy, this automatic physiological reaction to intimacy is preventing her from building healthy relationships.

Some physical reactions that result from sexual abuse can be extremely uncomfortable and make sexual enjoyment impossible. Another survivor explained her reactions:

Sometimes when my husband starts to touch me in a sexual way, I go through a tensing experience in my body. Weird feelings come in sporadic waves. Tense energy from my stomach moves out through my arms, creating a tightness. It feels almost like pain. I can't relax. It feels like a burning sensation, but, strangely, at the same time, I feel very, very cold.*

In contrast, other physical reactions can be extremely pleasurable and cause survivors to compulsively seek out sexual experiences. Sex can trigger high levels of excitement similar to those obtained by using alcohol or other drugs. Even the possibility of sex may produce an automatic feeling of euphoria. "When he ripped open the condom," a survivor said, "I felt the same excitement I used to feel when I was using drugs and someone was about to stick a needle in my arm." Although this automatic reaction is temporarily pleasurable, in the long run it can cause behaviors that lower self-esteem and prevent real intimacy from developing.

The following is a list of some common types of physical sensations that can be automatic reactions to sexual abuse. Check any you experience in situations involving touch, sex, and intimacy.

_____   I feel nauseated.

_____   I feel pain.

_____   I get a headache.

_____   My stomach feels tight.

_____   My heart beats rapidly.

_____   I feel chest pain.

_____   I feel genital pain.

_____   I experience an adrenaline rush.

_____   I sweat.

_____   I get chills.

_____   I feel cold.

_____   I feel flushed or hot.

_____   I feel euphoric.

_____   I experience unwanted or inappropriate sexual excitement.

_____   I experience spontaneous orgasm.

_____   I feel sleepy.

* After years of hearing survivors describe similar reactions to sexual touch, I suspect that the term *frigid* emerged from observations of what was essentially a delayed sexual trauma reaction, not necessarily reflective of a true disinterest in sex. It's a shame that many women suffered from this insensitive name-calling, instead of receiving compassion for the past trauma they experienced and help to overcome the reaction.

_____   I feel faint.
_____   I experience physical numbness.

Automatic reactions that are intrusive thoughts.   Sam is a forty-five-year-old heterosexual survivor of molestation by his older brother. He is bothered by thoughts of sexual abuse that creep into his mind when he is making love with his wife. In some ways Sam finds these thoughts stimulating—they add to his sexual arousal. But intellectually, he finds it upsetting that the content of his fantasies has to do with sexual abuse and exploitation. Sam is embarrassed and feels ruled by these intrusive fantasies. For Sam, these are not healthy thoughts that add to his overall sexual enjoyment and self-esteem. Rather, these fantasies take him out of the present moment and leave him less able to be sexually intimate with his wife.*

Intrusive thoughts can be very confusing and upsetting. After reading about sexual abuse in a newspaper, a survivor was disturbed and angry at herself for automatically fantasizing more details about the abuse and getting aroused. Another survivor said, "It pains me that even though I was used as an object for another person's gratification in the abuse, I still get the idea of using someone else the same way when I meet them for the first time."

Intrusive thoughts can cripple sexual enjoyment and satisfaction by causing survivors to shut down sexual arousal. One woman survivor felt so bad that thoughts of her offender's name kept popping into her head when she was about to climax in lovemaking that she wouldn't let herself become aroused.

The following is a list of some common types of intrusive thoughts that can be automatic reactions to sexual abuse. Check any you experience in situations involving touch, sex, and intimacy.

_____   I think abusive sexual fantasies.
_____   I think my partner is the offender.
_____   I think the past is the present.
_____   I think I am a child.

* Survivors of sexual abuse tend to have more disturbing sexual fantasies than their nonabused peers. For more information, read the article by John Briere, et al., and my book, *Private Thoughts*, coauthored with Suzie Boss (see Resources section). In one informal survey I administered at a large "Healing Woman" survivor conference in 1996, approximately four out of five female survivors indicated they were troubled by unwanted sexual fantasies.

_____   I think I am being victimized or abused.
_____   I think I am bad.
_____   I think I am inadequate.
_____   I think I am unworthy of being loved for myself.
_____   I wish I was someplace else.

EXPERIENCING AUTOMATIC REACTIONS

Some automatic reactions last for seconds, others for hours. Usually, reactions come in a series. They can be _linked_ so that one triggers another. One survivor said whenever she became aroused during masturbation, she immediately went numb and felt disgusted with herself. Linked reactions can frustrate and annoy, causing survivors to interrupt touch and sex activity. A survivor described her reaction:

> I find it hard to spontaneously initiate sex. I start to feel scared [EMOTION]. An incredible tape starts running in my head with real negative thoughts about my partner [INTRUSIVE THOUGHTS]. I get irritated with myself because my reaction doesn't make sense [EMOTION]. I then have to take extra time to talk things through with my partner before we can make love.

A _chain of automatic reactions_ can turn an otherwise pleasant experience into a nightmare. A man who had been molested by his mother and father recalled such an occurrence:

> My girlfriend and I had gone out for the evening. She came back to my apartment with me. We hugged and kissed for a while. Then she started taking off my clothes and proceeded to give me a blow job. I froze [PHYSICAL SENSATION]. I felt like I wasn't there [EMOTION]. I didn't want to be there [THOUGHT].

A chain of automatic reactions related to abuse can also cause a survivor to be drawn to self-damaging, compulsive sexual activity. Feelings such as depression, anxiety, fear, disgust, and loneliness may have become fused with an automatic reaction of sexual interest or arousal. Feeling bad about oneself can trigger a desire to engage in compulsive sexual behavior. "Whenever I'm feeling bad about myself, I am tempted to have an affair," a survivor said. Another survivor explained, "The days I'm likely to go to an adult bookstore are when a business deal falls through and I'm depressed and feeling lousy about myself."

For some survivors who experience sexual arousal in this way, having sex can be used as a way to end a chain of uncomfortable automatic reactions. Survivors attempt to bury uncomfortable mental and physiological reactions by escaping in powerful sensations of sex. Unfortunately, this pattern of seeking sex to end discomfort has negative consequences. It can lead to sexual experiences that harm one's self-esteem, endanger health, or hurt others. This kind of sex prevents real emotional and sexual intimacy from forming. A woman who had been raped on a date described her pattern:

I'll be out on a date with a guy. I worry that he might not like me or find me attractive. Suddenly I ache to be held and hugged. Then I become possessed with a desire to sleep with him. I manipulate the situation into a sexual one as quickly as I can. I end this panic by having sex, even though I know that later I'll feel miserable with myself.

Some linked automatic reactions don't simply flow in one direction. They can cause survivors to have *incompatible responses*, making them feel simultaneously a desire for sex and a desire to retreat from sex. "I'm scared to death, and I desperately want your body," a man told his wife. For him, two contradictory reactions—fear and sexual desire—were linked.

For some survivors a chain of automatic reactions can lead to an uncomfortable, uncontrollable fit of *anxiety*. They may feel consumed by fright—paralyzed and terrified. Panic reactions can be so extreme that they rob survivors of the comfort of nurturing, nonsexual touch, like the hug of a friend or the gentle, steady hand of a nurse during a minor medical procedure. A thirty-year-old deaf survivor was uncomfortable with any kind of touch.

My older brother molested me starting when I was about twelve. At the time I didn't wear hearing aids. I never heard my brother creep up from behind. He'd grab me and then proceed to feel, squeeze, and pinch my breasts. I have a sense his hands went lower, though I can't quite remember. What I do remember is the absolute terror of a big heavy man with big strong hands feeling me. I couldn't get free; I just froze. I have a "thing" about hands now. When anyone touches me I go cold. My stomach churns and turns over. I shiver and freeze—total panic. The whole area of touch, sex, and sexuality is a minefield.

What bothers me most is not that I can't make a sexual relationship—because I'm nowhere near that—but that I can't accept a nice comforting hug or cuddle. I can't let anyone hold me. I worry endlessly whether it's right, whether it's sexual or nonsexual. Where will it lead? Will I get hurt? Will I be able to cope? Invariably I just keep well away. But I'm dying of hunger—hunger for a cuddle or touch.

For this survivor, her fear of having a panic reaction makes her avoid any situations that could involve touch, sex, or intimacy. In essence, her fear cripples her life.

A chain of automatic reactions can induce an experience in which one's mind feels temporarily separate and split off from one's body, a sensation therapists call *dissociation*. Survivors can feel they are sliding out of the present moment, losing a sense of physical identity or emotional connection with a partner. "My partner used a certain tone of voice with me," a survivor said, "that pushed me back into a tunnel. I could feel myself falling away from him. He held me, but even his comforting touch felt very loud to me." Some survivors describe feeling as though their mind is in one part of a room (say, hovering near the ceiling), and their body is in another (lying on the bed, for example). These experiences of being split off from one's body can be strange, and even terrifying, at times.

Flashbacks are another disturbing but common manifestation of automatic reactions. More than sixty percent of the eighty survivors who filled out questionnaires to provide information for this book reported that they had experienced at least one flashback. Something in the present related to touch, sex, or intimacy triggers a number of strong automatic reactions at once. An intense flood of feelings, sensations, and memories rush forward as the original sexual abuse is re-created in the present moment. Survivors who were abused as children may feel themselves become younger and shrink in body size. Many survivors have vivid sensory experiences that cause them to relive what they felt during the abuse. "It was like being inside a videotape with every detail and color very vivid, with the addition of smell," a survivor said.

One woman survivor of a gang rape told me that the moment her present boyfriend put his penis in her vagina during lovemaking, she was immediately transported back to the abuse.

I felt like a young girl again. My brother's friend, Billy, was thrusting away on me. I could hear his friend, Donny (who was next in line to rape me), counting, "one, two, three, . . . a hundred fucks for a buck!"

Flashbacks often result when some aspect of present-day sex feels similar to what survivors felt in the abuse. An incest survivor recounted her flashback:

> I was performing oral sex on my partner. He began to tenderly play with my hair. Then I was back re-experiencing the first time I was forced to perform fellatio. I felt my uncle's hands on my head.

Once inside a flashback, survivors often see, hear, or feel things that happened in the abuse but aren't really happening now. They can have temporary sensory hallucinations, as these survivors explained:

> My partner touched my nipple when we were making love. Immediately, I *felt something push into my vagina*, though there was nothing there in reality. The sensation lasted several minutes and was very uncomfortable. I regressed emotionally to a very young age.

> Once when I was having oral sex with my husband I looked down at him and *saw my father's bloodshot eyes staring back at me*. I can remember him looking at me with that penetrating stare as if it were yesterday.

Flashbacks, panic reactions, feeling emotionally dissociated, and other combinations of automatic reactions can be extremely frightening and unpleasant. They usually happen without warning. In an instant, survivors can find themselves lost in another world, feeling things they don't want to be feeling and doing things they don't want to be doing. Automatic reactions can temporarily deny survivors a sense of being mentally and physically in control of themselves. They may feel they are losing contact with present-day reality. An incest survivor said:

> I was having sex with my partner. Suddenly I felt very young, helpless, and terrified. I started to cry, then I mentally left the experience completely. I went into the sheets and disappeared.

Because flashbacks and other automatic reactions are so upsetting, many survivors try to avoid them. Some survivors, like the deaf woman described earlier, simply stay away from situations that have anything to do with touch, sex, and intimacy. They shut down and steer away. The trouble is, this avoidance often becomes part of the problem. Staying away from touch and sexual experiences makes these experiences even more unusual and thus even more likely to cause an upsetting reaction when they unexpectedly occur.

Survivors may try to avoid unpleasant automatic reactions in many other ways: they may become very aggressive and controlling in touch and sex, they may actively use sexual fantasies and pornography to keep their minds off what is happening in the present, or they may develop a sexual dysfunction that prevents them from having certain sexual sensations that might trigger disturbing reactions. These ways of avoiding and handling intense automatic reactions often cause problems as well. They can inhibit healthy sex and intimate sharing. Later in this chapter we will learn about some new, alternative ways to handle automatic reactions that encourage healthy, positive sexual experiences.

Because automatic reactions can be upsetting, frightening, and annoying, it's easy to understand why many survivors come to hate or feel ashamed and secretive about their reactions. And they may even hate themselves for having them. Unconsciously, survivors often associate these sudden, unpleasant, disruptive, and overpowering reactions with the abuse itself. Automatic reactions may seem like an external threat, an outside force that is intent on inflicting harm. One woman said, "It feels like I'm being hounded by a plague of black flies."

When survivors maintain an antagonistic stance in relation to their automatic reactions, change can be difficult. We need to understand, respect, and in a way even accept our reactions before we can develop new ways to tame and diffuse their influence.

UNDERSTANDING HOW AUTOMATIC REACTIONS RELATE TO PAST ABUSE

Automatic reactions are not external forces. They are an understandable part of a survivor's legacy of past abuse.

Sexual abuse is alarming, traumatic, and strange. The abuse itself may last only minutes, but during that time victims are emotionally and probably physically overwhelmed. They lose their sense of safety, control, and individual autonomy. The abuse experience is too much to process, flooding victims with sensations, feelings, and thoughts that they cannot assimilate at once.

Sexual abuse affects survivors profoundly, like other intense events, such as having a life-threatening accident, giving birth, watching some-one die, or being kidnapped. Normal awareness is heightened, intensify-ing the experience down to the most minute detail. Most victims are unprepared to handle this situation mentally or physically.

To cope with the abuse while it's happening, victims learn to group together all aspects of the abuse. Everything—where they are, what they are doing, who they are with, and what they feel—becomes fused. A traumatic crystallizing of experience occurs, as if they have taken a three-dimensional picture of the abuse. Because survivors may be con-fused about what caused the abuse, this crystallizing records everything that might be a possible cause. When survivors feel more prepared to analyze what happened to them and why, they can retrieve this mental three-dimensional picture.

Automatic reactions are activated, or triggered, by something in our present-day reality that reminds us, either consciously or unconsciously, of the past abuse. The trigger can be almost anything: an object, a touch, a movement, a smell, a sound, a setting, a sensation, a physical characteristic, or a feeling such as fear, abandonment, or anxiety. When a trigger sets off an automatic reaction, within seconds touch and sex experiences in the present become contaminated with feelings, thoughts, and sensations from the past.

Any portion of the crystal image can become a trigger. If we were in a dark room and felt scared during the abuse, then darkness, fear, and sex become part of our crystallized picture. That's what happened to one woman, who was abused as an infant.

> Being sexual in a dark room can trigger a flashback. I say nothing. I have no words. I just feel abject terror and panic. My breathing becomes labored, and then I start to cry like a baby.

Many of our automatic reactions were learned as a way to cope with the mental and physical stress experienced in the abuse. Victims may begin dissociating, for instance, to sidestep anything from pain to plea-sure. "I didn't feel what was happening during the molestation because I was outside of my body," a survivor explained. Dissociating also allows victims to cooperate with the offender and thus avoid further violence and pain. "I coped with the abuse by mentally checking out," a survivor said. "It was a way of saying to the offender, 'You can do what you want, but you can't make me be here.'" This reaction can enable a victim to retain a sense of power and self.

For many survivors, especially those who were victimized repeatedly, the process of *dissociating* becomes something they do over and over again. Splitting off becomes an ingrained response to sex, a habit.

> I learned to separate myself from my body. I recall looking in a mirror when I was nine years old and hypnotically telling myself that the little girl in the mirror was not me. Now, every time I feel icky about sex, I head for the hills emotionally. I separate my mind from my body.

Other survivors may have learned to cope with the stress of abuse by *numbing their own physical sensations*. Numbing may have allowed them to endure the abuse.

> My abuse experiences were usually physically and emotionally painful. To take care of myself, I blocked out feelings and sensations as well as I could. One time in the abuse, I experienced some pleasure. I felt guilty and betrayed by my own body. It made me feel dirty like my abuser. Now if I happen to feel pleasure I automatically block it out as well as the pain.

A third coping strategy survivors may have learned in the abuse *is going along with what is happening*. Enjoying sexual feelings, experiencing pleasure, and having orgasms are natural, automatic responses to sexual stimulation.

> I coped with the abuse by going into it. I became aroused, flooded with sensation, overwhelmed, and orgasmic to get through it and to numb the psychological and physical pain. Now when I'm having sex I easily get flooded and overwhelmed. Then when I finally orgasm I feel frightened.

Some survivors learned that they could gain a degree of control over what they experienced if they went along with the abuse. Doing what a rapist tells you to do, and acting like you like it, can save your life or prevent you from further violence and pain. One man learned that he could avoid pain and injury by pretending to want what was happening to him when he was a ten-year-old boy being abused in an adult sexual orgy.

> After being tumbled, turned, and poked, I began to like it. At first I was only pretending to like it, but then I actually started to like it

in a weird way. I began to ask to be hurt. This made my abusers
touch me in less violent ways.

"Enjoying" abusive sex may have helped some victims to survive, but
meanwhile this was becoming ingrained as their way of responding
to sex.

Tragically, this life-saving method—going along with, encouraging,
or "enjoying" one's own sexual abuse—lowers self-esteem and endangers
a survivor's health and well-being. "It turns me on to think of being victimized," a survivor said. Survivors can feel ashamed of their sexual
interests and develop secretive, compulsive sexual activities. A man,
abused by another man when he was a teenager, expressed his reaction:

> Initially, I felt horrible about the abuse, but I was still attracted to
> the sexual feelings, the attention, and the excitement that was
> involved in it. With time I buried all my negative feelings and
> developed strong desires for the sexual stimulation.

His automatic reaction was to bury his anxiety, humiliation, and fear.
This protected him years ago from the emotional pain of the abuse. But
continuing to bury his negative feelings today only perpetuates the
damage.

Automatic reactions may have been important to you in the past.
You can respect yourself for having developed them in the first place as
a coping mechanism. Given what you went through, they helped you to
handle and survive your situation. But now that you no longer are in
extreme, traumatic situations, these protective measures no longer are
needed. You can learn to handle your automatic reactions in ways that
don't damage you or your sexual relationships.

IDENTIFYING WHAT TRIGGERS YOUR AUTOMATIC REACTIONS

As described earlier, triggers can be anything in your present-day reality
that reminds you, either consciously or unconsciously, of past sexual
abuse. Many survivors feel as if they're in a minefield, braced for an
explosion at any step. But it is possible for survivors to learn to antici-
pate these automatic reactions and to gain control of their responses
and even defuse the trigger.

You may already have some idea of what is likely to trigger your automatic reactions: a type of touch, a certain sexual activity, an object, feeling a particular way toward a partner. "I have always panicked when hugged from behind," a survivor said. The reaction of another survivor was triggered by a common word.

> I cringe and feel afraid when I hear the word *love*. My mom frequently spoke of what a loving person she was and how much she loved me. "Love" became the reason she could do anything she wanted to me and why I could not object.

Other triggers may lie dormant for years, then surface unexpectedly. A woman who had been molested by her cousin and later raped by a stranger said:

> I was having intercourse with my partner, and we decided to change positions. In the process he accidentally struck my jaw with his elbow. I cried out and became hysterical. I found myself in the corner, wrapped in the blanket. I was terrified. So was he.

Another survivor also discovered a trigger by surprise:

> My husband and I were having sex for the first time in our new house. I was focusing on the overhead lamp and realized it was just like the ceiling lamp in my bedroom as a little girl. Suddenly my husband became confused with my father. I became like a child, fighting back and weeping.

Sometimes survivors can easily see how a trigger connects to the abuse. "I have flashbacks whenever my arms or legs are restricted in any way," a survivor said. "My abuser used to lie on my legs in such a way I couldn't move them." For this survivor the restricted body position was a trigger.

Other times, the connection is less clear. Survivors may know only that something bothers and upsets them. Memory loss, a frequent repercussion of abuse, can keep survivors from understanding the reasons behind their reactions. Until he remembers past abuse in which he was encouraged to look at pictures of nude women, a survivor may not understand why he can't stop staring at women's breasts in public.

Some triggers may be difficult to identify because they are related to a highly specific aspect of a sexual experience. Josie, a married survivor, became distressed when she experienced the initial feelings of sexual arousal and excitement. But once past this stage actual intercourse and orgasm were very pleasurable. When Josie was a child her grandfather had fondled her breasts and genitals, but there was no penetration or orgasm. In contrast, Becky, a survivor of a brutal rape, was comfortable with affectionate touching and initial sexual arousal, but intercourse and orgasm triggered pain and fear.

Some triggers may be hard to identify because they at first appear to have nothing to do with sex, touch, or intimacy.

> I grew up with a strong revulsion about white handkerchiefs. I hated being around them. When I'd see adults use them, I became sick to my stomach. Handkerchiefs had a sexual connotation to me, and I didn't realize why. Recently I remembered my father having orgasms on top of me when I was a little girl. He'd use a handkerchief to clean up afterward.

Sandy, a survivor of molestation by her grandfather, made a similar discovery. For as long as she could recall, Sandy became hysterical when she saw mushrooms. Friends told her that her fear came from worrying she would eat a poisonous one, and they teased her for being unnecessarily afraid. In counseling, Sandy discovered that her reaction to mushrooms evolved because she associated them with the look and feel of the tip of her grandfather's penis. Lacking any language for the penis as a little girl, she had associated penises with an object she did know, a mushroom.

Since triggers can be almost anything, it's important to take seriously the reactions you have. Your reactions can clue you into particulars about your abuse and can facilitate your recovery. When you have a reaction you don't understand, you might ask yourself, What might have triggered my reaction just now?

It is possible to take an even more assertive approach to identifying your triggers. This approach, while often highly informative, can sometimes be unpleasant. Increasing your awareness of possible triggers will require you to think back on the abuse, in detail. You may not want to recall the subtleties of the experience. But if you try thinking back on the abuse, even if in little bits at first, you may find it helps you get a handle on what causes your automatic reactions.

Identifying triggers gives you power. Triggers lose their secrecy and mysteriousness once you understand them. Gaining this new awareness can be like learning how special effects work in horror films or finding out how a magician performs a trick. Once the mystery is explained, you may still react, but you will no longer be surprised or horrified by it. And you may find you can now put words to experiences that may have mystified you before.

The exercise Discovering Your Triggers can help you through this process. If you decide to skip it for now continue reading on page 152.

DISCOVERING YOUR TRIGGERS

This exercise is designed to gently guide you through a process of thinking back on the abuse. It helps you to slowly think through different aspects of the experience and find out what associations with touch and sex you might have made during the abuse.

As with all the exercises and techniques in this book, this is optional. You may be more comfortable doing this at another time or with a counselor. Or you might want to proceed, but give yourself permission to stop at any time.

Thinking back on the abuse can be difficult if you have little or no memory of it. Do as much remembering as you can with what you know or what you sense happened. If you have little or no memory of the abuse, give yourself permission to skip questions and guess at answers to questions you are unsure about. Be aware that your present feelings and reactions may get stirred up by this process.

Let's look at the factors that existed at the time you were sexually abused. If you were abused more than once, focus on your initial abuse experiences or experiences you think were most traumatic to you. Then repeat the exercise again later with other experiences.

Answering the questions below will give you clues to your present triggers.

What you were like at the time of the abuse

You may be sensitive to people and images that remind you of what you were like when you were sexually abused.

How old were you? _____

How much did you weigh? _____

How tall were you? _____

What did you look like? How did you dress? _____

How did you feel about yourself before the abuse began (insecure, successful, ignorant, innocent, and so on)?

_____

_____

Where you were at the time of the abuse

You may be sensitive to being in settings that remind you of the environment in which the abuse occurred.

What was the time of day? _____

What was the season of the year? _____

Were there any specific circumstances surrounding the abuse (holiday or special event)?_____

What were the weather and temperature?_____

Describe where you were._____

_____

What objects were there?_____

_____

What were the background noise, smells, and sights?_____

_____

Were you under the influence of any substances or unusual conditions (alcohol, drugs, illness, and so on)? _____

_____

What the offender was like at the time of the abuse

You may be sensitive to people, places, and things that remind you of the offender.

What did the offender look like?_____

How did the offender move?_____

What habits did the offender have (smoking, drinking, hobbies, interests)?

_____

What outstanding characteristics did the offender have (gestures, voice, posture, unusual body features, smells, sounds)?_____

_____

_____

What type of person would you describe the offender as?_____

_____

What your relationship with the offender was like at the time of the abuse

You may be sensitive to dynamics in a present relationship that are similar to the interpersonal dynamics that existed in your relationship with the offender.

How did you know the offender before the abuse (stranger, relative, acquaintance)?_____

How did you originally feel about the offender (friendly, afraid, respectful, creepy, and so on)?_____

_____

What did you most want and need from the offender (affection, respect, acceptance, love, and so on)?_____

_____

What were the main emotions the offender expressed in the abuse (anger, excitement, fear, "love," a lack of any emotion, and so on)?___

_____

How did the offender relate to you (violent, pleading, dominating, flirtatious, manipulating, and so on)_____

_____

What kinds of things did the offender say to you?_____

_____

How did you feel about yourself in relation to the offender during the abuse (chosen, betrayed, abandoned, scared, loved, and so on)?_____

_____

What touch and sexual experiences you had during the abuse

You may be sensitive to touch, activity, and sensation similar to what you experienced in the abuse.

What types of touching did you experience in the abuse (grabbing, hitting, pinching, soothing, stroking, rubbing, and so on)?_____

_____

What type of touching did you do?_____

What parts of your body were touched the most?_____

_____

What did the touching feel like (pleasurable, painful, ticklish)?_____

_____

What sexual sounds, smells, tastes did you experience?_____

_____

What sexual positions were involved?_____

_____

What sexual acts occurred?_____

_____

What injuries did you sustain?_____

_____

What sensations or lack of sensations did you experience in the sexual parts of your body (breasts, mouth, genitals, anus)? _____

_____

What sexual responses occurred (excitement, orgasm)?_____

_____

What was happening inside your body at the time of the abuse

You may be sensitive to physiological sensations in your body similar to the ones experienced during the abuse.

How did you feel physically in general (paralyzed, weak, not there, out of control, like fleeing, like fighting, excited, overwhelmed, powerful, hot, cold, sleepy, and so on)?_____

_____

What specific physiological experiences did you have (fainted, vomited, numbing, rapid heartbeat, bleeding, gagging, spitting, crying, sweating, shaking, and so on)?_____

_____

What your emotional feelings were at the time of the abuse

You may be sensitive to emotions that are similar to ones you experienced during the abuse.

What emotional feelings did you experience right before the abuse began (fear, sadness, confusion, shame, anger, disgust, terror, embarrassment, shock, humiliation, and so on)?_____

_____

What emotional feelings did you experience during the abuse? _____

_____

What emotional feelings did you experience immediately after the abuse? ____·_____

_____

Other outstanding sensations, feelings, or thoughts you experienced at the time of the abuse

_____

_____

   Any of the items you identified in this exercise have the potential to trigger automatic reactions. Because abuse is so traumatic, you may have unconsciously linked many items together or fused them in your memory. Now, as you begin to identify these triggers, you may find that one memory triggers another, just as one explosion can set off others in a minefield. But as you begin to defuse each one, you can learn to assume more control over how you react.

_____

AVOIDING AND DEFUSING TRIGGERS

Once you have identified possible triggers, review them and think about when they tend to arise. You'll probably notice that many triggers, such as heavy breathing and genitals, are natural parts of intimacy, sex, and even nonsexual life. These natural triggers can't be easily avoided without inhibiting your sexual enjoyment. You can avoid or minimize other triggers, however, such as those dealing with your environment, or words used in lovemaking. Reducing the number of triggers you have to contend with makes your sexual healing easier. You can focus more of your energy on learning to handle the triggers that naturally occur.

Jackie, a twenty-two-year-old survivor of incest by her older brother, had sexual difficulty with her fiancé. She froze and dissociated when he would approach her intimately. As a young girl, Jackie had been abused at night in her bedroom. After looking at her past abuse and identifying triggers, Jackie realized that her present apartment was furnished with the same furniture she had when she was abused—the same little lamp by her bed, the same drapes, the same pillows, even the same bedspread. Over the next several months Jackie changed the decor and furnishings in her room. This simple change helped. "I realized it was time to grow up," she said. "I feel a lot older and more comfortable when I'm in the room with my boyfriend now."

Another survivor, Josie, reviewed the abuse she had experienced by her grandfather. She realized that many of her husband's physical characteristics reminded her of her grandpa: her husband's hair was gray, he slurped his soup the same way, he had a similar body odor. Together Josie and her husband defused these triggers. He didn't change his hair color, but he did learn a new way to eat soup and began wearing a new cologne that Josie picked out.

Many survivors who feel drawn to potentially damaging sexual behaviors find they can minimize their urges and desires by avoiding stimulants that have provoked uncontrolled sexual responses. If using alcohol or other drugs encourages you to act out sexually, avoid them. If violence charges you up sexually, avoid movies, stories, and shows that associate violence and sex. Avoiding these stimulants is often easier said than done. Some survivors may fear that they will lose their ability to become aroused if they give up a particular trigger, even if it creates problems for them in the long run. Many survivors find they need special help to overcome their fears. Counseling, therapy groups, twelve-step programs such as Alcoholics Anonymous or Sex Addicts Anonymous, and sexual dependency treatment programs can be essential in avoiding and defusing triggers associated with compulsive sex (see Resources section).

GUIDELINES FOR HANDLING AUTOMATIC REACTIONS: A FOUR-STEP APPROACH

Automatic reactions can happen very quickly and take you by surprise. The key to coping with them is to bring them into your conscious awareness. You might say to yourself, "I'm having an automatic reaction." You can stop to acknowledge your reactions even when you are unsure what triggered them. Once you become consciously aware of your reactions, you can take time out to calm yourself and determine what may have caused them to occur. Then you can choose new ways of responding to the situation.

Robin, a forty-three-year-old single survivor, told of her success in changing an automatic reaction that had gone on for years:

> I went to visit my married sister and her family for a week in the summer. One day I entered the bathroom and saw my brother-in-law's swimsuit turned inside out to dry over the towel rack. Immediately, I felt scared, felt like I was a voyeur, and started to condemn myself as bad and sexually sick-minded.
>
> Before I got too far in that line of thinking I just stood there for a moment and relaxed myself. I thought, why am I reacting like this? I knew the suit somehow reminded me of my father's clothes. I thought about how this was my brother-in-law's swimsuit and how it made sense that he would turn it inside out and dry it in the bathroom. Then I examined the suit more closely. There really wasn't anything inherently disgusting or sexually suggestive about it. It felt so good to realize *I have choices in how I react.*

Robin was able to relax and stop her usual reaction, which would have been to feel fear, arousal, and self-loathing.

Robin followed a four-step process in responding to the swimsuit triggers. It is a process all survivors can use in present situations related to touch and sex. Here are the steps:

1. STOP and become aware.
2. CALM yourself.
3. AFFIRM your present reality.
4. CHOOSE a new response.

1. Stop and become aware

As soon as you find yourself reacting in a sudden, upsetting, irrational way that feels out of your control, *stop.* Acknowledge what's happening. Assume that you have hit a trigger and are reacting to past sexual abuse. Try to determine what triggered your reaction. Take this trigger seriously, even though it might seem silly or inconsequential. See if you can make a connection between the trigger and something that you experienced in the abuse.

2. Calm yourself

Tune in to your body. Are you feeling fearful or close to panic? Are you inappropriately sexually aroused? You may be responding with extreme physiological responses that go beyond the realities of the present situation. Calm yourself. Tell yourself some reassuring things such as, "I'm safe, no one can hurt me now." If your heartbeat is going wild, focus on slowing it down. Sit down. Sit up straight. Sometimes placing your right hand over your heart and applying gentle, slow massage can help. If you have stopped breathing or are breathing rapidly, concentrate on taking some slow, deep breaths. If you have tensed your muscles, relax them. By modifying your physiological responses, you modify your automatic reactions. You can't continue to feel anxious when your body is relaxed.

3. Affirm your present reality

Remind yourself that what you are doing and experiencing now is different from what happened to you during the abuse. Look around. Touch things. See where you are and who you are with. Look at yourself. Remind yourself who you are and how old you are. Affirm your rights. You have a right to positive, healthy sexuality. Remind yourself of the difference between sex and sexual abuse. Reaffirm that you have a true sexual self, separate from the influences of sexual abuse. Realize that your body belongs to you, that you can exercise choice and control in terms of what touch and sexual activity you engage in. A survivor said, "When I have a flashback, I remind myself that I lived through sexual abuse once and it was real then. It's not real now and can't hurt me." Another survivor said, "I recognize my reaction for what it is and tell myself, The abuse was then, this is now. Now is better."

4. Choose a new response

Once you've stopped and realized what's happening, calmed yourself, and affirmed your present reality, you have several options. You can *remove yourself from the trigger.* You can *alter the trigger in some way* so that it doesn't bother you as much. You can *approach the trigger slowly* so that it does not startle you. And you can *accept the trigger and experience your automatic reaction*, paying close attention to your thoughts and feelings in order to understand more about the abuse.

Removing yourself from the trigger.   In Robin's case, she could have removed herself by leaving the bathroom where the bathing suit hung. When touch or sexual behavior upsets you, you can stop. Breaking contact with the trigger brings relief. A survivor who was plagued with fantasies and flashbacks during masturbation said, "When they happen, I stop what I am doing, go make some tea, sit up in bed with my teddy bear, and wait out the night." She could also call a friend if she were in an incest survivors' support group to disarm the trigger by talking about it.

Altering the trigger.   You can choose to interact with the trigger in some way to change it. Robin did this when she examined the bathing suit more closely. The goal is to control and change your inner experience rather than avoiding the object or behavior that triggers your reaction. If an overhead light is a trigger, you might take a break from what you are doing to decorate it in some way you like. You might also choose to remove or replace it. If an automatic reaction is triggered during a hug, you might stop and practice hugging in different ways. If seeing a picture of a nude woman in a magazine triggers a desire to compulsively engage in sex, you might make paper clothes to tape over the woman's picture, or draw in some clothing.

Janet, a survivor of incest by her father, felt scared and sick when her partner said the words *I love you* to her for the first time. When Janet thought of saying these words to her partner, she imagined she would be saying, "Go ahead and beat me up!" Hearing them from her partner, it was as if her partner was saying, "Now I can do anything I want to you." Janet altered this trigger by asking her partner to change the phrase *I love you* to *Will you be my valentine?* With this change, Janet was able to exchange words of affection with her partner.

Some survivors, plagued with intrusive, abusive sexual fantasies, find that it helps to alter the content of the fantasy as it is occurring. Let's say a survivor fantasizes about a woman being tied up and raped by a man. The survivor might alter the fantasy so that the woman and man are good friends and lovers, playacting and being silly. The rope is a big spaghetti noodle, and the couple giggles through the whole experience. Changing the fantasy in this way starts to bend the unconscious thinking away from abuse and toward healthy sexual expression. If you can find humor, it's a great healer. Even if you can make only one small change in the direction of healthy sexuality in the fantasy, it is an important step: It will help you disarm the trigger.

Changing a sexual fantasy in small steps enables a survivor to hold on to the erotic power of the fantasy. Tory was troubled by sexual fantasies of an older man seducing a little girl. While she disliked the power imbalance and exploitation of her original fantasy, she did like the excitement found in the elements of innocence and curiosity it contained. Over time she revised the fantasy. She made the man younger and the female older so that they were both consenting adults, and she highlighted elements of sexual wonderment and teasing, which kept the fantasy arousing.

Realizing we have the power to revise and re-create our fantasies to suit our individual needs is empowering. As one survivor said, "Before, I used to feel like I had to surrender to my fantasies. Now I can go to fantasy and make it what I want it to be." *

Altering the trigger slowly can be especially helpful for survivors who experience fear and panic reactions. Have you ever noticed how a child overcomes his initial fear of a toy that at first frightens him? When my son, Jules, was a toddler, we got him a monkey doll that clapped its hands together, repeatedly clanging two cymbals as it jumped about. At first Jules hid from it, watching it carefully. Then he got a little closer and threw other toys at it to watch its response. Later he nudged it with a stick. And finally he kicked it about, picked it up, and pulled its arms apart. No longer afraid, he then set it down and laughed as it continued to jump around. Jules had discovered that he could overcome his initial reaction by interacting with the monkey—poking it, touching it, stopping it, permitting it to continue. He overcame his fear by experiencing his power in relation to it. Through his own actions he developed a new response to the trigger of the monkey doll.

A survivor told how she handled her reactions by altering the flashbacks that triggered them:

> When I have a flashback, I imagine that my experience is a video playing on the television. I use the control knobs on the TV to

* From *Private Thoughts: Exploring the Power of Women's Sexual Fantasies* by Wendy Maltz and Suzie Boss.

click the flashback on and off, depending on how ready I feel to handle it.

Approaching the trigger slowly. Survivors can learn to slowly approach some triggers, such as objects, places, or body parts. They can practice techniques such as slow breathing and muscle relaxation, so that they remain calm as they approach a trigger in small steps. For example, a survivor who becomes overwhelmingly sexually excited whenever he sees a woman's bra might practice standing at different distances from a bra. Perhaps when he is fifty feet away from a bra he is not sexually overwhelmed. From that distance, he can slowly move closer to the bra, stopping when necessary to maintain relaxation and calm. It may take practice on a number of separate occasions for him to begin feeling comfortable when he is close to a bra.

Accepting the trigger and experiencing your automatic reactions. Automatic reactions don't last forever. You can choose to experience and ride them through. This approach can be particularly helpful for survivors with compulsive sexual behaviors. Like pockets of hot, humid air floating in the wind on a cool summer's eve, uncomfortable sexual feelings last a while and then move along. You can learn to experience them without becoming upset at yourself and without acting in a destructive sexual way before they have a chance to pass.

You may choose to explore some automatic reactions which relate to withdrawing from sex, such as flashbacks and panic reactions, in a safe and supportive setting. Since these reactions can be quite disturbing, it's best to have the guidance of a skilled therapist or the support of an understanding partner. In chapter 9 partners will learn how they can assume a supportive role in this kind of active healing work.

Experiencing your automatic reactions can help you process feelings from the abuse, releasing emotions that may have been locked up for years, such as a survivor described:

> Sometimes when I'm having a flashback, I go into it, reexperience the feelings from the abuse, and scream and cry. Other times I choose not to go into them. I ask my partner to do specific things such as hold me, remind me to breathe, change positions, sit up and move around with me. I am safe with my partner. The more I reexperience flashbacks to the abuse, the less intense they get. It helps me understand that the past can't hurt me anymore.

Another survivor said:

> When I have a flashback my partner and I stop and let the flash-
> back continue. He holds me and later talks to me to bring me back
> to the present. For some reason I'm very accepting of these flash-
> backs. They feel like a release and remind me that I didn't make it
> all up.

Similarly, when experiencing an intrusive, abusive fantasy, a survivor can choose to look closer at the fantasy, watching what is going on
in it. Sexual fantasies are like dreams and nightmares. They can symbol-
ically represent unconscious psychological conflict. By analyzing interpersonal dynamics and identifying symbolism and imagery, survivors
can get clues as to how the abuse affected them on a subconscious level.

When David, a survivor of father-son incest, made love with his girlfriend, he would sometimes find himself fantasizing that his girlfriend
was shouting at him, calling him a prick. This fantasy became so upsetting that one evening David stopped in the middle of making love and
told his girlfriend what was happening. She listened attentively. In talking with his girlfriend about his reaction, David realized that he had
imbued his girlfriend with all the anger he felt toward his father, but had
never been able to express. David then imagined himself, as a boy,
shouting at his father, and he began crying aloud: "You prick, you bas-
tard, you prick! How dare you do this to me!" From that evening on,
David was no longer traumatized by the intrusive fantasies, and they
eventually disappeared. By voicing his inner outrage, David disarmed the
fantasy of its emotional power and made it psychologically unnecessary.

While it may be scary to think of riding an automatic reaction
through, survivors often describe a feeling of accomplishment at the
end. "I did it!" a survivor said. "I got through it, without slipping into
any of my old behaviors. I know that it will be easier to handle if I ever
have this reaction again."

OTHER TECHNIQUES FOR HANDLING
AUTOMATIC REACTIONS

Besides techniques for handling automatic reactions that survivors can
do on their own, several others can be done in a therapeutic setting
with the help of a therapist or intimate partner.

Adopting out the reaction

One such technique that I invented is called *adopting out the reaction*. In this approach a survivor describes a particular sequence of automatic reactions in minute detail to another person. You ask the other person to try to experience your reaction as you experience it. Obviously, the other person has to be someone who is psychologically strong and comfortable with this exercise. Sometimes, I encourage clients to do this with me. Here is an example of a female survivor's using this technique in a therapy session. Her automatic reaction was panic when her husband grabbed her around the waist and gave her a hug. I played her role as she described the automatic reaction.

ME: Where am I?

SURVIVOR: You are standing at the kitchen sink, looking out the window, washing dishes.

ME (*I stand and move to a window.*): I am standing at the kitchen sink, looking out the window, washing dishes. Then what do I experience?

SURVIVOR: You hear footsteps behind you, and you know they are my husband Fred's. Suddenly you feel his breath on your neck and his arms fold around your waist.

ME: Okay, I feel my husband Fred's breath on my neck and arms fold around my waist. Now what happens? What emotions do I feel? What's happening in my body? What am I thinking?

SURVIVOR: Fred squeezes you closer and says he loves you. You feel scared, but more than that a little angry that he surprised you, then you feel guilty for being so sensitive to his affections. Your body tightens, you lose your breath and suddenly feel hot and sweaty.

ME: Fred squeezes me close and tells me he loves me. Now I'm feeling scared, but I'm angry, too. Now I feel guilty for being so sensitive to his affections. My body tightens. Where do I feel it tighten in me the most?

SURVIVOR: Your chest and stomach tighten, like a knot.

ME: Okay. My chest and stomach are getting tighter, I can't breathe very well. I'm feeling hot and sweaty. Boy, this is uncomfortable. Then what?

This dialogue can be continued until the automatic reaction has ended. Survivors often feel relieved to share their reactions; the therapist, or partner, gains valuable insight into the details of the survivor's experience. Later the survivor and therapist or partner might brainstorm and practice different options the survivor could employ for handling the automatic reaction as it is occurring. For example, the survivor might practice stopping and talking with her husband, Fred, about how she feels when he approaches her that way, and how she would like him to approach her differently in the future.

Adopting out the automatic reaction allows the survivor to see his or her own reaction from a more distanced, psychological perspective. It validates the importance of the reaction. The survivor is no longer the sole person who has to experience the symptom. No longer do we have to be alone with our experience, like we were in the abuse: We share the burden of the reaction. The power and hold of the reaction are reduced.

Imagery rehearsal

Some survivors benefit from the therapeutic technique of imagery rehearsal. A survivor spends time in counseling generating a list of many possible touch and sex activities. Then he or she arranges the list in a hierarchical order with the least disturbing item at the top and the most disturbing at the bottom. Using slow, controlled breathing to remain relaxed, the survivor imagines progressively one of the listed situations at a time. When triggers are encountered, the survivor imagines successfully coping with the automatic reaction, for instance, by using the four-step approach described earlier. The imagining enables a survivor to rehearse and practice coping methods, gaining skills that enable him or her to comfortably experience the activities in real life.

Survivors can handle specific automatic reactions in an infinite number of ways. Give yourself permission to experiment with the different approaches mentioned in this book and to invent some approaches of your own. Aim for approaches that strengthen your self-esteem and help you take a step toward positive, healthy sexual experiences.

When we learn to handle our automatic reactions, we gain skills that enable us to move away from troublesome sexual behavior and eventually to create new, life-affirming sexual experiences.

8

Moving Toward Healthy Sexual Behavior

> My dysfunctional sexual behaviors make sense given the abuse. They helped me cope and expressed my pain. I honor them even as I acknowledge outgrowing them and cast them aside.
>
> —A SURVIVOR

Without even being aware of the connection, we may still be locked into sexual habits and routines that relate to past sexual abuse. Deva, a twenty-five-year-old survivor who had been raped by her boyfriend when she was a teen, frequently becomes sexually involved with men who exploit and abuse her, much like her high school boyfriend did. Ben, a fifty-year-old survivor of father-son incest, compulsively masturbates to pornography, a habit he started shortly after his father began abusing him.

Had they never been sexually abused, Deva and Ben would probably not be engaging in these behaviors today. Sexual abuse can influence some survivors to replicate behaviors they were first exposed to in the abuse, whereas others engage in new—but also harmful—sexual activities in response to the abuse. Deva continues the pattern by choosing partners who victimize her. Ben turns to degrading pornography to compensate for the humiliation and powerlessness he felt when he was abused.

These kinds of sexual behaviors that result from sexual abuse can feel familiar and habitual, even if they harm us or hurt others. Cross-country skiers know that it's easier to follow well-worn tracks than to blaze a new trail. But unless we dare to step out of old grooves, we can be sliding along in behaviors that make us feel bad about ourselves and emotionally isolated from others year after year. Many survivors do not take the first step to change until the pain of not changing outweighs the discomfort of forging a new path.

Making changes in sexual behavior requires a conscious commitment on the part of a survivor. For many of us, this is the most challenging territory of sexual healing. We need courage to look at the influence of abuse, and we need willingness to make new choices in behavior. We also need the commitment to stick with these changes, even in the midst of distress and insecurity. Though the prospect of change may seem overwhelming at first, over time these new sexual behaviors can become easy and familiar. It is possible to establish healthy, comfortable, and satisfying sexual behaviors free of the influence of abuse.

In this chapter you will have an opportunity to consider how your present sexual activities may relate to past sexual abuse. We will uncover reasons that survivors find it difficult to give up limiting and hurtful sexual behaviors, even when they consciously want to stop them. We will explore a variety of approaches and options you can use to help make the changes you want to make, when you feel ready. These options include stopping behaviors that are related to past sexual abuse, taking a healing vacation from sex, and establishing healthy ground rules for your future sexual encounters.

REALIZING HOW PRESENT BEHAVIORS RELATE TO PAST ABUSE

You have probably made some connections between your present sexual behavior and past abuse already (perhaps when taking the Sexual Effects Inventory in chapter 3 or when learning about your sexual attitudes and automatic reactions). By considering the following list, you can take a more detailed look at the many different kinds of sexual behaviors that can be a consequence of sexual abuse.

As you review this list, keep in mind that these behaviors can result from abuse in a variety of ways. Sexual abuse can introduce victims to many unusual and harmful practices: violent sex, child-adult sex, sado-masochism, pornography, prostitution, multiple-partner sex, and compulsive masturbation. And we may be drawn to certain behaviors because we feel bad about ourselves due to the abuse. Determining whether you have a serious problem depends on several factors: the level of risk and danger involved, the potential harm to yourself and others, the frequency in which you engage in the behavior, the intensity of the behavior, the context in which it occurs, and how it affects your self-esteem.

Although reviewing these behaviors may be upsetting or painful for you, you need to see your sexual behaviors clearly before you can make lasting changes. Put a check mark (√) next to any statements that describe behaviors you currently engage in.

BEHAVIORS THAT CAN RESULT FROM SEXUAL ABUSE

_____ I avoid or withdraw from sex.

_____ I fake sexual interest.

_____ I fake sexual enjoyment.

_____ I have allowed sex to be forced on me.

_____ I have unwanted sex (when you don't want to).

_____ I usually have sex while under the influence of alcohol or other drugs.

_____ I combine sex and emotional or physical abuse.

_____ I combine sex with emotional or physical pain.

_____ I engage in humiliating sexual practices (with animals, sado-masochism).

_____ I have sex while half asleep.

_____ I use pornography.

_____ I use abusive sexual fantasies.

_____ I engage in compulsive masturbation.

_____ I engage in promiscuous sex (many sexual relationships at the same time or in a row).

_____ I engage in prostitution.

_____ I visit a prostitute.

_____ I engage in medically risky sex.

_____ I have anonymous sex (in rest rooms, adult bookstores, telephone sex services).

_____ I have sex in relationships that lack intimacy.

_____ I have sex outside a primary relationship.

_____ I engage in secretive sex, which generates feelings of shame.

_____ I have sex with a person primarily involved with someone else.

_____ I have sex under dishonest circumstances.

_____ I have sex with near-strangers.

_____ I demand sex from a partner.

_____ I commit sexual offenses (voyeurism, exhibitionism, molestation, sex with minors, incest, rape).

_____ I visit topless bars, strip shows, and/or adult bookstores.

_____ I often watch X-rated movies or videotapes.

_____ I make sexual slurs or regularly use hard-core sexual language.

_____ I make sexually degrading jokes.

If you find your present behaviors described in this checklist, you may be unconsciously replaying or mirroring sexual abuse. Sometimes referred to as a *repetition compulsion*, this instant replay can be a survivor's unconscious way of trying to understand what happened and to resolve inner emotional stress by acting out the abuse again and again.

Staging replays may be a way of desensitizing ourselves to the shame, disgust, or pain we felt in the abuse. Replays may also be an effort to gain some mastery and control over even our worst experiences. "Shortly after the abuse, when I was twelve years old," a survivor said, "I did a striptease in front of the picture window in our living room. I had no idea why I was doing it."

Over time, replays can become ingrained, habitual, and reinforced by the pleasure of sexual excitement. We can be locked into the very sexual activities that first caused us anguish. During his abuse, Tyrone was exposed to X-rated movies; as an adult, he finds himself addictively drawn to watching the same kinds of movies when he masturbates.

Sexual abuse may have taught us to oversexualize our responses to affection and closeness. We may find it difficult to touch in our relationships without feeling sexually aroused, or without believing that touch will automatically lead to sex. And we may worry that an intimate relationship cannot possibly exist unless sex is a part of it.

Some of these behaviors may have developed as ways of trying to cope with deep emotions felt during the abuse, such as anxiety, rage, humiliation, and powerlessness. A survivor might have begun acting in a certain way in an effort to prove his or her sexual worth. A survivor who had been molested by her brother when she was a child described her behavior:

As a little girl I became preoccupied with my genitals and tried various experiments on them, like putting perfume on them. I was trying to make myself clean from the abuse as well as to make myself

more attractive. After putting on the perfume I would masturbate. I
think this was an attempt to use physical pleasure to resolve my
emotional confusion. Masturbation became something I felt I *had*
to do, rather than something I felt I *wanted* to do.

Some sexual behaviors may have evolved as ways of trying to avoid
negative feelings and prevent automatic reactions to sex. Survivors may
have begun using alcohol or pornography in conjunction with sex as a
way to dissociate and blot out painful memories of abuse during sexual
experiences. Similarly, survivors may avoid or feel drawn to certain sexual activities in an effort to mask sexual functioning problems such as
arousal or orgasm difficulties that developed in response to the abuse
(see chapter 11). For instance, a survivor may compulsively masturbate
to avoid the possibility of feeling embarrassed by an impotence problem
with a partner. Or a survivor may consciously engage a disturbing sexual
fantasy because it acts as a reliable way to boost sexual interest and facilitate orgasmic release.

Some sexual behaviors re-create relationship dynamics that survivors became familiar with in the abuse. A victim who was physically
abused and sexually molested may unconsciously be drawn to physically
abusive sexual relationships now. Hanna, a thirty-year-old survivor, told
of her history:

When I was a little girl my father would beat and rape me repeatedly. Once I saw him bruise my mother's breasts. Then, when I was
sixteen years old, I married a man who often beat me and humiliated me sexually. On one occasion, when I was getting ready to go
out with some friends, he saw that I looked attractive and tore my
clothes off. Then he shoved me outside the house and locked the
door. I was left huddling naked in the bushes in our front yard.

When we finally realize the connection between past sexual abuse
and our present sexual behaviors, we gain a powerful tool to help us
make positive changes. We can begin to understand why we are drawn
to or avoid certain sexual behaviors. At first we may want to hold on to
these sexual habits to satisfy psychological needs related to the abuse.
But once we examine these hurtful behavior patterns closely, we can
become more motivated to cast off the influence of past abuse. Then we
can establish new patterns free of associations with the offender and of
the trauma we suffered long ago.

All the behaviors in the last checklist are potentially damaging to you. They can generate feelings of unhappiness, loneliness, and self-loathing. They can prevent you from experiencing sex as positive and healthy, something that increases self-esteem and intimacy with others. Instead, these abuse-related behaviors tend to reinforce the sexual abuse mind-set in which sex is seen as a commodity, something uncontrollable, hurtful, secretive, and without moral boundaries. These behaviors can also perpetuate false and negative sexual self-concepts, leading survivors to continue to feel intrinsically bad or damaged, or to see themselves as sex objects.

Let's look more closely at how several of these harmful sexual behaviors may relate to past abuse and how survivors can develop a desire to change the behavior.

Avoiding sex

As a result of sexual abuse, survivors may have learned to withdraw from situations that have the potential to become sexual. A married survivor might sleep in a different room or bed from her spouse. A survivor who does not have an intimate partner might refrain from courtship and dating. By avoiding sex, survivors may feel that they are protecting themselves from harmful sexual behaviors, from unpleasant sexual experiences, or from being sexually abused again. Rich, a survivor who suffered multiple forms of child sexual abuse, feared that he would become an offender if he allowed himself to interact sexually.

> I have trouble getting close. I am very paranoid; I read into statements. On the slightest hint that I might get hurt, I bail out, I run. I have broken up with a number of women after sharing my feelings with them. I was afraid I would be hurt. I don't know how to make sexual advances. I don't even feel okay about advances. I'm afraid that if I make advances I'll become a perpetrator.

In therapy, Rich realized that his sexual advances would not, in and of themselves, make him an offender. He learned to distinguish between conditions that create sexual abuse and conditions that create healthy and positive sex. He reassured himself that his sexual intentions and consciousness were different from an offender's. "I'm not like an offender," Rich concluded, "because I'm committed to not wanting to sexually abuse anyone."

Social isolation can be self-perpetuating. Survivors can remain in a rut in which any social relating becomes more and more uncomfortable. Remaining isolated, they may fail to cultivate basic interpersonal skills. Feeling isolated, alone, and undesirable, survivors may turn to private sexual behaviors—such as compulsive masturbating or obsessive fantasizing about sexual abuse—that in the long run make them feel worse. While indulging in these sexual behaviors might allow for arousal and sexual release, it can also hurt self-esteem and interfere with the development of satisfying relationships. A woman survivor said:

> After the rapes I became extremely distant from people. I isolated more, fantasized more, masturbated more, and had fewer real relationships. Now, however, I am seeing that these behaviors keep me locked into emotional pain from the abuse.

Survivors with partners may withdraw from sex to avoid unpleasant automatic reactions and outcomes. They may fear betrayal, flashbacks, panic attacks, or a repeat of sexual abuse. A survivor in a committed relationship told of her fears:

> I am afraid of intimacy because it can lead to sexual contact, and sex remains too traumatic for me. I tend to avoid being alone with my partner and am hesitant to encourage or initiate touching. My partner and I are both hurting because we lack the intimacy that we both want so badly.

Survivors need to see that continuing these avoidance behaviors allows the abuse to cripple their ability to achieve healthy, positive sex on their own and with a partner. As we will see later in this chapter, and in the chapters in part three of this book, survivors can reach toward sex gradually, learning important skills and alternative ways of saying no to specific, troubling sexual situations. They can build healthy, intimate relationships while still protecting themselves from unpleasant feelings and reactions.

Faking sexual enjoyment

Monica, a survivor of sibling incest, used to pretend that she was having orgasms during sex with her husband. In the abuse Monica had learned to hide her true feelings. She became used to staying in a secret world, apart from the person she was relating with sexually. And she learned to squelch her own sexual needs and enjoyment. Monica feared that her husband would reject her if he knew that she wasn't easily sexually satisfied. Faking enjoyment was one way Monica believed she could control the sexual interaction: her husband would climax and stop sex when she faked an orgasm.

Recently Monica realized that by hiding her true experience by pretending to have orgasms she was continuing the abuse:

> It's becoming clear to me that if I'm really going to get over the abuse I need to talk with my husband and stop faking orgasms— stop re-creating the abuse every time we have sex. I want sex to be for me, too.

Having sex when you don't want to

Sexual abuse teaches submissive sex roles. Victims often learn that they will be assaulted and abused more if they assert their will. They may have felt terrified that they would be abandoned and unloved for not complying. One woman, who as a child had been forced to have sex at gunpoint, was irrationally afraid that her husband would kill her if she refused him.

Male survivors may have difficulty saying no to sex, fearing it will undermine their masculinity, which may have been threatened in the abuse. In fact, many survivors believe that saying no to sex is not an option open to them.

Katie, a twenty-eight-year-old survivor, realized that her recent involvement with a man who wasn't kind to her was an attempt to resolve feelings related to her father, the original offender. She desperately wanted the love her father was never able to give her.

> I was obsessed with this man even though he was unable to commit to a relationship and also was a sexual addict. I knew better, but I couldn't say no to sex with him. I was in incredible pain, turmoil, and confusion. I began writing about how I felt and realized that, through this man, my father was verbally, physically, and sexually abusing me. It all came down to a belief that if I have sex with my daddy, he'll see I need to be loved. He'll stop torturing me, and he'll love me. All of a sudden my behavior made sense. I decided I had to stop seeing the man.

Acknowledging the connection between her present behavior and her abuse was emotionally painful for Katie. She had to admit to herself that her father had been, and probably always would be, incapable of giving her healthy and caring love. Katie realized that she had to learn to give herself the love she had wanted from her father. Only then would she stop trying to get her need for love met through unwanted sexual behavior. "For me, having sex when I don't want to is not a solution," she said. "It's the problem!"

Another survivor, George, was abused by an older woman when he was a teen. She teased him about not being "man enough" for her when he hesitated in the sexual contact. As George explained:

> I used to feel that I didn't have a choice about whether or not to have sex with someone. If someone wanted me sexually, I'd go along with it. To refuse to have sex with a woman seemed unacceptable. I thought it would mean that there's something wrong with me. It seemed extremely rude and insulting. I was sure a relationship would end as a result. I believed that a man should never refuse a woman sexually. It wasn't until recently, in group therapy with other men survivors, that I realized how every time I have sex when I really don't want to, I am reliving the abuse and abandoning myself.

Like Katie and George, many survivors conclude that to break free from the influence of abuse, they need to learn to feel comfortable refusing sex. Many survivors find that being able to say no to sex during the healing enables them to say yes to sex later, when they feel ready and really mean it. Later in the chapter, when we discuss ground rules for healthy sexual encounters, we will talk about how to say no to sex when you need to so that you don't continue to feel like a victim or a sex object or continue unwanted behaviors.

Combining sex and emotional or physical abuse

In sexual abuse, the perpetrator forces the victim into a relationship characterized by secrecy, domination, humiliation, betrayal, or pain. As a result survivors may unconsciously be drawn to relationships in which they are again victimized. A survivor described his situation:

> I was married to a woman who would get angry with me because I didn't want to have sex with her as often as she wanted it. She never let me choose when we had sex. She always initiated it. She'd drink before we had sex. Afterward she made fun of me and put me down for not being like her other partners.

Survivors may get involved and stay involved with abusive partners because of their feelings of fear and low self-esteem. Survivors might tell themselves, "No one else but an abusive partner would want me," or, "I'm afraid someone better might want more from me than I can give." Some survivors who continue to feel responsible for the original abuse might be drawn to abusive relationships to punish themselves. "When I want sex and try to initiate it," a survivor said, "my partner always turns me down. He gets a kick out of seeing me suffer."*

If you remain in a relationship with someone who continually puts you down your behavior may be the result of a distorted effort to protect yourself from feeling the pain of betrayal from the original abuse. This is a damaging cycle: You try to prove to yourself you're bad by having partners who tell you you're bad; then you can fool yourself into thinking you caused the abuse. By blaming yourself you avoid thinking about the original betrayal. You don't have to feel bad about how horribly the offender treated you—because you never admit to that pain. Allowing a partner to hurt us in the present can feel more acceptable than admitting our father, sister, or friend hurt us long ago.

When survivors decide to break free from abusive relationships, it often means they have stopped punishing themselves for abuse that wasn't their fault. They acknowledge how horribly they were misused and betrayed in the past. And they start taking responsibility for protecting themselves from now on. A survivor said, "I realized that I'd never be able to feel good about myself so long as I was letting my boyfriend call me ugly names and threaten me with a beating. I had to set limits and spell out how he was to treat me if he wanted to stay with me—and I did."

Having sex when not fully alert

Sometimes sexual abuse takes place when a victim is half asleep or otherwise not fully present. A little boy may have been fondled in bed at night when he was asleep and then may have pretended to stay asleep until the abuse was over. A woman may have been plied with alcohol and then raped. Some victims of repeated sexual assaults learned that they could temporarily avoid emotional and physical pain by drugging themselves before being approached again by their offender.

* For information on abusive relationships and how to get out of one, see Ginny NiCarthy's book, *Getting Free*, listed in the Resources section.

Pam, a thirty-year-old survivor of father-daughter incest, had very little interest in sex. She turned from her husband, Lonnie, when he would approach her to have sex at night. Sometimes when Pam slept, Lonnie would fondle her breasts and genitals until she was sexually stimulated and aroused. Pam would awaken during the fondling and be very angry with Lonnie for touching her, but she would not tell him she was awake or ask him to stop. Pam said:

> I felt mixed about telling Lonnie to stop since it was hard for me to feel sexually turned on otherwise. But I was allowing Lonnie to treat me the same way my dad had when he would come into my room and touch me when I was a girl. I realized that even if it meant giving up rare moments of feeling sexually aroused, I had to stop this pattern. I didn't want sex to be like that anymore. It felt like I was sexually abusing myself. I wanted to be able to relate with Lonnie honestly and directly, and to stop seeing him as my dad.

Not being fully present may have been functional, and even preferable, during sexual abuse. But to continue tuning out now, in nonabusive sexual situations, robs survivors of being able to control their sexual experiences, to enjoy sensual pleasuring while alert and open, and to create real intimacy with a partner. For sex to be healthy and unlike abuse, we need to be all there.

Using abusive sexual fantasies or pornography

Carol, a twenty-five-year-old survivor, realized that the strong attraction she had to pornographic stories of adult-child sex related directly to sexual abuse by her father.

> I'm fairly sure that the sexual fantasies and books that I used to masturbate to while growing up were distinctly related to specific scenes with my father from the incest. Throughout my teens, my father and I carried on a secret relationship that involved sharing our pornography. He had a whole drawer of porn books in his room, and I had a drawer in mine. He would come take some of my books and exchange them for some of his. I'd use them for masturbation fantasies. We never talked about what we were doing. It was totally, completely unspoken.

The secret sharing of pornography was the primary way that Carol felt emotionally connected with her father. As an adult Carol found that when she stopped masturbating to abusive pornography, she also had to give up an emotional tie to her father. She felt trapped. Carol weighed the pros and cons of change.

> Reading incest fantasy stuff over and over as a way of sexual stimulation was like continuing the abuse. It made me feel I could be sexually stimulated only in situations that were secretive—with married men, with people of authority. I realized that unless I stopped I would never heal. I would never have a regular, normal sexual relationship with my partner, so long as all my stimulation came from abuse.

In time, Carol threw out her pornography and curtailed her abusive fantasies. Although it was painful, she realized that her father was incapable of connecting with her in healthy ways. As she healed, she grieved the loss of never receiving the love and bonding she needed from him.

Relying on pornography and abusive fantasies may have evolved as a way survivors learned to avoid feeling powerless, threatened, and fearful. Survivors may have learned to use fantasy and pornography to dissociate and avoid focusing on their own emotions and sensations during a sexual experience. For a long time, Gina, a survivor, used pornography to distance herself from past abuse.

> Pornography gave me an intense mental focus that kept my father out of my thinking. When my father intruded in my mind, I not only felt bad but lost interest in the sex.

Using pornography prevented one negative experience for Gina—the intrusion of her father's image. But as time went on Gina realized that the pornography was keeping her locked into mental images of sexual exploitation and degradation. There were too many undesirable side effects to this way of coping with her father's image. Gina decided to face her fear of her father's image more directly. She explored her feelings toward her father in therapy and began shouting "get out" at his image when it would intrude during sex. These new ways of coping worked better for her because they didn't inhibit her healthy sexual expression.

Some survivors use abusive fantasies as a way of punishing themselves. Because he still carries underlying feelings of guilt about the abuse, a survivor may fantasize that he is being whipped. Or a survivor may realize that her fantasies represent feelings that she is undeserving of healthy love and affection. A survivor described her abusive fantasy:

> My most arousing fantasy is that my partner is fantasizing about someone else. It's like a drug. It feels like I need it, and yet it makes me feel sad and lonely.

Some survivors realize they have been clinging to abusive fantasies because these fantasies offer opportunities for them to feel in absolute control of sex. In fantasy, survivors can design and change imagined sexual scenarios, and can attempt to compensate for feelings of helplessness and of being out of control that they felt during the abuse. As a survivor explained,

> Abusive fantasies have helped me feel the power and control that I didn't have when I was being abused. While this worked in the short run, now that I feel better about myself, I want to experience more in sex. I can't do it so long as I keep spacing out into these kinds of fantasies.

Abusive fantasies and pornography re-create and reinforce the original abuse experience. In sexual healing, many survivors realize they need to curtail these behaviors.* Then as they move further away from sexual abuse dynamics and the influence of the past, they can think in new and healthy ways during sex, such as by focusing on pleasurable sensations or loving thoughts of sexual contact with a caring partner.

Engaging in compulsive masturbation

When survivors feel drawn or "addicted" to masturbate, this behavior reinforces the abusive notion that sex is uncontrollable and overpowering. Unlike healthy masturbation, which we choose to do as an expression of self-nurturance, compulsive masturbation feels dirty, urgent, and driven.

In therapy, Dave realized that his compulsive masturbating related directly to having been sexually abused as a child by his mother. When Dave was a boy his mother would regularly demand to see his penis to determine if it was "the correct size." This led to Dave's anxiety and fear

---

* A variety of techniques for healing unwanted sexual fantasies can be found in my book, *Private Thoughts* (see Resources section).

about his sexual adequacy. Dave recalled his first experiences with excessive masturbation:

> Sometimes when I was an older boy I'd walk naked into the backyard at night. I tried on my mother's stockings and bras. I'd fantasize about seeing and touching my mom's breasts. I began masturbating to images of being sexually controlled by women. Once I got so upset with all the masturbating, I burned myself with a lighter. The secretive activity was a turn-on because of the secretive relationship I had with my mother. The sexual thoughts of her gave me a nonreality, a weird feeling that made me want to withdraw totally from people.

Survivors need to realize that this kind of compulsive behavior mistreats their own sexuality as an outlet for emotional pain. By exploiting themselves, survivors stay locked into abusive patterns while feeling isolated, detached, and different from others. Until they eliminate this compulsive behavior, they hinder their chance to build real intimacy.

Engaging in promiscuous sex

Some survivors, struggling with unresolved emotional conflicts from the original abuse, may have many brief sexual relationships in a row or have multiple sexual partners during a particular period. Isaac, a twenty-six-year-old gay man who had been repeatedly abused by his brother and uncles, realized that the pain of low self-esteem had been igniting his desire for many sexual partners. Through this kind of sex, he was unconsciously trying to "prove" or "show" how bad and disgusting he felt about himself as a result of his abuse.

> After I first came out, I had numerous sexual encounters in bookstores, bathhouses, and rest rooms. I used to try for large numbers—an even dozen encounters in a day. I was trying to cover for feelings of loneliness. Later I did massage for a living, which was basically masturbating men. I also made sadomasochism movies. It was good money and made sense at the time. For a while after the whole AIDS thing came out, I continued to practice unsafe sex. I remember thinking it was a real thrill that the sex could be what does me in. Since I've stopped those behaviors, gotten off drugs, and been in incest recovery, I can see now that what I was doing was acting out all my abuse stuff—keeping it alive while slowly killing myself.

Isaac's promiscuous behavior was a way of punishing and hurting himself for past abuse, like a child who bangs his head against the wall when he feels bad about himself. He had turned feelings of anger and betrayal meant for his offenders inward on himself.*

Because of the AIDS epidemic, survivors who realize the connection between their promiscuous behavior and past abuse, and who then decide to do something about it, may actually save their own lives and the lives of others.

Having sex outside a primary relationship

Having "love" affairs may be a survivor's way to replay the lost trust and the human betrayal inherent in the original sexual abuse. We may cheat on our partners, just as our abuser may have cheated on someone else or betrayed our trust. We may be dishonest about our actions, telling lies to our partners to maintain the behavior, just as our abusers told lies to us and others. The abuse may have taught survivors to feel addicted to the excitement of illicit sex. We may not admit how hurtful our actions may be to others, just as our abusers did not admit how they hurt us. Affairs can be miniature re-creations of the abuse. Like abuse, an affair is often a tantalizingly secret, "forbidden" sexual liaison. Many survivors conclude that they have to stop having affairs because affairs both keep them locked into patterns of deceit and secrecy and cause harm to others.

Acting in sexually demanding or exploitive ways

The repercussions of sexual abuse can lead a survivor to act in sexually aggressive ways. Survivors who act in these ways may not even consciously realize they are doing to others the same hurtful things that were done to them. This aggressive behavior can be overt, such as when a survivor commits incest or rape. It can also take on more subtle forms. Being nice to someone, sleeping with him, and then ignoring him is subtle abuse. So is demanding sex from a partner, using hard-core sexual language around people who don't want to hear it, and buying sex from a prostitute.

---

* For more on how victims of abuse may turn anger against themselves, see Alice Miller's book, *For Your Own Good* (in the Resources section), especially the chapter entitled "Unlived Anger," pages 261 through 270.

Sexually abusive behaviors may be unconscious attempts to align with the power that the survivor assumed the offender possessed. If I'm not doing it to someone else, then someone else will do it to me, a survivor might think, or, The best defense is a good offense. These behaviors hurt survivors by jeopardizing their legal, ethical, and moral integrity; they also deny survivors real intimacy and self-respect. You won't be able to feel genuinely good about yourself if you are treating other people as objects or betraying their confidence and trust.

Survivors may resist admitting that they have been acting in sexually abusive ways. They may be so focused on thinking of themselves as victims that the idea *they* are hurting someone else may never have occurred to them. But once reached this kind of awareness can pave the way for change. "It hurts me to realize that I have treated my wife as a toy, a machine whose orgasms could make me feel that I'm a man," a survivor said.

Once we identify the ways we replicate past abuse, we can begin to reduce the mystery and power our impulses have to control us. As we better understand the challenges specific behaviors may present, we can work more effectively toward lasting changes.

BREAKING FREE FROM ABUSE-RELATED SEXUAL BEHAVIORS

Sexual healing involves recognizing sexual practices that are associated with past abuse and then learning new ways of behaving that foster healthy sexuality and intimacy. Here are three different avenues survivors can follow to make changes in their sexual behavior:

1. Learn methods for stopping specific unwanted sexual behaviors.
2. Take a healing vacation from sex to develop a new orientation for integrating sex into your life.
3. Establish healthy ground rules for sexual encounters to improve self-caring and intimacy in sex.

I describe these avenues in a progressive order. They are complementary and can be combined and integrated with each other. For instance, a survivor may choose to take a healing vacation form sex to help him stop a specific unwanted behavior. Or a survivor may want to establish new ground rules for sexual encounters as she resumes sexual activity after a vacation from sex. You can decide to journey on each one to whatever degree you want, or you can travel them one at a time in the order they are presented. As with the rest of your healing journey, you need to create a program that fits your needs at this time. Become familiar with each of these avenues; you may want to take some steps now and plan others for the future.

Avenue 1: Stop specific unwanted behaviors

Once you've identified one or more specific sexual behaviors you want to stop, don't be surprised if you feel anxious about actually stopping them. Giving up old behaviors can seem overwhelming, even impossible, at first. This is natural. After all, your present sexual habits have probably become ingrained over many years. Even though they may be bringing you chronic unhappiness and reminding you of the abuse, you still know how to do them, and you know what happens when you do them. It's difficult to consider changing a behavior that feels familiar and secure, even if it's wrong for you. For no matter how a specific sexual behavior may be harming you, it may also be fulfilling some emotional needs.

Certain sexual behaviors give a survivor a sense of power and control. A survivor who retreats from sex may feel that this behavior helps her avoid unpleasant automatic reactions and potentially embarrassing sexual experiences. Stopping this avoidance behavior would mean developing alternative ways of self-protection and power. These might include building skills to handle automatic reactions and learning skills for communicating with a partner.

In contrast, another survivor may feel his aggressive sexual behavior gives him a sense of control and power in sexual situations. Stopping this aggressive behavior would require developing skills for feeling powerful and in control while being nonabusive and respecting the rights of a partner. Learning how to assert his feelings and needs directly and to build emotional trust with his partner may be the new tools that could replace aggressive behavior patterns. If you balk at losing something familiar, remember that you are gaining something much better.

Even if harmful, a particular sexual behavior may make you feel safe. Letting go of it will mean facing new feelings of vulnerability. Roxanne, a date rape survivor, was terribly lonely and wanted to date and be sexual again, but the thought of initiating social contacts made her shrink in fear. She worried that she would be abused again. Jake, a survivor who used abusive and degrading pornography to become aroused, desperately wanted to stop this habit, but he feared that giving up this behavior would make him vulnerable to sexual functioning problems. Jake described his dilemma:

> To eliminate my sexual fantasies would feel like getting out of a box. But it's hard for me to imagine anything being as stimulating as the fantasies. I worry that without the fantasies I won't be able to maintain erections and will humiliate myself with a partner, or that if I can still get erections, sex might become just plain boring.

Roxanne and Jake weren't able to stop their harmful sexual behaviors until they allowed themselves to take risks. Change involves accepting our intrinsic vulnerability.

A particular sexual behavior—even one you know is harmful—may have been serving a psychological function for you by keeping you from a painful realization about the abuse. When Roberta, a thirty-year-old survivor of father-daughter incest, began to take steps to stop promiscuous behavior, she ran right into an awareness that forced her to reevaluate her image of her father. Roberta realized that if she admitted she was capable of gaining control over *her* sexual impulses, her father must have chosen not to control *his* sexual impulses when he abused her. Finally Roberta realized that her compulsive sexual behavior had been sheltering her from feeling rage about being abandoned by her father. Roberta had to accept and mourn the fact that her father had intentionally abused her.

Some survivors are discouraged at the thought of stopping harmful sexual behaviors. Perhaps they tried to stop before and didn't succeed. Enthusiasm became disappointment, and they felt even more entrenched in their damaging behaviors.

Like quitting smoking or drinking, stopping old sex practices creates stress. You may fear that first day without the behavior, just as a soon-to-be ex-smoker dreads his first day without cigarettes. You may also wonder what repercussions stopping the behavior will have for you in the long run.

Because of all the resistance and fears, stopping a harmful sexual behavior will probably require a continued, long-term, concentrated effort. Keep in mind that the challenge is different depending on the kind of behaviors you decide to change: Survivors who retreat from sex need to continually challenge themselves to overcome their fears and to develop new skills to protect themselves during touch and sex. Survivors who are drawn to compulsive sexual behaviors need to continually challenge themselves to wrestle down and relax their desire for old behaviors, clearing the way for openhearted, whole-body sexual experiences in which they feel good sexually, emotionally, and ethically, all at once.

Here are some suggestions for how you can help yourself stop a particular sexual behavior that you have realized you want to stop.

Get clear on why you want to stop. Spend some time evaluating the particular sexual behavior you want to stop. Examining the negative behavior closely can help you remember why it's important for you to stop it and why stopping it is worth the time and trouble it takes. The following exercise may help you.

Serge, a survivor who was able to curtail compulsive masturbation to abusive magazine pornography, did so partly to protect his personal integrity. He realized that if he were to die suddenly, his family would find his stash of sadomasochistic pornography hidden in the garage. That possibility bothered him enough to help him change his behavior.

After you have thought through your own reasons for wanting to stop certain behaviors, you may want to rank which behaviors you want to stop first. Some behaviors—criminal sexual acts, medically risky sex, or degrading sexual practices—must be addressed immediately. Continuing any of these practices puts you and others at risk of serious harm.

Get support to stop harmful sex. Because stopping harmful sexual behavior requires long-term dedication, it is helpful—and probably essential—to have the support of individual counseling, therapy groups, or other recovery programs.* Without such help we can easily lose perspective on what it takes to change, unnecessarily blaming or shaming ourselves if we falter. A survivor said:

> It has been critical for me to find others with whom I can talk honestly and openly about my sexual experiences, feelings, compulsions, and attractions. I have been able to truly feel normal by just hearing that others have thought, felt, and done the same things I have, and by hearing about what had helped them to recover.

Survivors often need other types of support in stopping old behaviors. Taking classes about sex, obtaining social skills through training,

---

* See resource listing on how to find therapy groups, twelve-step recovery groups, and other treatment programs. Some hospital programs have been specifically developed to help people overcome sexually addictive and compulsive behaviors.

learning how to control anger, and developing assertiveness and communication skills can help you strengthen the personal resources that can assist you in making changes. In many ways, you are creating a new life for yourself out of the shadow of abuse. Changing your sexual behaviors will also probably entail relearning and redefining many old habits and attitudes—from how you view yourself to how you interact with the world around you. Realize that this is a big task, and find support to help you on your way.

Develop a realistic approach to stopping negative behavior.   Nurture yourself. Have compassion for yourself. Expect this healing process to take time.

You can't force yourself to stop fearing sex and withdrawing from it.

GETTING CLEAR ABOUT SPECIFIC SEXUAL BEHAVIORS

Review the abuse-related behaviors you checked at the beginning of this chapter, on pages 164–65. You may want to examine each behavior or focus on one or two. Then answer the following questions.

1. How does this behavior represent a way of thinking about sex in which sex is seen as sexual abuse?
2. How does this behavior reflect a false or negative view about myself as a sexual person?
3. How does this behavior reenact the relationship dynamics I was exposed to in the abuse?
4. How does this behavior hurt me?
5. How does this behavior hurt others?
6. Why is it important that I stop/change this behavior? (Consider the consequences if you continue this behavior: Could you lose an important relationship? develop a sexually transmitted disease? cause an unwanted pregnancy? be accused or convicted of a crime? lose a job? suffer years of loneliness, alienation, and remorse?)

You may want to expand on your answers in a journal, talk about them in a support group, or discuss them with a therapist. You may also find it helpful to write your answers to these questions on a card and keep them with you at all times. Refer to them frequently to remind yourself of the sound reasoning behind the changes you are making.

Withdrawal is a protective shield that you let go of as you feel safe in other ways. Conversely, making yourself be sexual when you don't want to is abuse of yourself. Take gradual steps. Focus on feeling safe and comfortable, asserting your needs, and handling your automatic reactions. You will stop withdrawing by slowly moving forward with other safe behaviors, such as exploring nonsexual intimate touch, communicating feelings and needs, and pacing sexual experiences. Proceed gently.

Stopping compulsions and addictions may require you to take a tougher approach. Survivors need to be alert to their tendencies to deny that their actions are problems. Denial sabotages our own sexual recovery. You may hear yourself making statements that rationalize and validate compulsive behaviors. Confront these statements. "Just one more time won't hurt," we may say, even though we know better. But you will always have another decision to make. We must find a way to say no each time. Because of the tendency to deny addictive and compulsive sexual behavior, support groups, twelve-step programs, and therapy may be essential to your recovery. We can't deceive ourselves so easily when we share our feelings with others who understand.

People make changes differently. You will need to find your own path. One survivor might stop having an affair all at once and never have another. Another survivor might find he has better success by gradually phasing out negative behavior.

One survivor caught in a pattern of sexual compulsion found that she was able to make progress by giving up her harmful sex habits one by one—easiest first, hardest last. One success encouraged the next.

> Sex had been a free-for-all. I had no boundaries to my behavior. I knew I needed to get control over my situation. After I decided I wouldn't sleep with anyone I worked with, I decided to have no more secretive sex. I had to have sex in the context of the relationship I was in or tell my partner about it if I was having an affair. That limited things quite a bit, which was good for me—*I needed limits*! Later I gave up affairs altogether.

If you choose to go slowly and gradually, don't fool yourself by making real goals too distant. In the movie *Uncle Buck*, actor John Candy plays the lovable uncle who talks about his five-year plan to stop smoking. He plans to first switch from cigarettes to cigars, then cigars to a pipe, then a pipe to chewing tobacco, then chewing tobacco to nicotine gum, and then to give up the gum. How likely is it that he'd ever succeed?

Abusive fantasies pose a different challenge. They function like automatic reactions, occurring spontaneously with sexual arousal. Don't expect your fantasies to stop completely even if you do stop harmful behaviors. Fantasies often persist, but survivors can stop feeling the shame and thwarted intimacy that often accompanies such fantasies. A survivor told of gaining control of her fantasies:

> I spent several years trying to stop my abuse fantasies during sexual intercourse. I was able to tame them down a lot, into less and less degrading images. But I was still frustrated and angry that I was drawn to them at all. They can so quickly pop into my mind. I got to a point where I stopped feeling bad about them. I just accepted they would sometimes be there. When they come up now I shift my mental focus away from them as much as possible. I ground myself in the present, think about loving myself if I am alone or loving my partner if I am with him. I don't let the fantasies interfere with liking myself or feeling close with my partner.

Expect to feel some mixed emotions when you stop engaging in negative sex. You may feel excited and encouraged one moment, discouraged and sad the next. Keep going. Don't quit.

Letting go is always a loss, even when you let go of behavior that hurts you. Cry about loss, but let go of the damage.

Learn how to prevent relapse.   In Alcoholics Anonymous there is a well-known saying, "Relapse is part of recovery." This is true as well for survivors wanting to escape from bad sex. Recovery isn't steady. You walk. You fall. You get up and walk again.

Some relapses are preventable. Ask yourself, *What need did this behavior fill? What is another way I can satisfy this need?* If abuse-related sex relieved stress, try relaxation training, exercise, or meditation. If harmful sex connected you with others, join a club, play sports, meet for lunch with a friend. Developing healthy alternatives reduces the tendency to see the old behavior as your only available response.

Relapses can be minimized and prevented when you establish certain guidelines for your sexual behavior. If you are stopping yourself from getting sexually involved too early in a relationship, you can limit your early dates to daytime settings with a group of friends. If you are stopping having sex when you are half asleep, you can discuss the situation with your partner and both agree that sex is not okay unless you make eye contact and verbally consent first.

We can reduce the likelihood of relapse by improving our self-esteem and releasing ourselves from shame. Acknowledge your accomplishments. Indulge your healthy desires. Develop a life-style that balances obligatory demands and satisfying activities.*

Another way to prevent relapse is to identify your triggers (see chapter 7). When a physical setting, a partner's behavior, or something else reminds you of sexual abuse, you may be aware by now that you are likely to react by withdrawing or behaving compulsively. By being aware you can control how you react.

I counseled a couple once in which the survivor, who had been withdrawn sexually, was making good progress. She was gradually feeling more comfortable with physical intimacy with her husband, making sure that she only had contact when she really wanted to. Then on the night of their fourteenth wedding anniversary, she began to feel guilty that she hadn't been overtly sexual with her husband for a long time. Without realizing it, she had begun to pressure herself to have sex out of a sense of obligation. She took their kids to her mother's house, bought a bottle of champagne, put on a sexy nightgown, and seduced her husband when he came in the door. Midway through the sexual act, she withdrew, emotionally distant and depressed. It took months until she felt like exploring any kind of physical intimacy again. Looking back on the experience, she could see that feeling guilty and acting out of obligation had triggered her relapse.

Some survivors plan ahead of time what they will do if they start to relapse. This might include getting out of a risky environment, talking with a support person, writing in a diary, or relying on a variety of alternative, positive behaviors.

When relapses do occur—and they probably will—remain positive. Relapses yield information that can help you. Ask yourself what triggered this relapse and how you could have prevented it. This hindsight can help you have fewer slips in the future. Don't hate yourself for slipping. Learn and get yourself back on track quickly.

Stopping your damaging sexual behaviors can bring about many positive changes. You become active in creating your life as you want it to be, instead of reacting to what others have done to you. You can protect

---

* See the Resources section for books on sexual abuse recovery as well as on related topics such as shame, stress reduction, and communication.

yourself from unconsciously assuming the role of victim in your relationships. At this point in your life you can assume responsibility for yourself and your future. When you become accountable for your actions, you accept and welcome your strength and power. Tom, a survivor of father-son incest, said:

> For most of my adult life my sexual expression was tied up with a desperate need to have someone love and approve of me. I had sex to get close. Later I felt used. I was sexually out of control.
>
> Lately I've been liking and trusting myself more. I realize that what I do, and have to give, is important. I've been setting limits for the first time.
>
> It's time for me to take charge of my life and to heal. I want to slow things down and learn to deal with my own reactions and needs by myself. To recognize my human value, I need to stop being sexual for awhile.

Many survivors feel a similar need to abstain from sex temporarily, to give themselves time to fully heal, and to learn new ways of behaving. Once you feel you have the skills to stop harmful sexual behaviors, you may want to take a vacation from sex. Just as a break from work can help you regain perspective and renew your energy, a vacation from sex can give you a chance to change the way sex fits in with the rest of your life.

Avenue 2: Take a healing vacation from sex

The emotional wounds of sexual abuse, like physical wounds, need time to heal. But like wounded soldiers who go right back into battle, many survivors never take an opportunity for rest and recuperation. Their wounds continue to ache. Survivors may feel opened up and raw, realizing how much they were hurt.

You need a healing rest, time to process your feelings and tune into your own being, apart from sexual demands. Slowly you can learn to trust, feel, and enjoy your sensual self.

A vacation from sex can free the emotional energy you need to heal from sexual abuse. During a vacation from sex you no longer have to feel anxious, threatened, or controlled by sex: You get a reprieve. Energy that was reserved for worrying and obsessing about sex can now flow into your sexual recovery.

Create your own vacation.   There are many different ways of taking a healing vacation. You will need to design a vacation that fits your present needs and situation. Here are some options to consider in planning your healing vacation:

1. Refrain from all sexual activity and intimate touch.
2. Refrain from sexual activities that involve genital stimulation, such as masturbation and intercourse, but allow other forms of intimate touch, such as kissing and hugging.
3. Refrain from sex with others, but allow self-stimulation.
4. Refrain from only some types of sexual activities. For instance, if you have an intimate partner, you may not want to be touched sexually or to be expected to touch your partner sexually. But perhaps you feel comfortable holding your partner while he or she masturbates.

Your healing vacation should last as long as you want it to last. While some survivors feel satisfied with healing vacations that last only several weeks to several months, I find that many survivors typically need at least three months of vacation to start to feel the benefits of the break. I recommend taking three months to one year. Some survivors, especially those who endured severe and highly traumatic abuse, may need more time.

Some vacations put the survivor completely in charge—no physical intimacy unless they initiate it. This can help survivors who feel overwhelmed when anyone tries to hug, cuddle, or kiss them. These survivors may have felt that all touch leads to sex. They need the vacation to learn to feel physically safe, in control, and relaxed.

Survivors who are not currently in a relationship may choose a celibate life for awhile. If you've associated dating with having uncontrolled sex, it may be best to refrain altogether from dating during your vacation. A single survivor of child molestation and date rape described her experience:

> I was celibate for eleven months after the rape while I first began to deal seriously with abuse issues. This time gave me space to release myself from the critical judgments and voices that had acted like boulders around my feet. I treated myself to only the touches I wanted. I began to consciously appreciate my own sexuality and to own it as part of me.

Survivors in committed relationships need the cooperation of their intimate partners for the vacation to work. Because of the impact a vacation can have on an intimate relationship, survivors need to talk with their partners about their desire and reasons for taking a vacation from sex. Obviously, the idea of stopping all sex for awhile can scare and upset a partner. Partners may fear the vacation will mean that their sexual problems are going from bad to worse. "Will we ever be sexual again?" a partner may worry. For a partner who is already feeling sexually rejected, the prospect of months and months of sexual inactivity can seem miserable.

But the partner need not feel forgotten during your vacation. The partner's role during this time is extremely important to sexual healing and to the establishment of future sexual intimacy. In the coming chapters we will look closely at the partner's feelings and examine how survivors and partners can work together on healing during a vacation. You will also learn a variety of progressive exercises for relearning touch and solving sexual problems. You can start practicing some of these during the vacation. Although taking a vacation may sound passive, it isn't. This can be the most active and productive period in your sexual healing.

If the vacation idea terrifies you, ask yourself why. Your answer may also help you understand your possible fears or addictions. When you compare three to six months or more on a vacation to your lifetime's suffering, it won't seem so long. Many survivors I have worked with tell me that a healing vacation has been the most important step they have taken to further their sexual healing.

How can a vacation from sex help you?   Let's consider some of the healing that can go on during a vacation from sex and why the break from sexual activity makes this process possible. Here are three main tasks that can be accomplished during the healing vacation:

- Healing your sexual self
- Resolving issues related to the abuse
- Learning new approaches to relationships and touch

HEALING YOUR SEXUAL SELF.   Survivors who were abused in childhood may not be able to recall a period in their lives when they were not sexually active. A safe and innocent childhood is a birthright you may have lost. By taking a vacation in adulthood, survivors can create an age of innocence, an experience they never had. It's a way of actively reclaiming a lost part of childhood, a way of putting sex into healthy perspective.

Rhonda, a thirty-year-old single survivor, was abused by her stepfather from the time she was eight until she was twelve. Since then she had been involved in one hot and heavy short-term relationship after another. She slept with men within days, sometimes hours, of meeting them. Sex was the main focus of her encounters. When Rhonda first considered taking a break from sex, she was terrified. It took her several attempts until she was finally able to do it. Six months into her vacation, something special started to happen: Rhonda started to feel sexually innocent. As she explained:

> I feel fresh and new. I think of myself as a virgin now. The other day I wore a white dress and white pearl necklace to a party. I felt special and good about myself in a way I never knew before. I've even started using *extra-virgin* olive oil for cooking.

Virginity is more a state of mind than body. It has to do with seeing yourself as presexual, pure, wholesome, curious, exploring, and self-protective. Regardless of your past abuse and experiences, with a breather from adult sexuality you can reclaim the experience of virginity for yourself.

Taking a healing vacation from sex creates an opportunity to repair the damage done to your social and sexual development. When children are not sexually molested, they typically go through stages in their growth that prepare them for relationships and future sexual contact. These stages include *feeling physically safe and protected from overt sex, feeling loved for themselves, enjoying touch and sensations, developing sexual curiosity, initiating social relationships, and establishing meaningful friendships and nonsexual forms of intimacy.* Later in life they can choose to have sex from a place of readiness, choice, and healthy excitement.

Healing vacations from sex can allow survivors to learn to protect themselves sexually. This is a good time to take assertiveness training and self-defense classes. Survivors get to know their personal needs and desires, and they can assert healthy boundaries that secure their autonomy. Survivors also learn how to slowly remove the unhealthy walls of fear they've hidden behind.

Healing vacations allow us time to become our own nurturing, protective inner parent who is capable of setting limits out of love and respect for ourselves. As one survivor discovered:

My first relationship has to be the one I have with myself. No one can make it up to me—what I went through. I need to learn to love myself and appreciate my sexuality myself.

During the vacation from sex, survivors have an opportunity to learn a new approach to touch. *Touch can be explored in gradual steps.* The techniques and exercises presented later in the book are designed to help you. Survivors can learn that touch can be pleasurable in and of itself, and not something that automatically leads to sex. Survivors can learn how to express their feelings through touch and can receive nurturance from the caring touch of others, as this survivor recalled:

Once I was secure that I didn't have to touch, I began to *want* to explore physical touch gradually with my partner. We started with simple things like holding hands, sitting close together, hugging, and cuddling. Then later, once I felt comfortable with these activities, we exchanged massages, did some kissing and petting. With each step I felt present, really there, expressing love and receiving it too. As I continue with exploring touch I know I'll need lots of time and plenty of patience.

The vacation gives survivors who have withdrawn from sex an opportunity to get in touch with their innate sexual drive and urges. No longer feeling constant pressure for sex, no longer having to defend against it, survivors can tune into warm and tingling genital feelings and healthy sexual fantasies that naturally come and go. Some survivors realize for the first time that they have sexual urges. They learn to identify their experiences as signs of healthy sexuality. Often they discover a world they've never known. A survivor of sadistic ritualized childhood sexual abuse who had been on a sexual vacation for a year explained how it helped her:

Yesterday I saw a man and woman riding bicycles together out in the country. It was cold and rainy, but they were smiling as I drove past. My mind wandered into a fantasy of how nice that would be if my husband and I were to bike together like that and then come home, take a shower to get warm, and then cuddle. The thought surprised me. That was my first positive sexual fantasy, ever.

The vacation can also provide a safe time to learn about sexual urges in a different, nonabusive way. Survivors who have been stuck in compulsions find they don't die without sex. They learn that sexual urges can be felt without being acted upon.

RESOLVING ISSUES RELATED TO THE ABUSE.   Taking a vacation from sex provides a good time for working on other issues related to the abuse. Without constant worry about having sex, some survivors find memories about the abuse surface more easily in dreams and therapy. It's as though the unconscious mind is no longer on guard—it can relax and let past sexual abuse experiences surface.

Strong feelings such as betrayal, anger, sadness, and grief often surface while survivors are resolving general issues related to the abuse. Survivors may become deeply depressed, want to hit things, cry a lot, or have nightmares. They may feel especially vulnerable. The vacation from sex enables a survivor to access and release these powerful emotions more easily. Later, when sex is resumed, survivors are then more capable of enjoying intimacy.

Because the survivor feels safe and protected during a vacation, this can also be a good time to learn to deal with triggers and automatic reactions. Knowing that you don't *have* to be sexual may give you the peace of mind to confront and analyze the triggers that may have upset or terrified you during sex.

Nonsexual healing work done at this time can also be essential to a survivor's long-term sexual recovery. When feelings from the abuse aren't resolved, they tend either to get turned inward on oneself or to be projected onto a partner, slowing down progress in sexual healing. If a partner continues to push for sex, the survivor may unconsciously confuse the partner with the offender. Anger meant for the offender may be directed at the partner. If the partner is willing to refrain from sex, the survivor may stop unconsciously thinking of the partner as an offender.

LEARNING NEW APPROACHES TO RELATIONSHIPS AND TOUCH.   In the safety and security of a vacation from sex, survivors can take a new turn in their sexual healing and start a rebuilding process. They can develop skills to approach touch and sex in a new way, and can learn how to replace the harmful sexual practices they've stopped with new, healthier behavior. As you enter this new phase in healing, you are in effect reinventing yourself. You are shaping new attitudes, new behaviors, and new responses. You want to be careful as you proceed that your new sexual self will be strong and sure. This time around, you get to be the person you want to be—not who the abuser said you were or who you came to believe you were because of the abuse. You also have a chance now to establish and nurture the kind of relationship you want.

I asked several survivors to describe their ideal relationship. Their wish list included love, laughter, tears, respect, friendship, trust, nurturing, and support. One survivor said, "I need to be treated gently." Another said, "I need a partner who is committed to personal growth and can share his problems, too. I don't want to be the 'sick one' in the relationship." Going beyond wishing, another survivor offered this:

> I feel that I'm in an ideal relationship now. My partner is loving and supportive. He is willing to hold me and listen while I talk of sad or painful things. He has stayed with me through my ups and downs as I work on healing. He has accepted my needs for aloneness and space. He has learned about abuse and healing. He has told me he loves and respects me more because I became the woman I am despite what I went through.

What would your ideal relationship be? During your healing vacation, take time to imagine the kind of relationship you want, and know that you are helping yourself make it a reality.

A healing vacation provides survivors with time to build relationships slowly and carefully. We can *establish friendships first* and avoid the problems that arise from rushing into physical intimacy. Whether you are single or already in a committed relationship, you need to get to know people as friends before even considering having sex with them. The healing vacation gives you time to do this.

In healthy, nonabusive sex, intimate relationships are *always* based on friendship. In a friendship, the focus of relating is on such things as common interests and a sense of trust. You get to know someone for who they are, and you let them know you for yourself. In friendships you learn to be vulnerable and share your feelings and thoughts candidly, without the added pressure of worrying whether you will still be seen as "attractive," "feminine," or "manly." Being able to feel relaxed and comfortable around others often involves feeling good about who you are and getting out from under the inhibiting influence of sex role stereotypes that were learned or reinforced in the abuse.

If you think that you easily fall victim to sex role stereotypes and other social prejudices, that they prevent you from "being yourself around a partner," you might want to try an exercise I call *putting on blinders* (see box, pg. 192).

PUTTING ON BLINDERS

You may have noticed that the horses who draw carriages often wear black blinders to keep them from looking sideways. Let's imagine that we have blinders too. Our blinders prevent us from noticing what sex we are and what sex another person is when we converse with them. Our blinders help us blot out sex bias, so we can express our thoughts and feelings directly. We learn to listen to others for *what they have to say*, rather than focus on the gender of the person talking. When we speak to others we express our individual ideas and values, not the fact that we are either male or female.

You might put on blinders when you meet someone for the first time. Imagine you are a heterosexual woman who has just been introduced to an attractive man. Instead of getting lost in how good he looks and the image he projects, you can put on blinders and listen to what he is saying, and watch what he is doing *as a human being*. Ask yourself: What if this were a 60-year-old woman? Would I agree or disagree? Does this person respect my ideas and feelings? Do I like how this person relates to me and others? Is this a caring and responsible person? Do I feel drawn to this person for the values and ideas he represents and expresses?

Putting on blinders helps us to be ourselves and see others for who they are, separate from sexual stereotyping. Try this exercise in your next conversation.

Relating with people as humans, instead of as objects or stereotypes, helps us feel better about ourselves. A survivor said:

> I am much more aware of what goes on in my head and my emotions when someone wants to get to know me. I can stop myself from tendencies to come on to people in sexual ways. Sex today is something I am in control of. I am able to direct my actions toward appropriate expressions of affection, friendship, and love.

Having friendships first lets us create relationships based on equality and mutual respect. A man who was abused as a child by his mother described his experience:

> I used to be nice to women to get sex. Now I have women friends. I can express my need for love and closeness nonsexually. I feel *equal*

with women and that makes me feel a lot better about my sexual
self. In the past I saw women as healthy and myself as not healthy.
Now I see women as fearful and needy too, as well as healthy and
adjusted.

Friendship is a good basis from which an intimate relationship can
grow. Without the confusion and expectations often generated by having sex, you can find out if another person accepts you as you are and
feels comfortable with himself or herself. As a woman survivor said:

In the beginning of our relationship, my present boyfriend and I got
to know one another through social functions with friends. Then
we spent time jogging on the beach, watching movies, walking
dogs, and doing other nonpressured, fun activities. We let things
happen on a solid and mutual basis as we got to know each other
better.

Once you have developed a friendship, you can use your vacation
from sex to give yourself permission to *date* and enjoy a period of nonsexual *courtship*. Whether or not you are already in a committed relationship, dating your partner without even considering sex can be
important to your sexual healing.

For survivors in long-term, committed relationships, "dating" again
now, during your healing vacation, can give you an opportunity to build
a romantic context for future sexual relating. Even in the best-adjusted
couples, individuals and circumstances change. Couples need to find
out more about each other's contemporary thoughts and feelings. Dating your intimate partner—even if you have known each other for
years—creates a special time alone together without the pressures of
household tasks and parenting.

Dating allows single survivors an opportunity to find out more about
a potential partner gradually, in progressive steps, over an extended
period. It takes many encounters with another person, under different
kinds of circumstances, to determine if he or she would make a good
partner for you. We can easily be fooled by our first impressions. Again,
the healing vacation gives you time to build your relationship carefully.

Though it may sound like a long time, I suggest that single survivors
invest three to six months on dating before they consider making love
with a new partner. This gives survivors time for building trust and
establishing open communication. You can mention your abuse history
a little at a time, when it feels appropriate, and see if the potential part-

ner has the capacity to be emotionally supportive about sexual abuse issues. Together you can find out if you share similar long-term goals for a future relationship, and whether your new partner can respect your needs to control the pace of and set limits on physical intimacy.

Single survivors should also be cautious because of our dangerous times. These celibate months can allow time for testing for AIDS and other sexually transmitted diseases. Find out whether the person you are dating cares about sexual health.*

Concluding the vacation from sex.   Healing vacations end when survivors feel ready to explore sex as an expression of self-caring and nurturing, or intimate sharing with a partner. You will need to *go slowly* and take gradual steps toward sexual intimacy. By going slowly you give yourself time to integrate new sexual experiences with other learning from sexual healing, such as developing a positive meaning for sex, improving your sexual self-concept, dealing with automatic reactions, and stopping old, harmful sex behaviors.

Sex needs to emerge from a growing desire to get *emotionally* closer to your partner. Liking who your partner is, enjoying touch with your partner, having fun when you are together, being able to discuss sexual issues and use of contraceptives and protection from diseases—all these are good signs that going to a deeper level of physical intimacy would be appropriate for you now.

It would be unrealistic to expect that things would go well if you jumped into full-fledged sex after having little or no sex at all. After a vacation from sex, it's best to ease into lovemaking gradually, taking one small step at a time. Don't push or rush. Start with simple, nonthreatening experiences, such as hand holding, hugging, and kissing. Work up to experiences that are more directly intimate and eventually sexual.

Vacations from sex can be repeated later if the need arises. At the conclusion of a vacation from sex, survivors may notice considerable differences in how they approach relationships and sex. Several survivors shared their experiences:

> Before, I viewed sex as essential to my attracting and keeping a
> partner in a relationship. I thought sex was the key to intimacy.
> Now I believe it is essential to build the relationship *before* getting

---

* For more information on establishing healthy sexual relationships, see the "Healthy Sex Skills" pages on my web site: http://www.HealthySex.com.

sexually involved. I see sex as the fruit of intimacy and intimacy as having many dimensions besides those that are sexual.

I used to pick my boyfriends first on how we did in bed together and then on if I liked them. That has changed. I'm willing to be with people I like and not be sexual with them until I get to know them better.

Sex is much less important to me now. I once thought that if I were unable to have sex for the rest of my life I wouldn't want to live. Now I enjoy emotional closeness more.

I place a different value on my sexual activity. I view sex as a way to communicate feelings. I separate sexual tension from the need for companionship, because I have enriched my relationships with friends to get the love I need rather than "sell" myself for attention.

Eventually, vacations from sex can lead to enjoying sex in a very different, much healthier context.

Avenue 3: Establish healthy ground rules for sexual encounters

Another way that survivors can make positive changes in their sexual behavior is by establishing new ground rules for sexual encounters. These ground rules can be a key to creating lasting, healthy behavior changes for survivors who have stopped specific, harmful behaviors or who have taken a healing vacation from sex. Ground rules establish limits so that you can feel safe in sex. They can be implemented at any time.

Here are some suggestions for healthy ground rules. (Feel free to add to or modify the list to suit your needs.)

Have sex only when you really want to. Examine your reasons for engaging in sex in the first place. Ask yourself why you want to have sex. If you get an answer like, "Because I should want it," "Because I have to have it," or, "Because my partner has waited long enough," then it's not the right time. You run the risk of rekindling old, negative behavior if you have sex while feeling pressured, responsible, or guilty. Sex when you are not ready can lead to anger, resentment, and shame.

Take an active role in sex. You need to be able to control your own sexual experience and initiate the kinds of sexual activities you want.

When your partner initiates sex, let him or her know what you feel comfortable doing. While some people may worry that talking could ruin a sexual experience, the truth is, for survivors, talk is always better than silence. Silence is what they remember of being a victim. We need to talk and make love, make love and talk.

Survivors need to take an active role in sex every time. Make sure you stay involved in a sexual activity only as long as you feel comfortable being involved in it. Direct how the experience goes, and end it how you want, when you want.

Some survivors benefit by imagining a sexual encounter before they engage in it. Perhaps a woman wants to engage in sexual petting without wearing clothes. She first might imagine the time of day and the place she would like to have this experience. Then she might imagine taking off only the clothes she feels comfortable taking off. Then she might imagine herself stroking and petting parts of her body and her partner's body. She thinks about how she is comfortable being touched. She considers how long she would like this experience to last, then she pictures herself hugging and cuddling with her partner at the end of their encounter. Now that she has an idea how she'd like it to go—from start to finish—she can talk with her partner. They can plan together.

While having an idea of what you want to do can help create positive experiences, it's important not to become fixed on a particular outcome in sex, such as you or your partner having an orgasm. In sexual healing, making orgasm the goal can easily lead to feeling pressured and to losing intimate contact with your partner. Focus instead on feeling warm, comfortable, close, and loving, whether or not orgasm occurs. With this approach sex is established as a way to nurture yourself or to share special time with your intimate partner.

Give yourself permission to say no to sex at any time. Sex needs to be your choice—not only every time but also throughout each encounter. Many survivors feel that once they've consented, they have to go through with it, all the way. "It wouldn't be fair to my partner to stop in the middle," or, "I said I would, now I must," we think. This is wrong. Survivors worry unnecessarily that it will physically hurt their partners or themselves to become sexually aroused and then stop. Denying yourself the freedom to say no to sex at any time will only hinder your sexual healing, rekindling all the old feelings of obligation or compulsion.

Remember this rule: *You can't say yes to sex until you can say no to sex at any time.* Let's say a male survivor is having intercourse with his girl-friend and realizes that he wants to stop, but he senses his girlfriend is moving toward having an orgasm. He needs to be able to give himself permission to gently get his girlfriend's attention and let her know what's happening with him. His girlfriend needs to be responsive to his need to stop.

You can follow this ground rule more easily when you and your part-ner both believe that agreeing to have sex means you are expressing your *willingness to explore sexual possibilities*, not your commitment to have sex from start to finish. Decide with your partner ways to stop that would make the experience of stopping easy and smooth. One couple told me they would shift into a gentle embrace whenever they needed to stop sexual activity.

By making changes in sexual behavior, sex can become a completely different experience than it was for you before. The before and after pic-ture can be striking. After a year of sexual healing a survivor described improvement:

> In sex previously, I didn't assert my needs. I didn't touch my part-ner, and I approached sex passively. We hardly ever talked during it. I felt disrespected, humiliated, and used. I thought of my enjoy-ment of sex as bad, making me bad.
>
> Now I keep my partner informed of how I'm feeling and what I need. I initiate touch and ask my partner to be passive at times so I can safely experience touching. I can stop and interrupt sex when I need to. I keep myself conscious of my partner's love and respect for me. I experience my enjoyment as something natural and posi-tive. These changes have been freeing: They have allowed me to feel better about myself and to establish a new and deeper closeness with my partner.

Healing involves the active support and involvement of an intimate partner. In fact, the partner's role becomes more critical as healing pro-gresses. Until now we have focused primarily on the survivor's experi-ence and needs. But for survivors involved in intimate relationships, the abuse has affected another person as well. In the next chapter we will look at how partners become secondary victims of the sexual abuse, and we'll examine ways partners can join with survivors to work together on healing. As an intimate team you and your partner can overcome the damage sexual abuse has caused to your sexual relationship.

For survivors not currently in a relationship, chapter 9 offers useful information about the dynamics that might arise in a future relationship. If you are a survivor who has seen relationships falter in the past, perhaps chapter 9 will help you understand what went wrong and show what you can do differently in the future.

9

Healing with an Intimate Partner

Healing with my partner has been one of the hardest things I've ever done. We've learned to transform the painful times—when we feel stagnant, depressed, and hopeless— into opportunities to grow personally and strengthen our intimate relationship.

—A PARTNER

Several years ago, when I was presenting a workshop for couples on healing the sexual effects of sexual abuse, I met Bill, a forty-year-old incest survivor, and Patty, his wife of ten years. During the lunch break, the three of us picnicked outside on a beautiful lawn. In low voices often cracking with emotion, Bill and Patty told me in detail of the problems sexual abuse had created in their relationship.

BILL: In the early years of our marriage, I felt emotionally distant from Patty. I rarely wanted sex, and when I did it was only when Patty would dress seductively. I couldn't express my love for her and have sex with her at the same time. It was like sex and love were in separate compartments. I couldn't pay attention to Patty during sex. I never kissed her; I just did the mechanics.

PATTY: I worried that I wasn't sexually attractive to Bill. I thought his lack of interest in me was my problem. He seemed unable to see me as a person: I remember once telling him that I felt like a knothole. Bill wouldn't talk with me openly or honestly. He would build walls. Both of us emotionally retreated from the relationship. We smoked marijuana and tried to forget our problems.

BILL: I didn't realize that my problems had anything to do with sexual abuse until three years ago when I began dreaming of having sex with my mother. After awhile, I told Patty about the dreams because I felt sick for having them. She encouraged me to seek counseling, which I did, and eventually I realized that the dreams were actual memories of the abuse.

PATTY: I was shocked and surprised when Bill told me what his mother had done to him. I felt sad for what Bill had endured as a child, and I was angry at his mother. I also got angry with Bill. Even though I realized that his memories of the abuse had been suppressed, I still wished I had known sooner. It would have explained so much. For years I had blamed myself for our problems. Once my anger subsided I filled with anxiety. I feared what this might mean to our sexual relationship and the whole future of our relationship.

BILL: As I continued in therapy to resolve feelings about the abuse, our family life became even more strained. I needed more emotional separateness from Patty. I didn't want to have sex anymore. I was afraid that if I did have sex I'd lose a sense of myself and my power. I'd never learned what it was like to have emotional or physical boundaries. If I wasn't putting up walls, I totally lost myself in Patty's feelings and needs. If she wanted a hug, I felt controlled, like it was a demand. I knew my yes wouldn't mean anything unless I could learn to say no.

PATTY: When Bill moved into a spare bedroom, I was devastated. I couldn't depend on him to be there for me in times when I needed him. And I did need him. My father died in a freak fire in his home. I had a miscarriage and underwent surgery for a breast lump. All that time, when I'd ask Bill if he still loved me, his response would switch from yes to no to I don't know.

I began individual therapy and started attending a recovery program to address codependency issues. I realized that because of experiences in my childhood I had been contributing to our problems. I grew up in a family where I was emotionally abused. I do not trust easily—it's all or nothing. I tend to focus more on Bill's feelings than on my own experience.

BILL: Now we're both working to develop a sense of separateness and inner strength.

PATTY: It hurts! I can't just come up and hug or kiss Bill. I have to ask first. I often get rejected. My sexual expression feels squashed. Masturbation takes care of only the physical part; it does nothing for my need for closeness. I'm sad every time I put Bill's clean clothes away in "his" room. I'm lonely when I go to bed at night. I don't feel married and I don't feel single.

I don't know how long it will take for Bill to heal. I don't know if it will be this year, next year, or five years from now. I hope I can last that long.

BILL: Our strength is that we're both intelligent people who are willing to keep trying and learning. Eventually we should be able to get it, right?

PATTY: What keeps me going now is this deep feeling I have. Bill seems to have it too. Even in the worst of times it keeps coming back. I think it's a deep love and caring for each other.

The story that Bill and Patty shared describes a common scenario for couples who are experiencing a crisis in intimacy because of sexual abuse. Both members of the couple suffer because of abuse: the survivor as a direct, primary victim, and the partner as an indirect, secondary victim. Both are affected by the distress that abuse causes, and both need to work on healing to overcome the crisis and enjoy a healthy relationship.

For some couples this kind of crisis proves too much to overcome. Sadly, relationships do break up because of the aftereffects of abuse. In these cases the couples don't heed the warning signs: they tend to stop communicating; they withdraw emotionally into their own worlds; the survivor doesn't involve or inform the partner in the healing process; or the partner refuses to cooperate or participate in a way that fosters healing.

But for most couples the crisis they encounter proves to be temporary and within their power to remedy. They adjust to the reality of their situation, make important changes, and strengthen their intimate relationship in many ways in the process. Bill and Patty were able to do this. I heard later that their story has a happy ending: They learned to work together on healing and eventually were able to create an enduring and satisfying sexual relationship, and to enjoy a strong marriage.

The crisis in intimacy that can result from sexual abuse hits at the very core of a couple's relationship. It disrupts the couple's ability to enjoy emotional and physical closeness. A partner told of his experience:

Sexual abuse has thrown a wet blanket on our lives. It feels as though our freedom to enjoy each other fully, our ability to revel in the happiness of our love, the inalienable rights of our relationship have been stolen and violated. As a couple we have to clear some sexual hurdles that wouldn't have been there otherwise.

Couples may find their relationships strained in other ways as well while they work on solving their crisis with intimacy. Daily events, household responsibilities, and family activities may suffer as survivors and partners go through periods of feeling angry, depressed, or withdrawn. Couples may be additionally stressed by the time-consuming and often financially draining demands of obtaining outside support and professional help.

Enduring this kind of crisis can be as hard on couples as when they encounter medical illness, physical injury, or the death of a loved relative. When a man discovers he has a low sperm count, *his* infertility can intimately affect the life of his female partner as well. When a woman suffers serious injuries in a car accident and is unable to have sex during a long recovery, her partner's sex life is also impacted. While one person in the couple may suffer the original trauma and pain, the daily happiness and expectations of both are affected.

A crisis in intimacy—whatever the cause—requires couples to acknowledge that the problems they are having are to some degree mutual problems.

HOW YOU CAN WORK TOGETHER IN SEXUAL HEALING

To overcome your problems you will need to develop a *mutual healing strategy*. You'll need to work individually on individual problems and together on problems that have to do with your relationship. You will both need to be active and involved to overcome the effects of abuse and eventually to establish new, healthy, mutually satisfying ways of relating sexually.

You will only make matters worse if either of you adopts a stand such as "These are *your* sexual issues—leave me out of it—fix it yourself." This kind of attitude ignores the reality of the situation, abdicates responsibility for healing, and only breeds more feelings of emotional distance and isolation in your relationship.

Similarly, you will both need to avoid tendencies to blame yourselves for the problems and stresses you are having. A partner might overlook the reality of the abuse and misguidedly blame himself for the couple's sexual distress in the past. And a survivor might feel guilty for "bringing this horrible crisis to the relationship."

Neither of you is to blame for the crisis you may now be experiencing. Your problems were caused by sexual abuse. They have surfaced now as a delayed repercussion of actions done in the past by the perpetrator.

In this chapter we will explore specific ways that couples can work together on sexual healing. We will find out how survivors and partners have each been affected by the sexual abuse and how they can develop an active team approach for creating new, positive experiences in sexual touch, enjoyment, and intimacy.

As you begin this process as a couple, you will need to accept a unique kind of partnership. Your individual needs in the healing process are not identical. Your roles in working toward healing will not be equal. Survivors, because of your need to control the pace of recovery from abuse, you must take the lead, for now, in improving physical intimacy in your relationship. Partners must be comfortable following rather than pushing. As a couple your roles will be complementary but necessarily unequal.

In this chapter I will sometimes speak to each of you individually, sometimes as a couple. It's important for each of you to know about and be sensitive to the other's needs.

While sexual abuse and sexual healing produce a crisis in intimacy, every crisis, no matter how upsetting at first, brings an opportunity to grow in positive ways. The skills you build in learning to work together in healing—empathy, honesty, trust, and communication—are skills that will benefit you as a couple for years to come. You can create something positive from your pain.

As we look at some specific ways you can work individually and as a couple, think of each one as an opportunity for change and healing. Although couples, like individual survivors, heal at their own pace and in their own unique way, we will work through these ideas in the order many couples experience them.

1. Accept the fact of sexual abuse.
2. Learn about sexual abuse.
3. Cope with heightened emotions.
4. Reach out for support.
5. Challenge your unconscious projections.
6. Adjust to changes in touch and sexual relating.

7. Open communication.
8. Work together as an active healing team.

Accept the fact of sexual abuse

When a survivor tells a partner about past abuse, the disclosure can rock their relationship. Tanya, a twenty-year-old incest survivor, had previously told her young husband, Brian, that she had been sexually abused by her father. During a counseling session, she decided to tell him the details.

When Brian learned that Tanya's father had fondled her breasts, had oral sex, and attempted intercourse over a period of five years, the reality of the abuse hit him hard. He leaped up, crouched on the armrest of the couch, and put his hand to his mouth. He then dashed out of the office and down the hall to the bathroom, where he threw up. When Brian came back, he announced that he felt like *killing* Tanya's father. Tanya told him not to kill her father, because that would hurt her even more. Brian would become a criminal and be sent to jail.

Brian's reaction was alarming to Tanya, but it also made her realize now how wronged she had been by her father. Individually and as a couple, Tanya and Brian had to resolve strong emotional feelings stirred up by the disclosure of the abuse and accept the reality of Tanya's past.

When partners learn about the survivor's sexual abuse history, they often feel shocked, unprepared, and unsure of how to respond. They may blame the victim, question the validity of the statement, or get upset and angry in other harmful ways. A survivor said:

> When I told my partner I had been raped, he said I was making it up. I told him I wasn't. Then he said it happened long ago and I could get over it if I'd only try harder. He made it sound like it was all my problem.

Resolving feelings from the disclosure.   When partners react insensitively to learning about abuse, tensions can flare. Survivors may feel very hurt and angry. Unless these survivors resolve their negative feelings about the partner's initial reaction, they will have difficulty developing a team approach to healing. Survivors need to realize that partners who respond in hurtful ways often do so out of ignorance and fear about sexual abuse.

In some couples the partner feels hurt by the news of the sexual abuse history. A partner in a long-term relationship may wonder, "Why wasn't I told earlier?" Some partners fear that the relationship was founded on deception or falsehoods. Love, honesty, and trust in the relationship may suddenly come into question.

When the survivor reveals the abuse story at a crisis point in the relationship, it's often accompanied by an admission that he or she has never really enjoyed sex or has found sex uncomfortable. The partner may feel betrayed that the survivor has had a secret world of feelings and experiences. The partner may wonder if he or she can ever trust the survivor again. A partner described her reaction:

> Up until the night several months ago that my husband told me that he had been sexually abused as a child and was a sexual addict, I thought we had a good sexual relationship. I never realized what was really going on with him: that he felt ashamed when he was naked with me, that he felt sad when he climaxed, that he fanta-sized about other women continually, and that he had been having affairs. I feel like an idiot for not being more sensitive, and I'm angry at him for not telling me earlier how he really felt. I saw our life together as being the way it was only for me, not for him. I trusted him before, when he wasn't being honest with me and didn't deserve my trust. Now I'm unsure how to start trusting him again.

Unless the partners who feel hurt resolve their feelings, they will have difficulty working as a team in healing. It can help them to realize that it is often difficult for survivors to get in touch with memories of abuse, to recognize that an experience was sexual abuse, and to share their sexual secrets (see chapter 2).

There may have been many understandable reasons that a survivor would have withheld the information. Survivors may have been told they would be killed if they ever disclosed the abuse. Survivors may not have realized that the abuse could have a significant effect on their rela-tionship, or perhaps they may have hoped that sexual problems would disappear on their own. In addition, these survivors may have feared that their partners would:

- Blame them
- Be disgusted with them
- Reject them
- Become overprotective

- Think there is something irreparably wrong with them
- Reject the survivor's family of origin
- Be unable to comfort them

Acknowledging the pain of abuse. Partners who have difficulty resolving their anger and sense of betrayal may be trying to protect themselves from pain. It hurts to face the reality of sexual abuse. Survivors already know this. Partners may find it easier to feel angry than to move on and confront even more painful feelings like injustice and grief.

To many partners sexual abuse can sound unbelievable, unlike anything in their personal experience. The husband of a woman who had been ritually abused and sexually tortured by her mother and brother said that the most traumatic experience he could remember was getting hit in the nose with a baseball bat. It was difficult for him to fathom the terror and violence his wife had had to endure.

When partners do accept the reality of their survivor's pain, it can trigger a spiritual dilemma. They may question the meaning of life and the existence of God. A woman who was dating a survivor was stunned by the story of the abuse.

> It was hard for me to face the reality of the sheer evil that he described. I prefer to see my world in a much safer, gentler light: I have never been exposed to such horrors. I had to integrate his experiences into my spiritual reality. I pondered such questions as, "How can I trust a God that allows such evil to happen to innocent children?" "How can I feel safe in a world where such things are even possible?" Ultimately these are questions any aware person must face, but my closeness to his pain forced me to face them.

The acceptance of a survivor's pain can connect the partner with a larger issue: Sexual abuse touches the lives of many innocent people in our society. When this sad reality reaches into our own homes, we can no longer ignore it.

Some partners empathize so strongly with the survivor that they feel directly wounded themselves. A partner said:

> The night after she told me she had been sexually abused, I had a nightmare in which she was being abused and I couldn't move to help her. The nightmare made me feel as if I was also being abused. Since then there have been times when my wife has talked about the sexual abuse and I actually felt pain and hurt inside myself.

Occasionally a survivor's willingness to talk about abuse can make the partner realize or admit that he or she is also a survivor. In such a double-survivor couple each person has a dual role: as a survivor and as the partner of a survivor. Their complex relationship is like a double-exposure photograph, with their separate histories of abuse overlapping in their relationship. Both partners need to accept the reality of the abuse history and be sensitive of their dual roles. These partners can have more empathy for each other, but at the same time face more difficulty in healing together.

Building trust. Regardless of how they might at first respond to the disclosure of abuse, many partners are eventually able to offer the survivor compassion, understanding, and support. Their validation of the survivor's abuse experience is a critical piece in the sexual healing process: it builds a foundation for trust and increases emotional intimacy. A woman survivor said:

> It was hard at first to speak of the humiliating, shameful, and abnormal acts of my abuser, but my spouse responded intuitively and intelligently. Gradually we learned together. I am certain that being able to speak freely to him has helped me greatly.

And her partner said:

> I always wondered why she was so unresponsive when she were having sex. But since I've become more aware of the extent of the abuse, I have a better understanding. Now we have hope for recovery.

When a survivor tells her or his partner about the abuse, it is often a sign that the relationship has reached a strong level of love, commitment, and trust. Couples should applaud disclosure *whenever* it happens.

Even though accepting the fact of the abuse may be difficult for a couple, most survivors and partners agree that it is better to have their problems out in the open, where they can learn about them and do something about them, than to keep them buried and festering. You can't undo what happened to your partner or yourself in the past, but you can take charge of how you respond and support one another in the present and future.

Learn about sexual abuse

In sexual healing, as in many other endeavors, knowledge is power. The more a couple understands about sexual abuse and how to recover from it, the easier it will be for both partners to direct their energies in ways that will promote healing. Together you can overcome old, false myths about sexual abuse and discover ways that other people have worked through the damage done by abuse. You can create a common base of knowledge and share a vocabulary for talking about personal growth and recovery.

Learning together.   Information can be obtained from a variety of sources. You may want to read books on sexual abuse individually or to read aloud to each other, then discuss what you have read (see the Resources section). Try underlining, with each person using a different colored pen, sections of a book that apply to you individually. This technique allows you to easily identify your personal concerns and learn which topics your partner finds sensitive.

You may want to attend seminars and workshops that address sexual abuse topics. Meeting other couples who are going through the healing process can help you realize that your situation is not uncommon. Perhaps you will gain helpful ideas from other couples.* You may also find helpful seminars on related topics such as sexual addiction or compulsiveness, dysfunctional families, codependency, relationship enrichment, and communication skills.

Increasing your understanding.   Learning more about abuse and related topics can help partners become more understanding and sensitive of the survivor's needs in healing. Partners can learn more about the particular type of abuse the survivor experienced. Knowing about the rape trauma syndrome can be important information for partners of rape victims, and knowing about how sexual abuse affects family dynamics can aid partners of incest victims.

Education about sexual abuse can help partners understand why survivors may react in particular ways. After attending a seminar on sexual abuse a partner told me, "I learned that a violated person thinks, acts,

---

* For an informative look at how survivors and partners can work together, see the videotapes *Partners in Healing: Couples Overcoming the Sexual Repercussions of Incest* and *Relearning Touch: Healing Techniques for Couples* (listed in the Resources section).

and reacts differently from an unviolated person." Another partner reported on his new comprehension:

> I realized why my offhand comments about sex have had such a profound negative impact on my wife. Comments and gestures that might be acceptable to someone who was never abused are unacceptable to a survivor.

To be more sensitive to their partners, survivors may want to read materials that pertain to the partner's experience as a secondary victim.* For both of you, learning more about sexual abuse and recovery offers a concrete, and relatively painless, way you can *do something* to strengthen your ability to work as a team in healing.

Cope with heightened emotions

The sexual healing process can tax your strength, emotions, and relationship. To build and maintain a team approach to sexual healing, you need to understand one another's needs and find positive ways to handle the extra stress that the healing process places on your relationship.

When one person in a couple becomes ill and needs bed rest, it puts a strain on the other person. The healthy partner must nurse the ill one, take care of his or her own needs, and do alone the work that the couple used to do together. This is difficult enough, but in sexual healing both of you are victims of the sexual abuse. Although neither of you is "sick," at times you will probably feel as if you both are hurting at the same time. Your reserves may feel depleted. Your focus is on your own needs. You each need special care and may find it difficult to have anything left to give to your partner.

To learn how you can cope with and master this situation as a couple, you both need to develop sensitivity and empathy for what the other is experiencing. You each need to learn healthy ways to take care of your individual needs as well.

Survivors: feeling more emotionally vulnerable.   It's not unusual for survivors to go through periods when they feel very emotionally vulner-

---

* Many of the books on sexual abuse recovery have special chapters for partners. For example, see the books by Bass and Davis, Davis, Gil, Ledray, Lew, Maltz and Holman, and Warshaw listed in the Resources section.

able. They may become depressed, angry, and sad; they may be preoccupied with recurrent thoughts of past sexual abuse; and they may suffer
from crying spells and nightmares. These reactions are symptoms of
posttraumatic stress, a temporary condition common to many survivors
of abuse both before and during their recovery.

In the early stages of her recovery, Rose, a thirty-two-year-old survivor of father-daughter incest, wrote this in her journal:

> In the last several days, I've been feeling lonely, scared, and terribly
> confused. My mind is constantly swimming and daydreams about
> the abuse come easily. I seem to be off in another world most of the
> time. I have the urge to cry, even when there is no problem. I am
> only aware of my strength when someone crosses me. Then, I'm
> quick to respond with anger. My sparks are easily set off. I some-
> times feel that my love for my husband has been buried so deep it's
> out of reach, or that it's gone forever.

For Rose, emotional changes and outbursts give her an opportunity
to release repressed feelings related to the abuse. It's a good sign of her
recovery that these feelings have surfaced. But Rose and her husband
may feel confused and upset unless they both understand what is happening to her and why.

Ideally, when such feelings emerge survivors will have a safe emotional
environment in which they can release and resolve them. Partners can
help create that safe place by being emotionally supportive and caring.

Partners: experiencing new challenges. Although partners may
intellectually understand the need to be more supportive, this adjustment can be difficult to make. Some partners may resent how they need
to restrict and inhibit their own actions in order to adapt to the survivor's recovery needs. Whereas they used to enjoy certain freedoms,
now they feel they need to be extra careful of what they say and do. A
partner who had been married for twenty-five years said:

> My wife is much more vulnerable to my comments than I had ever
> imagined and more needy than I expected also. I find myself analyz-
> ing myself before I respond to her. Before, I just responded. Now I
> have less freedom and more guarded responses in our relationship.

Partners may be unaccustomed to giving the amount and type of
emotional support that the survivor now needs. If the survivor had pre-

viously tended to care for the emotional needs of the partner, the whole dynamic of the relationship can come to feel reversed. Now the partner feels he or she must be in a more giving and supportive role. The relationship can feel imbalanced, with the partner expected to be supportive without asking for much in return. A lesbian partner told of her frustration:

> My lover wants me to be there to cuddle, rock, and essentially mother her. But when I feel tired or needy, she says she can't handle being there for me, in that way, now. I don't want to resent her needs, but I don't see how I can be expected to go on indefinitely like this.

These new dynamics can strain a relationship. The survivor feels especially vulnerable and wants extra care. The partner is asked to give more emotional support while suffering from a loss of old, enjoyable connections. Partners may feel they are walking a tightrope, balanced precariously between passive disinterest and active demands for change. Partners will find their footing by being supportive and encouraging, yet not dominating or domineering.

As a result of these new demands to be emotionally supportive yet patient in sexual healing, many partners feel powerless. They may feel like their hands have been tied, as these partners did:

> I used to think that if I did this or that differently I could make things better. I felt tender and protective of her, she had been through something pretty awful, yet I wanted her to get going so we could be sexual in a more ordinary way. But as time went on, I realized that progress was out of my control. She could make changes only when she felt ready to make them.

> I felt controlled by my wife's need for me to empathize with the hurt and shame she was going through. I wanted to face the issue head on, solve our intimacy problems quickly, and get on with our marriage. I learned the process of sexual healing doesn't work that way. The hurts of her sexual abuse were deeper and more profound than I had originally imagined.

It can be difficult for partners to realize that for now they have to sit in the passenger seat and let the survivor drive. They can't change the past, erase the survivor's present pain, or even make immediate changes to repair the damage. They are dependent on the survivor to initiate recovery and make it happen.

Without a sense of control over the recovery process, many partners begin to feel pessimistic about the future. One said:

> I can do no right other than not leave, and I can commit numerous sins. The recovery process moves at a snail's pace, and there is no apparent end to the tangential issues related to the abuse. I have no control over what's happening. I have no idea that the healing is in fact going to occur at this point. I doubt that we will ever be able to return sexual freedom to our relationship again.

In response to these feelings of powerlessness, some partners may attempt to push, control, or dominate the healing efforts. "If you don't heal soon, I'll leave," a partner might threaten, out of frustration. "You're not trying hard enough!" a partner might shout in anger. These kinds of comments can hurt the relationship. Survivors may rebel and, in protest, stop sexual recovery work. Often these feelings of anger are only smoke screens for feelings of sadness and powerlessness that the partner finds more difficult to express. If you are a partner, look for deeper issues beneath the feelings you're experiencing on the surface.

The challenge to partners is finding positive ways to overcome their sense of powerlessness. They may remind themselves that they have a choice to remain in the relationship. They can learn to express their feelings and fears directly but sensitively. Sometimes, if a partner can express his or her needs clearly, without blaming or coercing the survivor, the partner's comments encourage the survivor to keep moving along in recovery. This is what happened for Susan and her partner:

> After about six months of being patient and nonpressuring, I sat down with my partner [the survivor] and told her that even though I loved her I was having thoughts of leaving the relationship. I told her that lately she didn't seem to be doing anything to promote sexual healing. The reality was that I couldn't wait forever. The next day she called a therapist and began getting help. Looking back we agree that it helped that I told her honestly how I felt at the time.

Even the most supportive partners may occasionally wonder if they have what it takes to hang in there during sexual healing, as this partner expressed:

As I realize the tremendous grief and pain that my wife is enduring, and the toll this is taking on both of us, I begin to question my own abilities to deal with the abuse. Am I emotionally strong enough? Sometimes I fear that healing will require too much and that I'll end the relationship, but I stay with it. I don't want our relationship dissolving because of something done to her in the past!

Even when partners trust that healing can occur, they may suffer anxieties. They may fear that healing will take too long. They may battle with fears that the survivor will leave them once the healing is done. And they may fear what will happen if they share how they really feel. The crisis caused by abuse challenges both the partner and the survivor to talk openly and share their feelings in depth. It's scary to talk about issues that cut to the heart of their relationship. While this crisis gives a partner and survivor an opportunity to grow together the growth process can cause them pain.

Personal issues arising for partners.   Sexual abuse and sexual healing recovery work can trigger personal issues for the partner. These emotional issues often relate to unresolved feelings from the partner's past and may arise now because the partner feels vulnerable from the stress involved in sexual healing. A partner who felt sexually rejected in a previous relationship, for example, may be extremely sensitive to feeling rejected now.

The lack of comfortable physical intimacy seems to affect all partners to some degree, making them doubt their sexual attractiveness and adequacy. Even when they know intellectually that the survivor's sexual issues relate primarily to past abuse, many partners have to constantly battle inner tendencies to feel that they themselves are personally being sexually rejected.

Many partners are also pained by witnessing the survivor's emotional suffering and struggle. They may worry about the survivor's mental health and physical welfare. In time partners may become more keenly aware that they are secondary victims of the survivor's abuse. "I find myself absorbing a lot of the pain and ugliness of his abuse," a partner said.

Partners themselves may have been physically or emotionally abused in the past. Many partners come from dysfunctional families, failed to get the support and nurturance they needed as children, or suffered earlier traumatic experiences. Now they may feel they lack knowledge and skills to respond to survivors in recovery. Or they may be lost in unresolved or unmet needs of their own. Partners may question their self-worth and wonder whether they will be accepted or loved for who they are.

Partners who were victims of sexual abuse may feel uncomfortable with the whole issue of sexual abuse. They may not feel motivated or ready to address sexual healing, for themselves or their partners. As Denise, a forty-year-old survivor-partner, explained:

> Before, I had been reasonably content with being in a sexually unsatisfying relationship. I used to avoid sex and be glad if my husband went to other women for it. When we had sex I could divorce myself from my emotions and service him sexually. Things are different now. He has done a lot of healing and wants real intimacy in our relationship. He feels more capable of it and feels he deserves it. I feel I've lost my old buddy. I'm trailing behind. His recovery has forced me to look at my issues.

Jerry, Denise's husband, believes that his progress in sexual healing is hampered by her unresolved issues. Excited about the changes he has been making, he finds it difficult to be sympathetic to her slower pace.

> My feelings are opening up. They're threatening to Denise. I'm becoming a much less defensive person, and I feel more desirable. Her issues are more repressed than mine. Here's an example: I used to not take good care of myself physically. I wouldn't bathe much. Denise used to say she didn't want sex with me because of my hygiene. Now I bathe and shave frequently, but she finds other reasons not to want sex. I dropped a defense, and it threatened her.

As a double-survivor couple, Jerry and Denise both had personal issues that were raised by sexual healing. Not only did they need to challenge themselves as survivors to address their individual concerns, but they also needed to become more sensitive to each other's feelings and reactions.

The survivor's dilemma.   For many survivors it hurts to acknowledge a partner's pain. Survivors may worry about a partner's ability to handle needed changes. Because of feelings of low self-esteem, some survivors may doubt that the partner would want to stay with the relationship. One survivor shared this concern:

It's hard for me to accept that my partner would want to put herself through all this just to be with me. I feel like I'm asking too much from her. It's like I'm saying, "I'm going to step out here in the void and things are going to get real strange, and you can come with me." It doesn't seem fair to her.

It can be a difficult yet important accomplishment for a survivor to realize that he or she is deserving of the patience, love, and support required of a partner.

Some survivors may be tempted to jeopardize their own sexual recovery to protect the partner from feeling further emotional pain. Consider the case of Paula, a forty-five-year-old survivor.

I'm sad that helping me recover has been hard on my husband, Richard. He doesn't complain, but I know what he is going through. For him sex is something beautiful. I fear my continued celibacy is destroying something he enjoys.

Paula is in a bind. If she overrides her present need for celibacy to please Richard, she would neglect herself and in time probably feel resentment toward him. Paula needs to find ways to remain true to herself and her sexual healing program while still being sensitive to her husband.

Teaming up to cope together.   Each of you in the relationship needs to realize that you are in a temporary crisis. This crisis can put you both under additional stress. You will each need to find ways to take good care of yourself and cope with the additional burden of stress. Eat well, exercise, and rest. The healthier you feel, the better you will handle the psychological challenges of sexual healing. Find activities that are good for you and pleasurable—playing a sport, going to the theater, doing a work project, or expanding a hobby. One partner reported that taking up Zen meditation was especially beneficial to him. A female survivor found that getting a weekly facial helped her relax.

During this time it's likely that tensions will build and result in emotional outbursts. Each of you needs to be sensitive to what the other can handle. If you feel angry, talk about your anger rather than lashing out.

The time you have put into learning about abuse will help you be less afraid of these emotional outbursts. One partner said that when he learned to respect his wife's anger he stopped expecting her to be over it completely. Once partners have learned that moodiness is common in survivors, they can take the survivor's expressions of anger or rejection less personally. A partner said:

> I've developed a sense of realism—I know the abuse is part of the past and that we may need to make appropriate adjustments to get through an occasional bad day.

Partners will only threaten the survivor if they put unreasonable time limits on recovery or erroneously suggest that healing can be done by an act of will. The reality is that healing usually involves a tremendous amount of unlearning and relearning how to be in a relationship and how to enjoy physical intimacy. Healing needs to go slowly, and couples must build emotional trust and safety before they attempt physical intimacy.

Since partners have a tendency to feel unloved and unattractive when sexual intimacy is curtailed, and survivors have a tendency to feel alone and guilty for pulling back from physical and sexual closeness, both members of the couple can help ease emotional tensions by finding new ways to express positive, loving feelings. You may want to tell your partner directly how much you love him or her, give your partner a special card, plan an outing to a place your partner enjoys, or get your partner a gift which symbolizes your understanding of the situation and commitment to the relationship. In one couple, the partner gave the survivor a stuffed animal and the survivor gave the partner a gift certificate for a therapeutic massage.

As you work together to heal, cheer for each other's personal growth. Mention positive changes and progress. Share your respect for each other, and, when you feel it, share your optimism about your future together.

Reach out for support

Sexual healing is a time to reach outside your relationship for emotional support. Survivors may be too close to the issues and too preoccupied with their own healing to be able to give their partners the support they need, and partners may be too personally affected by the crisis to be the sole or primary emotional support person for the survivor. Either of you may want to pursue individual therapy, which would give you a private time with someone who is focused on your issues alone. A support or counseling group for survivors or partners can also help you find comfort outside your relationship.

It can be very powerful to learn you are not alone. Many others have survived abuse, and many other partners have experienced feelings similar to what you may be feeling now. One partner said counseling enabled him to let go of guilt he was feeling about sexual dreams and fantasies involving other people. The therapist explained that his fantasies were understandable, especially given his current lack of sexual activity. This partner realized the difference between having thoughts or fantasies and acting on them.

Focusing on your own issues can help you get clearer about your priorities. What is most important to you? How crucial is sexual relating to your overall happiness and well-being? What strengths exist in the relationship? Why do you continue to choose to remain in the relationship? With conscious values and self-awareness, you are better equipped to handle those times when you may feel pessimistic.

Obtaining emotional support may make it easier for partners to handle the temporary changes and adjustments demanded by their situation. At times your personal growth may directly help the survivor to heal. A survivor told of her husband's involvement in her healing:

> My husband started a support group for partners at a local counseling center, and already he's more supportive of what I'm going through. When I feel he understands and supports me, I feel I can trust him to be here for me and not put me down anymore. He's truly accepted not having sex, and that alone has made it possible for me to approach him comfortably.

If you are a partner who is also a survivor of sexual abuse, outside support can be critical to your relationship. Each survivor in a double-survivor couple needs to work on individual issues and to learn new skills for emotional and physical intimacy. Without the influence of people outside your relationship, you risk triggering each other's fears and negativity. A survivor-partner described her experience:

> Before we both got into therapy we felt stuck in a situation of the blind leading the blind. Neither of us knew what it meant to be normal. We didn't know what healthy sexuality meant to us as individuals. I think we both avoided sexual issues by unconscious mutual consent. We would often collide in our fears of intimacy. Rather than pushing through like another couple might, we were happy to stay locked in our fears.
> I believe that since we have both worked hard on these issues

the commonality aids us in understanding what we each go through. We both know that sexual abuse is for life and that we have a recovery process we can put into effect if we slide back. We both understand the valleys and are willing to work together to get out of them.

For all couples, couples therapy can provide a time to focus on sexual healing issues that pertain to your relationship while giving you the extra support and guidance of a trained professional. You can concentrate on strengthening your relationship by building trust, developing empathy, and improving communication. Therapy sessions can give you check-in time for tackling any concerns that may arise as you proceed with developing new skills in relearning touch and improving sexual experiences. A survivor said:

> I found long-term couples counseling the most helpful activity I participated in for my sexual healing. I learned that I wasn't the only one who was hurting. My husband was finally able to understand how some of his actions were destructive to our sexual relationship. He learned what not to do, and that has enabled me to become freer.

Challenge your unconscious projections

Couples face a host of challenges in recovering from abuse. One of the more subtle ones is a tendency for each person in the couple to project emotional feelings really meant for someone in their past onto the present-day partner.

For example, survivors can unconsciously associate their current partners with the offenders of the past. A partner may also unconsciously associate the survivor with someone in his or her past, such as a former lover who was sexually rejecting, a parent who withheld physical love and affection, or a close acquaintance who was emotionally needy and self-preoccupied. Because these associations and projections can occur unconsciously, it is important that you each develop an ability to identify them and bring them out in the open so that you can relate to each other without being encumbered or misled by these unspoken feelings.

How survivors feel.   I used to think that only survivors who were still in abusive relationships tended to subconsciously associate their current partners with the original offenders. I was wrong. It seems that to some degree all survivors tend to confuse the partners with the offenders. I've seen this happen no matter how loving and kind the partner is and no matter how different from the offender the partner is. The partner's desire for sex and intimacy can often be enough to automatically trigger the response, as this survivor explained:

> Sometimes my spouse becomes my abuser in my mind. The abuser completely used up my husband's credit, like a stranger making withdrawals from your bank account. If my husband accidentally pinches me during sex, the pain feels exactly like the pain during childhood sexual abuse—his act becomes abuse. He can't make any mistakes or act parental toward me without my thinking he is behaving just like my abuser and therefore is *becoming* my abuser.

Unbeknownst to them, many partners act in ways that remind the survivor of the offender. "When my lover strokes my face in a certain way, I immediately feel that it's my father stroking my face," Tess, a lesbian survivor of incest, told me during counseling. "I get angry at her and want her to stop touching me." Although her lover may feel she is being affectionate in stroking Tess's face, for Tess the lover's behavior serves as a trigger for automatic thoughts of her past offender. Another survivor said, "My husband used to push sex on me when I didn't want it. He was always nicer to me after sex, just like my father."

Other factors may lead the survivor to associate the partner with the offender. A survivor may notice that the partner and offender have similar physical characteristics such as a hairstyle, common personality traits like being shy or outgoing, or similar habits such as smoking or drinking. One survivor's boyfriend had a distinctive widow's peak hairline—just like the offender's.

Sensing any of these similarities, survivors may erroneously assume that the present-day partner is just like the offender, with the same ways of thinking and the same intentions to control, exploit, or harm. The survivor may assume the partner also sees sex as sexual abuse, just as the offender did. Therapists call this kind of association *unconscious projection*.

Without realizing it, survivors may often target their intimate partner to receive the anger and resentments they have about the abuse and about the offender. The partner presents an available, relatively safe person to release those feelings onto. As this partner described, a partner may be directly accused of actually being an offender:

I have become the target for my wife's anger. In recent months she has gotten extremely upset and sometimes confused me with her abuser. She has become violent, accusing me of raping and killing her. I fear her anger and other strong emotions. *I didn't do it, but I suffer for it!*

Many survivors also have a tendency to confuse their current partner with a nonoffending parent or caretaker from the past. One day Betsy, a twenty-seven-year-old survivor, screamed at her boyfriend, "I'm hurting and you're not doing anything to help me!" Later, once she had calmed down, Betsy realized that she was projecting onto her boyfriend her own anger at her mother for not protecting her from her father's sexual advances.

How partners feel.   When unconscious projections happen, partners can become disturbed and upset. It's painful for partners to realize the survivor they love thinks of them as an uncaring supporter or, worse, as an offender. "I feel nauseated when I think about how my wife interprets my sexual advances as a desire on my part to sexually abuse her," said a partner. Some partners may feel trapped:

When I touch her even casually I never know whether she will accept me as her chosen mate or reject me as the reincarnation of her abuser. My attempts at foreplay are regarded as an assault. When we do make love, I worry that she feels like she's doing me a favor rather then expressing and receiving love.

Partners can begin to feel strange about their own healthy sexual needs and desires. A partner said:

My own sexual wants now seem weird and demanding. I feel ashamed for wanting to mess around when I know how appalling the abuse was to her. I have to remind myself that I'm okay and not the problem.

As a result of this kind of projection, some partners may develop problems with sexual desire and functioning. They may begin to doubt their own healthy sexual drives and desires. "Maybe I am just an animal like she says I am," a partner said. Partners may start to condemn their natural passions, and they may feel guilty for enjoying sexual release. As a result some partners may want to withdraw from sex.

Diana became afraid of her own sexual feelings. She believed that she had become the target of a sexual sabotage effort by her partner, Kate, the survivor of father-daughter incest.

> When she was a little girl Kate learned to sense when her father wanted sex. If she couldn't avoid him then, she tried to make his "sexual adventure" with her as awful as she could by doing things to interrupt his concentration or interfere with his orgasm. Now, though she doesn't mean to, she does the same things with me. I have become apprehensive about feeling sexual, getting aroused, and reaching orgasm.

Partners often feel insulted, knowing that on some level they are being seen as an offender. They may feel their individual identity and good intentions have been ignored. Partners may feel they have been reduced to an object—a penis or a vagina—and are seen merely as horny and willing to do anything for sex. Most partners hope that their relationship is built on love and sharing; they feel sad when they realize the survivor believes their desire for physical contact is simply a desire for sex.

What partners can do. Partners need to remind themselves that their sexuality is good and positive. Talking about healthy sexuality can enable partners to explain to survivors how their ideas about healthy sex differ from an offender's abusive attitudes.

Partners also need to stop any behaviors that might mimic sexual abuse or that might trigger a survivor to associate the partner with the offender. If a partner has taken time to become educated about abuse and to learn specifically about the abuse his or her own partner survived, these triggers and behaviors will be easier to avoid. Ask yourself if you are doing things associated with sexual abuse, such as:

- touching without consent
- ignoring how the survivor really feels
- behaving in ways that are impulsive, out of control, or hurtful*

If you are, your behavior might be slowing down or even preventing sexual healing.

I recommend that partners seek treatment for drug, alcohol, or sexual addictions if they have problems in any of these areas. These behav-

---

* Partners may want to take the Sexual Effects Inventory in chapter 3 for yourself. It can identify attitudes and behaviors that relate to sexual abuse.

iors are so closely related to sexual abuse that they will surely undermine progress. Partners need good judgment and physical control during the sexual healing process. Either can be impossible when a partner is under the influence.

Survivors need to be able to control how much contact the partner has with the offender. If a partner has developed a friendship with the offender, it is best to stop or cool the relationship if it's uncomfortable for the survivor. A partner who likes and associates with the person responsible for sexually victimizing the survivor reinforces the survivor's tendency to see the partner as an offender too. The partner can take an active role in diminishing these unconscious projections by the survivor.

Just as importantly, partners need to avoid making unconscious projections onto the survivor. Justin, a partner married to an incest survivor, described his experience:

> The more my wife became involved in her sexual abuse recovery, the more I saw her differently. In my mind she went from being a warm and loving person to being cold and uncaring. I resented the fact that she was so focused on herself. It seemed that no matter how hard I tried, I still couldn't please her and bring her loving attention back to me.
>
> When I was eight years old, my mom and dad divorced. I lived mainly with my dad, because my mom got involved quickly with another man who had a family of his own. Although I never told my mom, I felt she had abandoned and stopped loving me. Nothing I did seemed to be able to get her to want to be with me more. She was all caught up in her new life and didn't seem to care about me anymore.
>
> In individual counseling I realized that my feelings toward my wife were related to unresolved feelings I had toward my mother when I was a child.

For Justin and his wife to continue to work effectively as a team in sexual healing, Justin needed to become aware of how he was tending to associate his wife with his mother. He needed to stop projecting his anger and fear onto his wife. Realizing what was being triggered for him, his wife was able to understand Justin's reactions better. Her understanding helped her give him reassurances of her love and caring in ways she felt comfortable with during that time.

What survivors can do. Survivors can help reduce unconscious projections by sharing their thoughts and progress with their partner. This talking helps survivors relate to the partner as a friend, not as an offender, and it helps partners reduce their tendencies to see the survivor as distant or uncaring.

Once survivors realize they are confusing the partner with the offender, they can use skills for handling automatic reactions (presented in chapter 7), such as stopping, calming, affirming, and acting to defuse the projection. Survivors can also reduce projections by learning to direct anger meant for the offender away from the partner. For example, they might write about this anger, engage in role-playing or talking with the offender in therapy, or confront the offender and express their feelings directly. Survivors who have dealt with feelings toward the offender through direct confrontation or other methods in therapy have often regained a feeling of strength and autonomy.

With these unconscious projections—by either of you—out in the open, you both can learn to respond to one another more effectively and can work to heal rather than hurt your relationship.

Adjust to changes in touch and sexual relating

You will never resolve physical intimacy problems by merely wishing things were different. As a couple you both need to work together to overcome automatic reactions, stop behaviors that mimic sexual abuse, follow through with a healing vacation from sex, and establish new ground rules for touch and sexual intimacy. These changes are major, and they can be difficult. Both of you will need to make adjustments. It can become frustrating at times. You may feel stuck or wish you could go back to an earlier time when sex and touch may have been easier for you.

When sex continues. When sexual intimacy problems that relate to sexual abuse come to the surface, some couples attempt to deal with the situation by continuing to have sex. They may hope that by making a few adjustments, such as becoming more sensitive to automatic reactions, their sexual intimacy problems will heal. Sometimes this works, but sometimes it's not enough to foster healthy changes. For some couples, continuing to have sex when sex is problematic can produce negative consequences. "Sex has become associated with struggle rather than pleasure," a partner said.

When sex continues some partners feel like they are walking on thin ice, trying to avoid triggers and automatic reactions. While they may see the value in becoming more sensitive to the survivors' needs during sex, they may also feel their own sexual needs are being ignored by the survivors. Sexual activity may lose a sense of being relaxed and free. A partner expressed his dismay:

> When I perform oral sex on her I might say something during a momentary passion that she finds upsetting. Suddenly her mood will change to a negative one. We have to stop sex. Experiences like these leave me feeling that I'm being more responsive to her needs than she's being to mine.

It's a rough situation. Intellectually partners know that survivors can jeopardize their own recovery if the focus is switched to meeting the partner's sexual needs. Still, partners may feel left out in the cold. The lack of comfortable reciprocity hurts. When sex continues, restrictions on sexual activity may seem endless. A partner said:

> We can be sexual only in bed, never elsewhere. I can't use my tongue when I kiss her because she gets scared. I can't joke about sex because she takes offense and feels scared. In the rare times when we do have sex, I have to be extra gentle, slow and easy, and never vary from this. Relaxed sex play is too threatening for her. She won't participate after climax. We're not able to carry over sexual arousal from other activities, like having fun or a close talk. Sex is isolated and not a part of anything else.

The idea of sex as fun, playful sharing, or an expression of love can get lost in power struggles over whether to have sex. The sense of mutual giving and receiving may seem lost as well. A partner of a survivor who withdraws from sex expressed frustration:

> Sometimes we snuggle. Sometimes she pushes me away. No sex. She won't rub or massage me, but she wants me to rub and massage her. I've thought about getting a lover, but it's more than sex. I want the intimacy with *her!*

For healing to proceed when sex continues, the survivor and partner need mutual commitment and cooperation. Both of you need to make adjustments and accept changes. Both of you need to support and respect limits on touch and sex. Survivors need to respect these limits so that they can take their own self-worth seriously, enabling sexual healing to progress. If survivors keep breaking their own limits, healing will take more time and cost more frustration in the long run. Partners need to understand the importance of physical limits and not get angry when touch or sex is interrupted or has to stop altogether. The survivor is not being inconsiderate but is actively involved in healing.

Partners of survivors who compulsively seek sex may experience frustrations in other ways when sex continues, as this partner explained:

> My girlfriend wants affection and sex more than I do. I feel like I have to put out more than I want to. I often end up feeling sexually inadequate because I'm expected to fill her every emotional need through the sex act. It never works.

For these partners, adjusting to the situation and helping to foster the survivor's healing may mean that they will need to set limits on sex. It is unproductive for any couple to continue sex when it is constantly causing problems.

Because of the many problems and stresses that can occur, an individual member of the couple or both partners may reach the conclusion that continuing sex is not working at all or not working well enough to facilitate positive changes. Continuing sex may be generating negative feelings for both partners, or reinforcing behaviors associated with sexual abuse. A couple may decide, often regretfully, that for healing to occur, it's best that the survivor take a healing vacation from sex.

During a vacation from sex. Probably one of the most difficult challenges for partners is supporting and respecting agreed-to limits on physical and sexual activity during a vacation from sex. While many partners understand the theoretical importance of a survivor's healing vacation from sex (see chapter 8), the experience nonetheless throws the partner into a state of forced celibacy. The partner has to give up an important shared activity, perhaps be denied contact he or she believes is needed, and has to adjust to solitary sex. A great deal of emotional suffering can result, as a partner explained:

> We now have no sexually intimate relationship. When the abuse came up, her sexuality and sex drive was put into a cold storage unit. While she knows some things she *does not* want—which is

okay with me—she has no idea yet of what she *does* want. Her
entire sexual history is dominated by the patterns she learned in
the abuse. The challenge to me is to keep going with masturbation
and close physical contact without sex.

As a result of the lack of sexual activity, some partners begin to question who they are as sexual persons, what sex means, and how important sex is to them. As mentioned before, they often find themselves
questioning their attractiveness and sexual desirability.

Since traditional cultural roles portray masculinity as linked to sexual activity, some male partners have to revise their views of what it
means to be a man.

I've had to reshape my self-image as a man and as a sexual person
in adapting to my partner's reactions as an incest survivor. We have
learned to be companions and friends without much sexual intimacy.

Some partners make matters worse by erroneously believing that the
survivor must not love them if he or she doesn't want to be sexual with
them. They may need to remind themselves that sex is just one expression of love. The survivor's willingness to take major, often painful,
steps (such as a vacation from sex) to eventually increase sexual intimacy and satisfaction is itself a significant expression of love for the
partner.

Survivors can help by reminding their partners of their affection and
attraction. One partner was delighted when his wife called him in the
middle of the day to say she felt like having sex with him. They both
knew they wouldn't act on the desire, but hearing it expressed felt good
to both of them.

Honoring the vacation.   If a partner continues to press for touch and
sex, even subtly, the survivor's progress in sexual healing can come to a
halt. Survivors whose partners are unable to respect limits on touch and
sex during a vacation may themselves reach a false, self-damaging conclusion: I have to be sexual to be loved.

Even though they desire sexual intimacy, partners may need to assert
the ban on sex at times. Let's say you both agreed that it would be best
not to have sex for three months. Two weeks later, your partner, the survivor, lets you know she senses you are irritable and feels bad you've
been sexually deprived. "It's okay if you want to do it, really it's okay,"

she says. Don't fall for it! Tell her that you made an agreement and you intend to stick with it. If she starts to want you more sexually, that's fine, but don't act on it. When it comes to sexual healing, *if in doubt, don't proceed.*

There are many reasons why a survivor might test sexual limits in this way. These reasons often relate to subtle views the survivor has of herself or himself as a sexual object and victim, you as an offender, and sex as a commodity. A survivor might be stuck in old attitudes and think: All my partner really wants me for is sex anyway. I have to give it to him or he'll leave me to find it elsewhere. He won't ever be able to last that long. If we have sex now, I won't have to feel the pain of him not following through. The only way I can keep him is by giving him sex. I don't feel loved unless we have sex.

Respecting sexual limits enables a partner to show the survivor that you can be trusted. You will protect your partner and not sexually exploit and abuse her or him. This helps distinguish yourself as separate from the offender. By refraining from contact, you allow the survivor to build a desire to have physical and sexual contact with you. The limits followed now will make your relationship more genuine in the future. You'll know your partner wants to be relating with you out of desire, not duty, guilt, fear, or poor self-image.

If a survivor tests the limits, a partner might respond, "I want you to want me sexually *because you want me*, not because you think I want you." When limits are secure and consistent, the survivor gains an opportunity to learn to reach out for sexual intimacy.

To cope with long periods without sexual contact, many partners turn to masturbation for sexual release. They may worry that they will be condemned for masturbating. Survivors can help partners make this adjustment by learning to respect the time and privacy partners may need for self-sex. Survivors need to see masturbation as a healthy way to cope with the situation, and they need to remember that the partner's sexual feelings are healthy.

Even without sexual intimacy, couples can find an infinite number of ways to express physical affection and emotional caring. Survivors can initiate touch that does feel comfortable, such as a back rub or foot massage. Together you can come up with ideas for nonsexual activities that would bring fun and pleasure to your relationship now. Work on a project together, go to the theater, ride bicycles, go out to eat, or just spend relaxed time being together and enjoying each other's company.

During this period remember that you've put sex on vacation—not retirement. Physical intimacy will eventually return to your relationship. Continue to see yourself and your partner as loving and sensual even though you may not be having as much contact as you did before. A healing vacation can be an opportunity for both of you to find out more about yourself sexually—your sexual feelings, your insecurities, and your ability to accept and respond to your own sexual needs.

Open communication

Communication is the key to healing together. So many of the problems and difficulties that couples encounter can be remedied by talking out feelings honestly and brainstorming ideas for change together.

Communication neutralizes the effects of sexual abuse. It runs counter to the dynamics that existed in sexual abuse, such as silence, secrecy, shame, and victimization. When you're talking, what you are doing is not secret like the abuse was. You are asserting aloud what is important to you. Shame doesn't have a chance to build. A male survivor told of his progress:

> Talking has helped me tremendously. I told my new partner how I felt uncomfortable being naked. She was understanding and said she had similar fears. We kept talking about this and experimenting with taking off our clothes with each other. Now we take showers together regularly. This is the first time I feel good being naked in front of a partner.

Communication takes survivors out of the passive victim role, where things are done to them without their having any say in the matter, to an active position where they are setting limits, directing actions, and negotiating with a partner about how things will proceed. You both are important. A lesbian survivor said:

> My partner and I tell each other how we feel about things. She respects my feelings; I respect hers. We avoid power struggles. Instead of manipulating each other in a way to try to get what we want, we put forward what we want and we negotiate. It's healthy and very supportive.

By communicating, you build emotional intimacy with your partner. This is a prerequisite for healthy physical intimacy as well. Author-therapist Sharon Wegscheider-Cruse explains:

Intimacy is a basic human need, and it shouldn't be confused with the need for sex. Sex can be an important aspect of intimacy but sex is not the only—or even the most important—kind of sharing. . . . Before we can find and *maintain* sexual satisfaction with a partner, we must develop our ability to achieve and maintain "emotional intercourse." . . . It grows from the desire to connect with someone else—to learn what that person thinks and feels, and to share, in return, your innermost self.*

You can use communication to help you maintain a strong sense of yourself as you pursue emotional and physical closeness with your partner. A survivor said, "We strive for open communication: It leads us to safety, which leads us to positive sexual encounters."

Communication can also strengthen your sense of being part of a healing team. "When we talk, we share the experience—we are together," a partner said.

Listening to learn. Because communication is so important to sexual healing as a team, both partner and survivor need to learn to do it well. You and your partner will need to create a climate in which communicating feels safe. Many resources are available to help you establish good communication.†

Remember that sex and sexual abuse are sensitive topics. The types of issues you will be discussing are very personal. Many people fear that their partner will judge them negatively or reject them if they share honestly in these areas. They may believe that their feelings and experiences are unique or abnormal, when in reality many people are in similar situations and feel the same way. Your sensitivity to how vulnerable your partner may feel will allow communication to move forward.

Here are several guidelines for how to make communicating with your partner safe and productive.

- Find a mutually good time to talk.
- Focus on one topic at a time.
- Start discussions from your own experience, stating "I feel . . ." rather than making statements about your partner ("You think . . .").

* Sharon Wegscheider-Cruse, *Coupleship: How to Have a Relationship* (Deerfield Beach, Fla.: Health Communications, 1988), 4.

† See the Resources section for general interest books on couples communication.

- Avoid blaming, name calling, and labeling.
- Listen actively. Don't interrupt.
- Repeat back what you hear your partner saying.

If you don't understand your partner, ask for clarification. Major difficulties in communication can arise when you assume you know what your partner is feeling or thinking. When I was in college a marital studies professor of mine used to quip, "When you 'ass-u-me' you make an ass out of you and me." The message to couples: Don't assume—*ask*.

Listening can be improved when you and your partner understand that you are both "in process." This means that your feelings, perceptions, and ideas reflect how you feel at this point. Nothing is fixed. You can develop a new and different sense of a situation as time goes on.

Although these guidelines enable communication to proceed more smoothly for all couples, they are especially important when partners discuss sexual healing (see box).

Applying what you learn.   Partners need to know about the survivor's experience so they don't feel isolated from what's happening during healing. When they are unaware of the progress that is going on, their feelings of anger, despair, or powerlessness may worsen. Communicating is one way the survivor can help keep the partner informed and involved.

Knowing details about the abuse can help a partner know what to do to help the survivor feel more comfortable with touch and sex. A survivor said:

> Since I told my partner exactly what happened in the abuse, he understands why certain body areas and types of touch can trigger reactions in me. He doesn't touch my breasts without being careful to ask me first, and he remains sensitive to my feelings and responses.

Many partners complain that they don't know what to do to be helpful. They need instruction and direction. Survivors can help by telling partners specifically what they do and don't want them to do.

I suggest couples talk at least several times a week about progress or setbacks in their healing. How much you share and what you share is up to you. A survivor explained her situation:

> During the beginning and middle stages of my healing, most of the changes I made went on in my head. My behavior stayed pretty

much the same. Though it was hard, I would explain to my partner how my thinking was going through major changes.

The survivor can't assume that the partner will be aware of progress. Changes may not be apparent to anyone but the survivor. Survivors may want to share such things as: what issues you are dealing with, what short-term goals you are working on, what you are feeling better about, and what your concerns and hopes are for the future. This type of sharing helps you avoid tendencies to withdraw from your partner in secrecy, silence, and private pain. Remind yourself that your partner is

---

DISCUSSION TOPICS FOR HEALING TOGETHER

Here are some ideas for topics you might want to discuss with your partner to improve your teamwork in healing. Remember to follow the previous suggestions for good communication to ensure that your efforts will be productive. The goal is to develop trust and understanding. If the idea of face-to-face communication seems too difficult at this time, you and your partner may want to write your responses to each other in letters. This process can be a step to communicating more directly in the future.

Take turns asking each other these questions. Focus on only one or two at a time. It's okay to skip a difficult question and come back to it later.

1. How do you believe the sexual abuse has affected you personally?
2. How do you believe the sexual abuse has affected our relationship?
3. What is your greatest fear of what will happen to us in the future?
4. What does sex mean to you?
5. How would you like sex to be for us as a couple?
6. How do you feel about yourself as a sexual person?
7. What do you need from me to help sexual healing go more smoothly for you? (Note: A good way to respond to this question is by beginning with the phrase, "It would be helpful to me if . . .")

Remember that there are no right or wrong answers. Your goal as a couple is to learn about one another's needs, whatever they may be, and plan together for future intimacy.

also affected by the present situation and can benefit from knowing more about what's going on. Share even when you are afraid. Silence is your enemy.

In these regular discussions, partners can ask directly—but without pressures—about the survivor's experience and how they could be more helpful. Partners often have valuable insights and awareness about the survivor's family of origin, past experiences, or present behavior that can be of help to survivors in sexual healing. When a partner has some insights to offer, it's best to share the information when the partner knows that the survivor feels ready and interested in hearing it. "I have an idea about that," a partner might say. "Do you want to hear it now?" Following this format in offering information respects the survivor's need to control his or her own recovery process.

When the survivor feels ready, he or she needs to learn more about the partner's feelings and needs. Partners often bottle up their feelings. They may fear upsetting or bothering the survivor with them, even though this holding back often increases their own feelings of isolation. When partners don't communicate their feelings, they run the risk of feeling not only physically rejected but also emotionally rejected.

The survivor needs to check with the partner, asking questions like, "What feelings has this healing work brought up for you?" "What are your fears?" "What are your concerns?" "What are your needs?" As you listen to your partner's response, remind yourself that *your ability to hear what your partner has to say is more important than responding in a particular way.* You may not be able to fulfill what your partner needs and desires right now, but your attention and concern are gifts in and of themselves.

Robert, a partner, was extremely concerned that his wife, Jane, was letting her father, the offender, come to visit their home when he was not around. Robert worried that the father might interact in manipulative or abusive ways and that he would not be able to intervene and stop the father. But he hesitated telling Jane about his feelings and asking her to do things differently. Robert feared she would think he didn't trust her to protect the children or herself and that he was trying to tell her what to do.

As his anxieties increased, Robert realized that to take care of himself he had to share these feelings and needs with Jane. He talked with Jane, making sure to focus on how *he* was feeling and what *he* was needing, rather than on Jane's behavior. Though Jane was at first a little defensive, she was able to see that this was a *personal need* of Robert's based on his insecurities as well as his positive desire to protect his family from possible harm. His request was not an effort intended to control her. She checked in with herself to see if responding to his request would infringe on her own recovery in any major way, and she decided it wouldn't. Together they agreed to let her father come to the house only when Robert was there also.

In time, effective, open communication helps a couple bridge their gaps in understanding each other. The more able partners are to listen to one another, without either blaming themselves or giving up principles, the more freely each one will be able to share things honestly and directly. Communicating becomes the main way to bond in the relationship. Later, sexual relating can become another intimate way for the couple to communicate.

Work together as an active healing team

Survivors and partners can actively work as a team on certain key areas in sexual abuse recovery and sexual healing. These include resolving feelings related to the abuse, developing new attitudes about sex, handling automatic reactions to touch and sex, and developing a new approach to physical intimacy.

By actively working in these areas, healing is more likely to proceed smoothly and consistently. If partners do not cooperate and support each other, emotional distance can grow in relationships, and survivors' healing attempts can get stymied. Many survivors attribute their success in sexual healing to the special relationship they were able to establish with their partners. Because the crisis creates problems for both members of a couple, *both the survivor and the partner benefit from participating in the solutions together*.

In many ways partners can help only as much as survivors allow. Survivors have much to gain when they invite the partner to become more directly involved in the recovery process. Working as a team provides the survivor with an opportunity to actively challenge any unconscious tendencies to view the partner as an offender and helps offset the partner's feelings of frustration and rejection.

Partners do themselves a favor and their relationship a service when they become involved in sexual healing in a positive way. Involvement can help partners overcome feelings of powerlessness, frustration, and depression. Involvement can foster greater intimacy and caring.

Resolving feelings related to the abuse.   Partners can become involved in helping the survivor resolve feelings related to the abuse. They can create a safe, supportive, nonjudgmental atmosphere so the survivor can risk talking more freely about the abuse itself, relationships with members of the survivor's family of origin, feelings toward the offender, and sexual behavior that stemmed from the abuse. By listening openly and compassionately, partners validate the survivors' perceptions and thoughts. The survivor is comforted by the healthy love that exists in the present relationship.

Partners can also do special things for survivors to show their support during times when the survivors are immersed in abuse issues and feelings, such as offering words of encouragement or preparing a meal. One partner cleaned the house to show support when his wife felt vulnerable after talking with her mother about the abuse. He knew his wife always felt better when the house was clean. His wife was delighted.

Confrontations.   When survivors want to disclose the abuse to members of their family of origin or confront their offenders, partners can help.* While it's up to the survivor to initiate, design, and control disclosures and confrontations, partners can listen to the survivor's concerns, accompany the survivor to a meeting with the family member or offender, wait nearby, and be there afterward for emotional support. The quiet, calm presence of a partner during such a stressful time can be extremely important to building trust and intimacy in the relationship.

Developing new sexual attitudes.   Survivors and partners can work together to develop new sexual attitudes. A couple may want to share materials—poems,† stories, or articles—that present a healthy model for sex, in which sex is based on consent, equality, respect, trust, and safety. As a couple you can avoid talking about sex with words or in ways that reinforce a sexually abusive way of thinking.

Partners can help survivors develop a more positive sexual self-

---

* For information on preparing for a confrontation and about confrontations in general, see *The Courage to Heal* by Ellen Bass and Laura Davis, pages 133–148, and *The Courage to Heal Workbook* by Laura Davis, pages 340–366, both of which can be found in the Resources section.

† I have created two collections of poems that inspire and celebrate healthy sexual intimacy, *Passionate Hearts: The Poetry of Sexual Love* and *Intimate Kisses: The Poetry of Sexual Pleasure*. Both anthologies are published by New World Library and feature many well-known poets. See Resources section or call (800) 972-6657 to order.

concept by reminding the survivors that their basic sexual self is good and healthy. Kent, a survivor who had engaged in compulsive sex practices since being molested as a child, told his wife that he "felt like dirt" and that he couldn't believe anyone would really love him. His wife replied, "You can go on feeling that way about yourself if you choose. But I want you to know that, regardless of your past and regardless of your present tendencies, I think you are a beautiful person, and I sincerely love you." While Kent was not able to take in all that his wife told him in that moment, her words helped him to heal in the long run.

Handling automatic reactions.　　As we discussed in chapter 7, partners can help survivors identify triggers to automatic reactions that relate to the abuse. Together the couple can plan ways to handle automatic reactions, such as panic attacks, flashbacks, and dissociating. Couples may want to work up a list of strategies for handling automatic reactions that will inevitably occur. This might involve discussing what the survivor needs from the partner during a flashback: to be held, to be talked to, to be encouraged to express feelings, and so on. Couples can creatively brainstorm ways to avoid or alter triggers.

One survivor said she and her boyfriend developed a plan where he would stop sex and talk with her as soon as he noticed she seemed "off in another world." This encouraged the survivor to stay present and maintain feelings of emotional closeness during sex.

Another partner, after talking with his wife about triggers and automatic reactions, said, "I've learned a great deal about why my wife was so sensitive to certain sounds and touches, and about what I can do to promote sexual intimacy in gradual stages." His wife responded, "My husband is helping me learn that touch can be good and that enjoying touch is a key to overcoming my sexual my sexual problems."

Relearning touch.　　Partners can help the survivor learn that the focus of touch is not sex. Touch can be pleasurable by itself. A partner said, "I make it a point to cuddle and hold my boyfriend, without sex as the end result. I want him to know that sex is not an ulterior motive."

As a partner you can support and become involved in relearning touch and sex exercises, and in helping the survivor overcome sexual functioning problems. When survivors need to do exercises on their own, partners can help by creating a secure, quiet, private time and place for survivors to work on healing. You might protect the survivor from interruptions such as phone calls and children. Later, in the exercises that are done with a partner, you can join the survivor in building new skills and creating positive experiences with touch and, later, with sex. Your support gives the survivor both permission to explore new territories and a loving partner with whom to explore them.

In double-survivor couples, working together on healing can trigger feelings for each of you about your own sexual abuse. Progress can seesaw if one partner's healing puts pressure on the other. These couples need to be especially creative in finding healing activities both feel ready to work on together.

THE REWARDS OF WORKING TOGETHER

Sexual healing can build a deep emotional bond between the two of you. The skills you build to heal are the same skills that help relationships thrive. A partner reported on progress that had been made:

> Sexual healing has been a challenge for us, to say the least. We have grown stronger as a couple because it has forced us to be honest with what we want in an intimate relationship. We communicate openly. We respect ourselves. This has been a lesson in mutual understanding and trust.

The results of being involved in sexual healing can be individually rewarding. As a partner said:

> I have been able to make a distinction between intimacy and sexuality, and I have realized that I used sex as a vehicle to achieve "wholeness." It was difficult, but I learned not to take this all personally and to remind myself that I'm okay. I learned not to get angry with my girlfriend for withdrawing and feeling disgusted when I'm opening myself and being sexually vulnerable. I have developed patience, trust, and self-confidence.

"Maybe this whole thing has been a blessing in disguise," another partner said. "We now know for sure that our relationship is not based on sex alone." Sexual healing can have many positive side effects. It can help both partners improve self-esteem. It can teach you to work more effectively as a partnership. And it can bring richness and depth to your relationship. A survivor related her experience:

Our situation has been one of mutual change. We read, write, and talk with each other about the abuse and its effects. We experiment with touch in a slow, gentle, and accepting way. There's open understanding and kindness on both sides. We offer each other a safe place to share ourselves and a fertile ground for healing and love.

The challenges facing couples are indeed great during sexual healing, but the changes you make will benefit your relationship long after healing has been accomplished.

Now, as you learn to rely on your partner for understanding and encouragement and to involve your partner more in recovery, let's move on to some specific techniques and exercises you can do to promote sexual health, pleasure, and intimacy.

PART THREE

Getting There

Creating Positive Experiences

10

Techniques for Relearning Touch

To touch and be touched intimately means exposing my underside like the belly of a porcupine. I feel vulnerable. Step by step, I'm learning to replace the pain of sexual abuse with the joy of being alive and a sensual person.

—A SURVIVOR

When I was a little girl and couldn't sleep at night, I would sit up in bed and call to my father, "Daddy, I want a drink of water!" He'd come into my room, bringing a glass of water, sit down next to me, and wait as I took a few sips. Then I'd scoot back under my covers, and he would stroke my head for a while. He would gently run his hand above my ears, combing my hair with his fingertips, over and over again. I'd relax immediately, and often I fell right asleep. More than the water, I needed his touch.

Warm childhood experiences, like the one I had with my father, teach a child to enjoy touch. We learn when very young that touch is a source of comfort and security. We learn to touch as a way to share commitment, trust, and love. Without fear, worry, or discomfort, we come to value touch for the security and sensual pleasures it brings.

Tragically, sexual abuse can interfere with this lesson. Many survivors fail to learn that touch is a healthy form of communication. In abuse, touch becomes a way to dominate and control another person. When we're sexually abused, we may learn to experience touch as mechanical, unemotional, often a painful manipulation of our bodies. Because of abuse, we may associate touch with pain, betrayal, and fear. It can become difficult or even impossible for us to imagine touch as healthy and desirable. "How could anyone want to be touched in an erotic way? Wouldn't they automatically feel taken advantage of?" a survivor asked.

Many survivors feel this way. If survivors had no choice about who touched them sexually, or when or how or where, they may automatically assume that all touch leads to sex. Survivors may avoid touch that is sensuous and intimate but outside the sexual context: a friend's hug, a coworker's handshake, a nurse's massage. A woman who had been abused by her mother, father, and brother described the dilemma:

> I grew up without nurturing touch and with lots of inappropriate sexual touching. Now I am confused about touch. I'm afraid to trust someone to touch me and unsure that my touch will be received with pleasure if I touch someone else.

Survivors can't erase the past. They were sexually abused and may never have had a chance to learn to enjoy being touched. But it's not too late to begin learning to enjoy touch now. It is possible to build a new mental file, a place to tuck away fresh, enjoyable memories about touch, like saving snapshots from a wonderful trip. By creating new experiences, survivors can take off in directions they never dreamed they could travel.

You have reached a new frontier on the sexual healing journey. In parts one and two, the focus was on understanding past and present experiences, on undoing negative beliefs about our sexuality, on gaining control of automatic reactions learned in the abuse, and on making changes in our sexual behavior and relationships. Building on this foundation, you are now ready to begin to make changes on a physical level—experientially, with touch. You can reach out for new, positive experiences instead of withdrawing from or desperately seeking touch because of the damage done by the abuse. You can learn to experience touch as a source of comfort, caring, and pleasure.

First you'll be asked to look at the relationship between touch and sex. Second, you'll be introduced to several important skills that can be used in relearning touch. Finally, you'll be guided through a series of seventeen practical exercises that will provide you with hands-on opportunities to safely, gently, and playfully explore your sensuality. In small, progressive steps, you will learn how to feel relaxed and present during touch, and how to alter your experience in response to your individual feelings and needs. You can work on many of these exercises alone, whether or not you are currently involved with an intimate partner.

These skills and exercises will allow you to compensate for the learning you may have missed because of sexual abuse. This is a chance for you to relearn touch in a positive way and to develop whole new avenues for enjoying sensual pleasure.

PUTTING SEX WHERE IT BELONGS

Human beings touch one another in a wide variety of ways. Most touch is not sexual at all. Sexual touch is only one possibility of sensual touch experiences. To illustrate how different touch experiences interrelate, we can imagine a continuum of sensual touch, listing experiences progressively from less sexual to more sexual kinds of touch.

Ideally, we learn to enjoy touch in stages, feeling comfortable with the more primary, soothing kinds of touch before we ever experience touch in a sexual context. Each experience, while satisfying in and of itself, also prepares us for the next step. We gradually build a foundation of pleasing touch experiences.

For most survivors, however, touch has not been learned under these ideal conditions. They may have been forced to experience sexual touch too early in the touch continuum, before they had a chance to build a foundation of other, less sexual touch experiences.

To enhance sexual healing, survivors can now go back and rebuild a healthy continuum of touch experiences. The key to remember is that *sexual pleasuring comes after—and not until—you have learned to feel safe and comfortable with nonsexual touch.*

The illustration on the following page shows one example of a touch continuum. Yours might look somewhat different, but it should show a progression from nonsexual to more sexual touch.

Survivors need to feel well practiced in their ability to relax, stay present, and guide the touch activity before they can enjoy the unique pleasures inherent in sexual touch. Start with touch experiences that you perceive as easier to do and that occur earlier in your touch continuum. One survivor may feel more secure if she begins with a hug than if she begins with a kiss. Another survivor may want to hold hands during a movie before he's comfortable receiving a back rub.

Relearning touch involves moving step by step toward touching in more sexual ways. Having sex and developing sexual bonds fit naturally

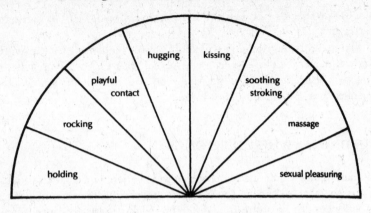

An example of a touch continuum

into the progression as survivors heal, but these activities should occur only after they have a foundation of pleasant touch experiences. Once the survivor feels secure with this foundation, he or she can invite the partner in to share at each stage along the continuum, building shared sexual experiences gradually.

CRUCIAL SKILLS FOR RELEARNING TOUCH

Before you begin the exercises for relearning touch, let's go over three important skills that can help you overcome difficulties that may arise:

1. Relaxation and rest
2. Active awareness
3. Creative problem solving

Relaxation and rest

Giving yourself permission to stop and relax when you feel the need is a prerequisite for all of these exercises. Don't start a relearning touch exercise until you feel that when needed you would be able to stop, rest, calm yourself down, and feel safe.

Relax first.   How can you create a mood in which this is possible? Try some preliminary relaxing before beginning an exercise. Unwind in a hot bath. Read about the exercise. Take a few minutes to imagine yourself doing it.

Some survivors find they can relax further by using a relaxation exercise, slowly stretching and massaging their muscle groups. Others may use yoga, dance warm-ups, or self-massage.*

Here is a simple exercise I use that involves tensing and relaxing different muscle groups in succession: Take time to lie down awhile on your back. Breathe and rest. When you're ready, begin to alternately tighten and release the muscles in your feet, then legs, then stomach, then chest, then hands, then arms, then shoulders and neck, and so on. Breathe slowly and deeply. End this activity by tensing and relaxing your whole body at once. Breathe slowly. Imagine your muscles becoming heavy, as if your whole body is sinking into the floor. Relax and continue breathing slowly.

There is no one prescription for relaxing. Each of us needs to find what works best. Other relaxation methods could also work well for you.†

Rest when needed.   During the exercises, whenever you feel like it take a few minutes simply to breathe. Inhale and exhale fully, reminding yourself that you are in charge, that you are doing this by your choice, and that you can stop whenever you want. The techniques described in chapter 7 for gaining control over automatic reactions can help you now, applied to relearning touch exercises.

When sensual experiences with her partner became too intense, Dee, a survivor, would put her hands in a T signal for time out.

> I stop for just a little bit until I can realize it isn't the abuse all over again. I concentrate on my needs, which helps me move beyond my reactions.

The nonverbal signal Dee used was an easy way to remind herself and her partner she wanted a break. Remind yourself to stop, move around, go to the bathroom, get something nonalcoholic to drink, or talk about

---

* A therapeutic technique of deep tissue massage and muscle stretching has been used successfully in helping victims of sexual torture to restore positive consciousness to the body and to regain feeling to sexual parts of the body. For an interesting article on this topic, see H. Larsen and J. Pagaduan-Lopez, "Stress-Tension Reduction in the Treatment of Sexually Tortured Women: An Exploratory Study," *Journal of Sex & Marital Therapy* 13, no. 3 (Fall 1987): 210–218.

† See Resources section for relaxation books and tapes.

your feelings if you're with a partner. Another survivor described a particular incident:

> One time my partner and I were kissing. We stopped and checked
> in with each other. I realized I hadn't really been "there" while kiss-
> ing my partner. I opened my eyes, looked at my partner, and
> reminded myself who I was kissing. That helped. It gave me a sense
> of power.

Taking a short break reinforces your choice and makes you aware you are in control. You can also stop the exercises sometimes when you feel fine. If you stop only when the going gets tough, you can make stopping itself seem traumatic. It need not be. Resting is natural. It's better to stop than to push too hard. Take it slow, adding two or three time-out breaks to each exercise. Stop and go at your own pace.

If you find that stopping becomes so frequent that it interferes with your progress, you may not be ready to do the particular exercise you have chosen. If you are feeling intense anger or panic, attend to these feelings first. Back up a little, and review the aspects of the healing journey covered in part two. Don't push yourself to move forward until you feel ready.

When you stop the exercises, do something you find calming. Find your own reassurances. You may want to hold your hand over your heart, listen to music, meditate, hold a teddy bear, pet your cat, or simply breathe and nap.

Find a home base.   When doing exercises with a partner, it may help you to find what I call a safe home base—a spot on your partner's body that feels safe and comfortable for you to touch.* By touching this spot, the survivor remembers that this person is the partner, not the offender. The spot is a *home base* to which the survivor can come back and feel comfortable.

While doing relearning touch exercises, Charlotte, a rape survivor, felt calmed and reassured by stroking the smooth underside of her boyfriend's arm. This was a part of the male body that had absolutely no association with assault for her. Home base touching can be a source of reassurance when some other touching may feel uncomfortable.

---

* This technique was originally developed by Karla Baur, a sex therapist in Portland, Oregon.

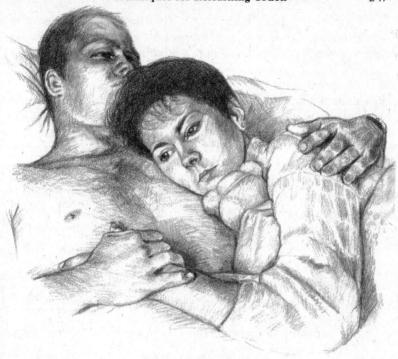

Listening to heartbeats

Listen to heartbeats.   Similarly, some survivors are comforted when they stop and listen to their partners' heartbeats. For almost everyone the sound of the human heart is primordial. We heard it in the comfort of our mothers' wombs long before we were abused. The sound can make us feel secure again now.

Active awareness

Our goal now is to help you feel conscious, safe, and in control. It's not "how far you go" in the exercises but how comfortable you feel. You must be able to tune in to your feelings at all times. Being aware of your feelings during touch is not easy. It takes time and practice to learn.

Practice completing the sentence "I am aware . . ." What comes to mind? There is no correct answer; whatever you think of is right. Ask yourself again, "I am aware . . ." What comes to mind this time? Active awareness means tuning in to your thoughts and feelings constantly.

I'll do it now to give you an example: "I am aware that my fingers are hitting the keys on my computer keyboard. Now I;'m aware that I made a typing error. Now I'm aware that it will be funny when it gets printed this way. Now I'm aware of wanting to concentrate on the exercise. Now I'm aware that I have an ache in my shoulder. Now I'm aware of the sounds of my children playing outside. Now I'm aware what a beautiful day it is outside. Now I'm aware of feeling sad that I'm indoors. Now I'm aware that I want to go outside. . . ."

Notice how my awareness includes all experiences: body movements (fingers on keyboard), thoughts (humor in imagining a typing error purposefully included in the book, wanting to go outside), physical sensation (ache in my shoulder), sensory experiences of the environment (hearing the sound of my children playing, seeing how beautiful a day it is), emotions (sadness at being inside on a lovely day), and desires (wanting to go outside). Practice active awareness. Ask yourself more specifically:

- What do I see, hear, touch, taste, and smell right now?
- What am I doing?
- How do I feel physically (muscle tension, heart rate, stomach sensations, aches, pains, calmness)?
- What am I feeling emotionally (anger, fear, joy, peaceful, sad, excited, confused)?
- What do I want and need right now?
- (If with a partner) How do I feel about my partner? What is my partner doing? How do I feel about the two of us?

Active awareness can keep us from mentally leaving what we are doing. Awareness is a skill you can practice before, during, and after a relearning touch exercise. At first, you may find it hard to acknowledge, even to yourself, what you are feeling. Keep practicing. You may wish to try saying your awareness sentences out loud. This reaffirms your experience. If you are with an intimate partner, you may want to share your awareness sentences with your partner. If you are a single survivor, you may want to share with a therapist, support group, or friend. Do you find this difficult to imagine? Remember, you are in charge. Share only what you feel ready to share for now. The more you let your partner in on your experiences, the more intimate your relationship can be.

Watch out for the tendency to judge yourself for your feelings: How can I feel this way? Why am I thinking of that? Don't judge. Accept whatever you are experiencing. It's real, and it's a valid feeling; it's what you are aware of in a particular moment.

As you become more practiced in active awareness, you may notice that you don't have to make a conscious effort to tune in. Your awareness will come more naturally. Like learning a new language, learning to be actively aware takes conscious thought at first, but eventually you begin to "think in the language" of active awareness automatically.

Creative problem solving

We all have individual responses to relearning touch exercises. It is common for survivors to have problems with learning touch in a new way. You may run into emotional blocks, such as a feeling of anxiety or fear, in doing one exercise or another. When this happens, don't give up. Evaluate these emotional blocks. Understanding why something makes you uncomfortable can help you become aware of ways you may need to change the experience to help you feel more emotionally secure. This is itself an important part of relearning touch. Your feelings are your guide. Believe in them, and proceed to create more enjoyable sexual experiences in the future.

Creative problem solving means *adapting exercises to your personal needs.* When you run into a block ask yourself, "What can I do to feel more comfortable with this exercise?" As you adapt you stay active in your healing while respecting your personal feelings. The following are several techniques you might find helpful when you hit a block.

Shift back.   Because the exercises coming up are arranged progressively, running into a block may indicate that you are going too fast. You may need more time to practice skills in familiar touch activities. By shifting back to an exercise you did earlier, you can maintain your sense of control and safety while setting your own pace.

Jenna, a twenty-seven-year-old survivor, had been teaching herself to feel more comfortable touching her own body. She started by focusing on remaining calm and present while taking a shower. She found this cleansing exercise relatively easy to do. She decided to try another exercise which involved lying on her bed and rubbing body lotion into her skin. Suddenly she got scared. Jenna felt exposed and uncomfortable.

She went back to the shower the next day. By the third time she did her cleansing exercise, Jenna began to feel curious and more confident about doing the next exercise. She was ready to move on. When she got out of the shower, she dried off and went directly to her bedroom. This time she felt relaxed applying the lotion. Shifting back to the cleansing exercise for a while had given Jenna the time she needed to get more comfortable touching herself.

You can adapt the shifting-back technique however you wish. Let's say Jenna felt fine with putting lotion on her legs and arms, but became fearful putting lotion on her chest. Jenna could then take time for several sessions of applying lotion only to her legs and arms before she even considered putting lotion on her chest area again. Adapt. Set your own pace.

Bridging.   Another technique of creative problem solving is making interim steps in an exercise. By adding steps to an exercise, you create a bridge from one touch experience to another. Suppose we are hiking through the woods and come to a river we want to cross. We spot a few big rocks in the water, but our legs are too short. We can't comfortably reach from one rock to the next. What do we do? We add more rocks to make smaller steps in between the bigger ones. Now we can hop across easily, and we do.

When you reach a block in relearning touch, you might ask yourself, "What little rocks can I add to cross this river?" Perhaps you could *decrease the amount of time* you spend on an activity. For example, do the exercise for three minutes instead of twenty minutes. This allows you to expose yourself a little at a time. You might try a different way than suggested—*change the setting or position yourself differently.* Jenna could have bridged by adding a session or two where she remained in the bathroom after her shower, dried off, and applied lotion there instead of in the bedroom. This would have allowed her to retain a body position and environment similar to those during showering. Her success with the cleansing exercise might bridge her to the lotion application.

Therapist Jill Kennedy of Sacramento, California, described how a client of hers used clay molding as a bridge to overcome a fear of kisses. A survivor of father-daughter incest, the woman had done some healing work and had reached the point where she could comfortably have sexual intercourse. She felt safe until her husband, aroused, moved to kiss her on her neck near her collarbone. Her father had kissed her just this way. She discussed her feelings with her husband and he agreed not to touch her in this way. But the woman felt sad about the restriction and decided she wanted to overcome her fear of being kissed. Kennedy wrote:

The woman was a potter and bought some plastic molding clay
with which she began what she called her "mouth and lips cam-
paign." She started by sculpting mouths and lips during sessions
and smashing them with her fists, or throwing them against the
floor to destroy them. This phase moved to one in which she began
to make affirming statements such as, "This is not my father's
mouth, . . . everyone's mouth is not my father's mouth." Gradually,
she began to experiment with pressing the mouths she molded to
her neck and collarbone, always affirming that she was in control of
this contact. Eventually she took the models home and in carefully
controlled exercises with her husband, she allowed him to touch
her with the models she had made. Over time, she was able to feel
pleasure in receiving her husband's kisses on her neck.*

This creative solution worked. By using the clay lips, the woman was
able to erase old associations to the abuse. She relearned the experience
of being kissed as healthy, within her control, and enjoyable.

A common type of bridging that can be used in relearning touch
involves *varying the amount of clothing you wear*. Amy, a survivor, was
extremely uncomfortable going to bed nude. After talking with her
partner, Amy suggested they both go to bed with clothes on when she
started relearning touch. Knowing they were both dressed, touch was
less threatening for her. After a few sessions Amy began to suggest they
remove one article of clothing at a time. For awhile they went to bed in
underclothing. They were both surprised to discover their socks were
the last thing to go!

Another survivor, Tanya, used eye makeup as a bridge. She and her
partner were experimenting, giving and receiving massage. Suddenly
Tanya felt afraid and stopped. Tanya realized she needed a way to show
her partner clearly where she felt okay being touched. Rummaging
through her purse, she found some eyeliner and drew a line around her
breasts and genitals. Touching inside the line was off limits. In future sessions Tanya stopped using the eyeliner and instead used her finger to draw
imaginary borders. Her forbidden areas grew smaller and eventually disappeared. These inventive bridging techniques enabled Tanya to relax.

With some creative thinking my clients have been able to find effective, enjoyable bridges for themselves. A few favorites: rubbing egg
whites between the fingers as a step toward feeling comfortable with

* Questionnaire response, 1989.

vaginal secretions or semen; holding the little fingers together as a step toward holding hands; giving and receiving butterfly kisses (blinking eyelashes against partner's cheek) as a step toward kissing with lips; having a squirt gun fight in the shower as a step toward feeling comfortable with a male partner's ejaculation.

We can make great progress learning to solve touch problems creatively. Like the couple with the squirt guns, you can sexually heal while having a lot of fun.

Relearning touch is gradual. It requires creativity and gentle persistence. You can't rush it, because doing so will probably stir up fears, anxiety, and overexcitement. A survivor who slowly taught herself to masturbate described her approach:

> I treat myself to only the touches I want. I never push myself to do more than I can handle. I listen to my inner voice, what I want and need in the moment.

Hurrying can lead to being overwhelmed, and that can make you give up on relearning altogether. You need to expect that you will experience some difficulty and anxiety with this process. Changes always bring temporary discomfort. To find the balance and allow yourself to succeed, you might follow this survivor's suggestion:

> Do what feels comfortable, but stretch a bit beyond the comfort level. It's worth it to keep on going even when you think it's harder than possible to achieve.

RELEARNING TOUCH EXERCISES*

You can think about relearning touch as a process of making many bridges from easier to more challenging touch activities. Many survivors spend at least one week doing each exercise three or four times before moving on to another exercise. All the exercises have variations that can be used as bridges to exercises that come later. Use the exercises and their variations to create a sequence that fits for you. Stay flexible with

---

* My video, "Relearning Touch: Healing Techniques for Couples," features sensitive demonstrations of the exercises, and discussion by three couples who benefited from the techniques. For information and to order, call: (800) 678-3455.

the order and variations of exercises you do. Your needs will probably change as you proceed and make progress with touch.

For exercises you do with a partner, remember that the survivor initiates all exercises, sets the pace, and controls the process. Either survivor or partner can stop an exercise at any time, or can suggest a way to adapt the exercise to make it more comfortable.

Remove the relearning touch exercises from any expectation of sexual release or interaction. Of course, sexual arousal may happen, but it's not the purpose now. In fact, if you are not currently taking a vacation from sex (as described in chapter 8), I recommend that you wait at least several hours after doing an exercise before engaging in sexual activity. Many couples find it works best to refrain from sex on the days when they do the exercises. In the early months of healing, these exercises are not to be viewed as a prelude to sex. There must be no demand or pressure. Remember your goal for now is to begin to experience touch for its own sake, free from old sexual associations.

Relearning touch can eventually help you create better sexual relations, but you'll need to be patient. Let your curiosity guide you and your laughter accompany you.

Here are the relearning touch exercises listed progressively, according to learning categories:

PLAYFUL TOUCH

Sensory basket
Hand clapping
Drawing on body

BUILDING SAFETY

Safe nest
Safe embrace
Safe embrace to touching
Hand-to-heart

INITIATING AND GUIDING CONTACT

Magic pen
Red light–green light

BODY AWARENESS

Shampooing hair
Cleansing
Reclaiming your body
Getting to know your genitals
Genital exploration, with partner

PLEASURING

Body massage, with partner
Genital pleasuring
Genital pleasuring, with partner

If you are a single survivor, you can practice selected exercises without a partner. A program for single survivors could look like this:

RELEARNING TOUCH EXERCISES FOR SINGLE SURVIVORS

Sensory basket
Safe nest
Cleansing
Reclaiming your body
Getting to know your genitals
Genital pleasuring

Let's take a closer look at the exercises.

PLAYFUL TOUCH

SENSORY BASKET*

PURPOSE: To awaken senses, to remain relaxed and present during touch, to recognize preferences, to play and experiment with touch

SUGGESTED TIME: Ten to twenty minutes

* A special thanks to Miriam Smolover of Oakland, California, and Joyce Baker of Eugene, Oregon, for introducing me to similar versions of this exercise.

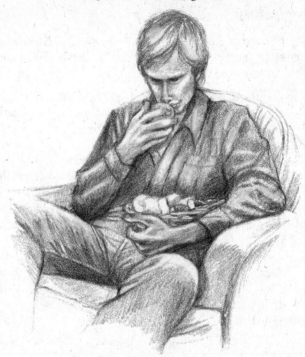

Exploring a sensory basket

In a basket collect a variety of objects to awaken your senses. Choose objects that you think you would find pleasurable to touch, smell, taste, listen to, or look at. A sensory basket might include such things as velvet cloth, feathers, rattles, bells, fruit, spices, jewelry, polished rocks, rubber bands, and stuffed animals.

Spend a few minutes interacting with each object. Practice relaxation and active awareness skills to keep yourself calm and present. Hold the object up to your ear; shake it. Put it under your nose; smell it. Rub it against your cheek or the back of your hand; feel it. Arrange your objects in a line, putting your favorites at one end and those less favored at the other. Make a design or a face using all of your objects. Have fun, experiment. Feel free to add or subtract items from your sensory basket.

FUTURE VARIATION: Hold, pet, and play with an animal such as a dog, cat, or hamster.

HAND CLAPPING

PURPOSE: To practice designing and implementing playful touch, as well as developing cooperation and communication with a partner

SUGGESTED TIME: Varies

Sit in facing chairs or cross-legged on the floor at such a distance that you can comfortably press the palms of your hands together with those of your partner. Develop a hand-clapping routine to teach your partner. This is similar to hand-clapping games you may have learned as a child or seen children do. The one I learned was to clap both my hands once with my partner's hands, clap my hands together, then right hand once with my partner's right hand, again clap my hands together, left hand to my partner's left hand, and again clap my hands together. I used to sing a song like "Take Me Out to the Ballgame" or "A Sailor Went to Sea" in rhythm with the clapping.

After you decide on your hand-clapping routine, teach it to your partner. Practice it several times together. This exercise is complete when you are able to run through your hand-clapping routine three times with your partner, singing a song to go with it, without either of you making a mistake.

FUTURE VARIATIONS: Do the exercise sitting in bed, wearing swimsuits, or, later, without clothing.

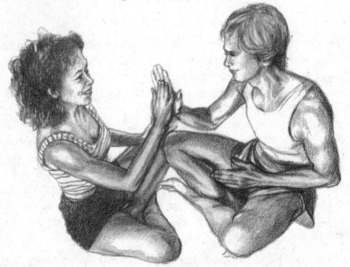

Hand clapping

DRAWING ON BODY

PURPOSE: To learn touch as a form of communication
SUGGESTED TIME: Varies

Sit facing your partner's back. Using your finger, send a written message to your partner, drawing one letter of the message at a time on your partner's back. The partner remains still and tries to guess each letter as it is written, and says the message out loud when you are done. You might write "I like you" or "It's your turn to do the dishes" or whatever you like. When you feel ready switch places with your partner, and let your partner write a message on your back.

FUTURE VARIATIONS: (1) Write messages on other parts of your partner's body such as the palms of the hands or bottoms of the feet (likely to get a laugh). (2) Do the exercise with bare backs.

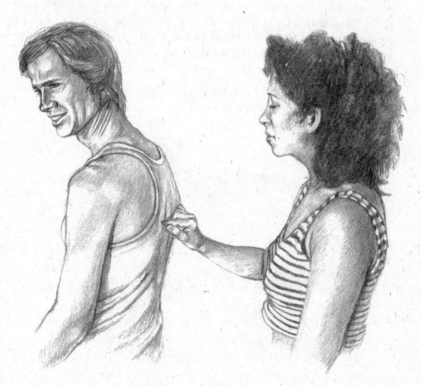

Drawing on body

BUILDING SAFETY

SAFE NEST

PURPOSE: To create a safe setting for experiencing sensual touch; to identify and respond to your emotional and physiological needs

SUGGESTED TIME: Twenty to thirty minutes

Create a safe, warm environment in which you can physically and emotionally feel relaxed alone. Secure your privacy; take the phone off the hook, tell housemates not to disturb you, and so on. Wear soft, loose-fitting clothing. Using blankets, pillows, and other bedding, form a nest for you to rest in. Use relaxation skills to calm yourself and awareness skills to focus on being with yourself in the present moment. Breathe consciously. Focus on your body and your environment. You are aiming for comfort and relaxation. Ask yourself what you could do to make the situation more comfortable: turn up the heat, open a window, lock a door, have a friend in the next room, play soft music? Tune in to your needs and take them seriously, even if they seem silly or insignificant at first. Rest comfortably.

FUTURE VARIATIONS: (1) Hold and hug yourself. Rock yourself gently.
(2) Over time you can practice with less and less clothing.

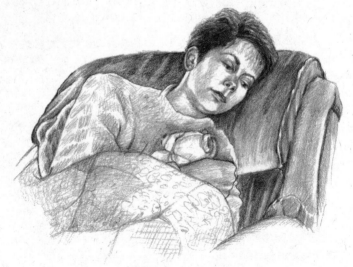

Resting in a safe nest

SAFE EMBRACE

PURPOSE: To relax and feel safe with a partner

SUGGESTED TIME: Twenty to thirty minutes

Invite your intimate partner to join you in your safe nest. Both wear soft, loose-fitting clothing. Find a sitting or reclining position in which you feel comfortable having contact with your partner. You might hug gently or rest your head on your partner's chest, listening to heartbeats. You might want to wrap your arms around your partner or have your partner wrap his or her arms around you. Breathe slowly together. Relax and rest together. Occasionally share your awareness of how you feel in the present moment. Gentle rocking is okay, but avoid hand exploration and stroking.

FUTURE VARIATIONS: Over time you can practice with less and less clothing.

SAFE EMBRACE TO TOUCHING

PURPOSE: To experience touch that has movement and direction in a
relaxed, safe setting

SUGGESTED TIME: Ten to twenty minutes

Start with safe embrace. While being held, survivor initiates small
touches; partner remains passive. Touch your partner's body, exploring
texture of clothes, softness and hardness of body parts near to where
your hands are resting. Take little steps, maintaining relaxation and present consciousness. Stop at any time, and focus on holding partner or
being held by partner.

FUTURE VARIATIONS: (1) Broaden the areas that you touch. (2) Over time
you can practice with less and less clothing.

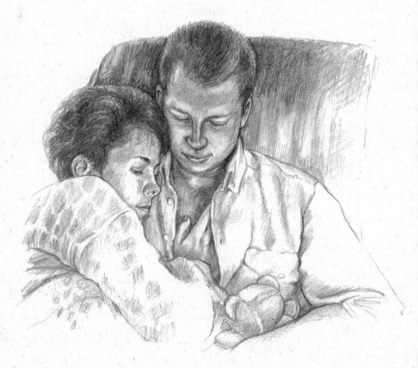

Exploring touch in a safe embrace

HAND-TO-HEART

PURPOSE: To associate touch with the exchange of positive, loving, respectful feelings

SUGGESTED TIME: Ten to twenty minutes

Wearing soft, comfortable clothes, you and your partner sit in chairs or on the floor facing each other. Get close enough so that you can each comfortably place your right hand on your partner's shoulder with your elbow slightly bent. Make eye contact with your partner. Take a few deep, slow breaths. This exercise is designed as a silent sharing, unless either of you needs to talk. Each of you now move your right hand from your partner's shoulder and rest it securely and gently, palm down, over your partner's heart. Look into each other's eyes again. Now look at the circle that you and your partner are forming, hand to heart and heart to hand.

As you remain in this position, bring your awareness to the feelings that you have toward your partner. Focus on what you like about your partner and the things you appreciate your partner for. Think of past

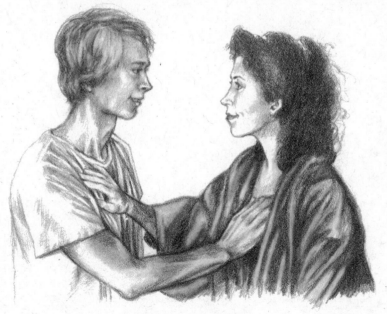

Sharing hand-to-heart

times you spent together that were fun and pleasant to you. Let these thoughts collect together and become loving feelings resting in your heart.

Now imagine these loving feelings traveling from your heart over to your right shoulder, down your arm, and out through the palm of your hand, into your partner's heart. Your partner receives your love and combines it with the love feelings he or she has for you and sends them through his or her shoulder, arm, and hand, back to you. You receive them, add to them, and send them back, and so on. Together you create a circular flow of loving feelings, from heart to hand and hand to heart.

FUTURE VARIATIONS: (1) Move your right hand to rest on shoulders, cheeks, knees, and so on, creating a flow of loving feelings to other areas of your bodies. Most advanced version involves genital parts. (2) Do the exercise with less and less clothing.

INITIATING AND GUIDING CONTACT

MAGIC PEN

PURPOSE: To develop skills in initiating contact and controlling movement with a partner; to practice communicating needs verbally
SUGGESTED TIME: Five to ten minutes

Sit at a table or on the floor, facing your partner, about two feet
apart. Put a pen on the table or floor between you and your partner.
Firmly but comfortably take hold of one end of the pen. When you feel
ready, ask your partner to hold on to the other end of the pen. Move the
pen up and down and around in circles. Lead your partner, creating different movements. You might think of a conductor directing an orches-
tra or a child making designs with a 4th of July sparkler. Move in ways
that your partner can comfortably follow without losing contact with

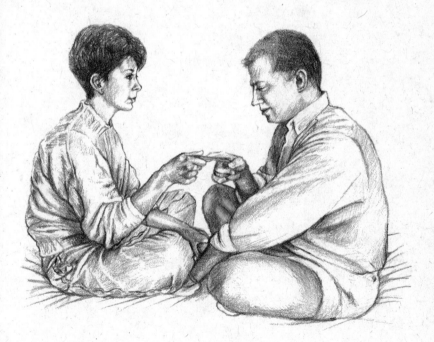

Guiding the magic pen

the pen. The partner holds on securely yet doesn't lead. The partner needs to allow the survivor to be in charge of the movement at all times.

When you feel finished (this might be after only a few seconds the first time you do it), ask your partner to let go of the pen. Don't let go of the pen first. An important part of the learning is to practice telling your partner when you are ready to start and stop contact.

FUTURE VARIATIONS: (1) Dispense with the pen. You may want your partner to hold on to your pointer finger in the same manner as the pen, or simply hold hands with your partner in a comfortable manner. (2) Later do the exercise with less and less clothing.

RED LIGHT–GREEN LIGHT

PURPOSE: To develop comfort and control in giving and receiving touch
SUGGESTED TIME: Fifteen minutes

Begin in a relaxed, comfortable position such as safe embrace or sitting close to your partner. Spend a few minutes looking at your partner. Remind yourself that all the parts of your partner's body connect together. Look at one of your partner's arms. See how the hand is part of the arm, and the arm part of the body, and the body part of the head. Look into your partner's eyes. Relax and breathe.

Indicate to your partner when you are ready to begin. Make sure your partner is ready to begin as well. When you both feel ready, your partner says, "Green light." Begin touching the partner's arm that you had just looked at. Explore how it feels. Gently rub and massage it, if you like. During this time, your partner is to count slowly to ten. When your partner reaches ten, he or she says, "Red light." As soon as you hear this, stop touching and instead hold your partner's arm. Repeat three times, then switch roles so that your partner is touching your arm and you are the one saying "green light" and "red light." Remember to stop the exercise at any time if you should need to—just say "red light" earlier than planned.

When you feel ready, repeat the exercise changing the count to twenty seconds. Switch roles again. Continue expanding the length of active touching until you reach one minute.

FUTURE VARIATIONS: (1) Dispense with counting and use the words *green light* and *red light* to indicate to each other when to start and stop touch. (*Note to partners:* Don't let more than a minute or two go without saying "red light." Better to say it more often than you feel like than less.) (2) Later versions can reduce the amount of clothing and extend the touch exploration and massage to other parts of the body such as head, face, back, and legs.

BODY AWARENESS

SHAMPOOING HAIR

PURPOSE: To create a mutually pleasurable and fun wet touch experience
SUGGESTED TIME: Ten to twenty minutes

This exercise is like creating a mini–hair salon in your own home (or backyard). Have your partner sit in a chair with a towel draped around his or her shoulders. Wet your partner's hair with warm water, add shampoo, and work the shampoo into the hair until you get a nice lather. Experiment with different ways of massaging your partner's head, making different designs with the hair and the lather. Rub your fingers gently over your partner's head, making sure to touch those areas that are hard to reach. Explore the different sensations to your fingers as you shampoo the hair with the lather. Invent ways to shampoo that are fun for you. When you are done, help your partner rinse, comb, and dry his or her hair.

FUTURE VARIATIONS: (1) Exchange positions so partner shampoos the survivor. (2) Both of you wear less and less clothing.

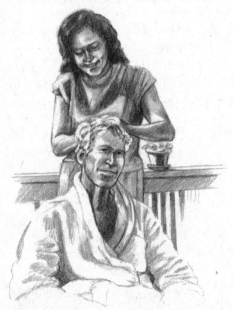

Shampooing hair

CLEANSING

PURPOSE: To enhance your awareness of your body and skin
SUGGESTED TIME: Twenty to thirty minutes

Secure privacy and uninterrupted time. Take a long, relaxing shower or bath. While you are in the water, rub soap on a bathing sponge or washcloth and wash your body all over with it. Experiment building lather in places and making designs and swirls with the soap. Try different kinds of strokes: long, short, light, firm. Remind yourself that this is your body—*you* own your body.

Look more closely at your skin. Did you know that your skin is an organ of your body? Did you know that you are constantly shedding the surface cells of your skin? The skin that you feel now is not the same as it was weeks, months, or years ago, when the abuse occurred. The skin on your body now is new and different. Your skin possesses very powerful, self-healing abilities. As you cleanse your skin think about how fresh and new it is. When you are ready come out of the water and dry yourself with a soft towel. Get dressed right away, or rest in bed under warm covers for awhile before getting dressed.

FUTURE VARIATIONS: (1) Use your own hand instead of a bathing sponge or washcloth, paying attention to the sensations you receive in touching yourself. (2) Cleanse your partner's body or have your partner cleanse your body.

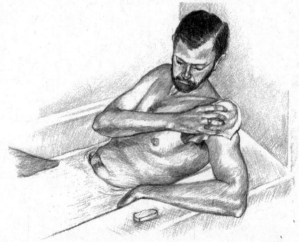

Experimenting with cleansing

RECLAIMING YOUR BODY

PURPOSE: To increase feelings of body ownership and body awareness
SUGGESTED TIME: Ten to twenty minutes

Begin with the cleansing exercise. Look at your body without clothes on in a full-length mirror. Turn sideways to view parts of your body that you can't ordinarily see. How do you feel about the different parts of your body? What parts of your body do you like the most? What parts do you tend to judge negatively or ignore? Identify each part of your body by saying out loud, "This is my hair," "This is my arm," and so forth.

Touch yourself, excluding your nipples and genitals. How do these different parts of your body feel? Which are the softest places? Which are the roughest? Which are the most sensitive? Remind yourself that your body belongs to you.

Rub body lotion into your skin. Notice how the texture of your skin softens and your skin becomes moist. Experiment with different types of touches to your skin: smooth gentle strokes, deep muscle rubbing, circular strokes, feathery touches, and so on.

FUTURE VARIATIONS: (1) Touch yourself with the goal of increasing pleasurable sensations. (2) Eventually include nipples and genitals in the exercise.

GETTING TO KNOW YOUR GENITALS

PURPOSE: To increase feelings of ownership and awareness of your genital area

SUGGESTED TIME: Twenty to thirty minutes

Begin with the safe nest exercise. With a light on and using a mirror, look closely at your genital area. Can you identify the different parts of your genitals?* If you are a woman, find your outer vaginal lips, your inner vaginal lips, your clitoris, your urethra, your vaginal opening, and your anus. If you are a man, find your scrotum, your testicles, the glans of your penis, your frenum, and your anus. Touch each part gently as you say its name. Notice the differences in skin texture and color of the different parts. Pay attention to what you feel. Remember to breathe. Experiment with different types of touches, such as pressing, gently tugging, tapping, stroking, or massaging. What parts are most sensitive? What parts are least sensitive? Focus on remaining present-centered and relaxed, not on arousal. Remind yourself that your genitals belong to you.

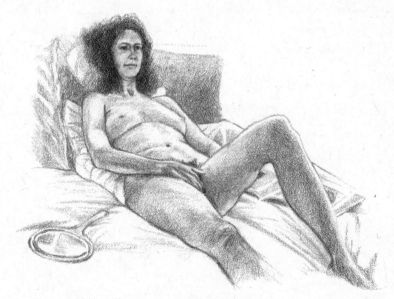

Concluding genital exploration with a hand hug

* See the Resources section for sex education books. They have diagrams that can help you learn the names and locations of genital parts.

End this exercise with a "hand hug." Securely and comfortably rest your hand over your genital area. Remind yourself of the love and protection that you can give this special part of your body.

FUTURE VARIATIONS: (1) Draw a picture of your genital area. Use different colored pencils to represent how sensitive different areas are to touch (for example, a red pencil means intense sensations, a blue means few sensations). (2) Use modeling clay to sculpt your genitals, paying close attention to shape and texture.

GENITAL EXPLORATION, WITH PARTNER

PURPOSE: To share knowledge and reduce anxiety about genitals
SUGGESTED TIME: Thirty minutes

Both you and your partner need to have done the getting to know your genitals exercise before doing this exercise. First do the cleansing and safe embrace exercises with your partner. Taking turns (survivor decides who goes first), move into a position in which your partner is able to see your genitals easily. Point to and name the different parts of your genitals for your partner. Feel free to share what you learned about the different parts of your genitals with your partner, such as what areas are sensitive to what kinds of touches. Ask questions of each other about your genitals. When you are done end the exercise with a safe embrace.

FUTURE VARIATIONS: Touch and name out loud the different parts of your partner's genitals.

PLEASURING

BODY MASSAGE, WITH PARTNER

PURPOSE: To explore touch sensations with a partner
SUGGESTED TIME: Twenty to forty minutes

Wearing loose clothing in a warm room, start with a safe embrace. Let your partner know when you feel ready to begin massage. Have your partner undress to a degree that you choose, such as to underwear or no clothes. Direct your partner to lie down on a comfortable surface—on the bed or on a blanket on the floor. Position your partner lying on his or her back or stomach, depending on what you feel more relaxed with. Begin touching your partner from head to toe, excluding breasts and genitals. Start with parts of your partner's body that are most familiar to you. Touch in ways that feel comfortable to you. Eventually have your partner roll over, and touch the other side of your partner's body.

In general your partner is to remain receptive and relaxed. However, your partner should speak up if you are touching in such a way that is uncomfortable or unpleasant. If this occurs, it's best for the partner to

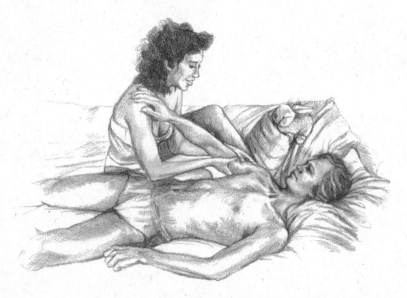

Body massaging with a partner

suggest a different kind of touch. A partner might say, "I feel uncomfortable when you touch my elbow. Rubbing higher up on my arm would feel better." The partner states his or her experience and then *gives specific directions* for how the survivor can make the touch more comfortable. When these communications are in practice, the survivor can focus on touch sensations without having to worry about the partner's experience.

Focus on the sensations that you receive to your hands as you touch. Let yourself experiment with different ways to touch, such as rubbing, stroking, and caressing. Notice the different textures in your partner's body—hairy, smooth, hard, and soft. What places do you find most enjoyable to touch?

End the session in a way that feels comfortable to you. You might want to cover your partner in a blanket, do a safe embrace, or sit and talk for awhile.

FUTURE VARIATIONS: (1) After touching your partner switch roles so that you are lying down and your partner is the one touching you. Use red light–green light exercise to remind you of your ability to control the experience, and stop and communicate frequently. For a bridge you may want to place your hand gently over your partner's hand while your partner touches you. This way you can guide your partner in touching you until you feel more comfortable. (2) Include genital and breast areas, but touch them only as you would any other part of the body. (3) Massage each other simultaneously. Survivor decides whether to wear clothes and when to start and stop.

GENITAL PLEASURING

PURPOSE: To discover pleasurable ways to touch your genital area
SUGGESTED TIME: Twenty to thirty minutes

Begin with the safe nest and getting to know your genitals exercises. Experiment with different types of touch to your genital area. Use a personal lubricant* to create new types of sensation and make genital touch easier. Try circular movements, stroking, light and hard touches. Breathe consciously. Pay attention to what you feel. Stay present and mentally relaxed. Gradually shift from experimenting with touch to touching yourself in ways that increase pleasurable sensations. If orgasm occurs, that is allowable but not your goal for now. End each session with a gentle hand hug to your genital area.

FUTURE VARIATION: Do the exercise while being held by an intimate partner.

---

* Several brands of personal lubricants are available in drugstores, such as Astroglide, Probe, Sylk, and K-Y Liquid.

GENITAL PLEASURING, WITH PARTNER

PURPOSE: To explore genital touch and pleasuring
SUGGESTED TIME: Thirty to sixty minutes

Begin with cleansing exercise with partner and safe embrace. Shift into the body massage exercise, variation 2, in which you include breasts and genitals in exploratory touch. Decide which role you would like to begin with, either you touching your partner's genital area or your partner touching your genital area.

When you are in the role of being touched, place your hand gently over your partner's hand for a while, directing your partner in the places and style you like to be touched. Communicate with your partner frequently. Indicate which touches you like best. Stop at any time. You may want to end with your hand resting over your partner's hand as your partner's hand hugs your genital area.

When you are in the role of touching your partner's genital area, feel free to ask your partner questions as you touch: "Does this feel good? How hard can I press here before it would be uncomfortable? What does it feel like when I pull at the skin here?" Touch only as much as you feel comfortable touching in any given session.

FUTURE VARIATIONS: Explore touching the genital area with other parts of the body, such as the feet, cheeks, mouth, or tongue.

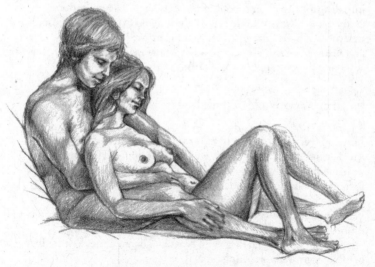

Genital pleasuring with a partner

Relearning touch exercises make it possible to gradually move from playful, friendly touch to sexual touch. We stay present, relaxed, and in touch with our feelings. If we run into blocks, we have an opportunity to employ techniques, such as resting and relaxing, active awareness, and creative problem solving, as well as the four-step approach to handling automatic reactions described in chapter 7. The new experiences we have help our old fears subside. A male survivor who wasn't in a relationship gave his reaction:

> It was fun creating and playing with a basket full of toys and other things to touch. I also bought some bubble bath and body lotion. Using them was nurturing. My inner child had a nice soothing time. I became aware that there is a large part of me that wants to be held. These exercises are a nice break from the struggles of abuse recovery.

For survivors currently in an intimate relationship, the relearning touch exercises offer an opportunity for continuing self-awareness, as well as for establishing a new format for physical intimacy and sharing with your partner. A survivor described her experience:

> I had a difficult time with all levels of touching with my partner initially. Just the plain touching was new to me as a sensation to enjoy. I had always told myself that if somebody touches me, especially touches me "there," then that means we have to have sex, and sex was not fun. Touching was a whole new area for me. It was scary and difficult, but it was worth it in the end.

Another survivor told of the advances he had made:

> I used to feel afraid and uptight. I worried if I touched my wife, she'd accuse me of not knowing what I was doing. The exercises gave me permission to slowly explore her body. I'm overcoming my fears and realizing how much we are alike, even though we have different bodies. It's amazing to have lived with my wife for ten years and only now be aware of those freckles and funny little hairs on her body. I felt like I was fumbling in the dark for so long, wrapped up in fear and fantasies. Now I've opened the door and am actually learning something new.

Yet another survivor said:

> In the past, when I'd think of my husband's body, I'd picture him
> with a big hole in his genital area. I hated to think about his penis.
> It was as if his penis was a barometer for my fears. If it was small,
> my fears were small; as it got larger, fear rose inside me. Whenever
> my husband's penis would touch me, I'd feel small, scared, and like
> I was expected to have sex. Now, after doing these exercises, I'm
> not afraid of his penis anymore. It's a part of his body, connected to
> who he is and to the love in his heart for me.

When you relearn touch, you increase your ability to experience
pleasure on your own and, eventually, with a trusted partner. After several months of exercises a survivor described her progress:

> I've reached a place where my desire to have fun is stronger than
> my fears. I can feel safe, without turning off or blocking out. I'm
> feeling better about allowing sensations of pleasure to occur. Each
> time I do and it goes well, I've come to believe more and more that
> nothing bad will happen if I do feel pleasure.

As you have worked through these exercises, you have begun to acquire
a new, healthier collection of memories about touch. In the future
repeating these exercises may help you solve specific problems with sexual functioning or may simply reinforce what you have learned—that
touch is a source of comfort, security, and pleasure.

As you become more comfortable with touch, you may enjoy
inventing new exercises to expand on these healthy feelings. Remember
to emphasize safety, nonpressured exploring, and graduated success. Let
those be your guides as you continue on your healing journey.

11

Solving Specific Sexual Problems

Traditional sex therapy techniques for sexual dysfunctions
may actually be harmful to survivors, unless they are well
down the road to overall recovery from sexual abuse.

—MIRIAM SMOLOVER, *Therapist*

Practically everyone experiences a troublesome sexual problem sometime in life. Some sexual problems are temporary and go away on their
own. Others persist. The sexual problems that result from sexual abuse
are usually persistent problems. Solving them requires our active attention.

Problems with sexual functioning, interest, and relating often plague
survivors over the course of many years. Some survivors have never felt
a strong interest in having sex. For others sexual problems may have surfaced only recently, as a result of their sexual healing work. A survivor
who has learned to stop fantasizing about sexual abuse, for example,
may now have difficulty becoming aroused.

Now is a good time in the sexual healing journey for survivors to
address specific sexual problems. Survivors have gained new under-
standings about the relationship between sex and sexual abuse, made
important changes, and have developed new skills for relearning touch
and sex. By this time in the journey, many survivors feel less apprehen-
sive about sexual activity, having learned that sexual touch is just one
expression of physical intimacy.

In this chapter we will examine the causes of a variety of sexual
problems and learn specific ways to solve each of them.

FINDING THE TRUE CAUSE OF A SPECIFIC SEXUAL PROBLEM

Sexual problems have a wide range of causes. Some can result from organic causes, such as medical conditions, physical injuries, and the effects of certain drugs.* Others stem from psychological causes or specific life events, such as stress, inadequate sex education, rigid parental attitudes against sex, interpersonal problems, and bad experiences like sexual abuse. While there may be good reason to believe a current problem stems from early abuse, it is unwise to assume that sexual abuse is the only, or even primary, cause of all our sexual problems.

A good first step is to see a medical professional and, perhaps, a certified sex therapist† to determine if the sexual problem might have an underlying cause other than sexual abuse. Without accurate diagnosis you run the risk of spinning your wheels in trying to heal a sexual problem.

Wanda, for example, was plagued by vaginal discomfort during intercourse. A twenty-five-year-old rape survivor, she assumed this problem resulted from sexual abuse. During intercourse she would focus on relaxing and reminding herself that her present partner was not an offender. She and her partner would begin intercourse slowly, and Wanda would stop frequently to reassure herself that she was in control of her experience. But her discomfort continued. Finally Wanda went to her gynecologist, who examined her and suggested that a minor yeast infection might be causing the problem. Wanda got rid of the infection, and, to her amazement, intercourse felt fine.

When Chuck, a thirty-five-year-old survivor of childhood molestation, entered a sexual abuse survivor support group, he began having difficulty with erection and ejaculation. His erections didn't seem as firm as they used to be, sometimes he ejaculated quickly, and on a few

---

* The most common organic causes include diabetes, alcoholism, spinal cord injury, multiple sclerosis, infections, injuries to the genitals, hormone deficiencies, circulatory problems, prescription drugs (such as for high blood pressure and depression), and street drugs (such as amphetamines, barbiturates, and narcotics).

† In the Resources section, see American Association of Sex Educators, Counselors, and Therapists (AASECT) to obtain a list of certified sex therapists in your area. Before setting up an appointment, interview the therapist to make sure he or she has specialized training in sexual abuse treatment. As with finding any therapist, you may also want to talk with people in your community, such as physicians and people in referral agencies, who are familiar with the therapist's approach and work.

occasions he felt pain at the base of his penis. Chuck assumed that these symptoms were expressions of unresolved emotional pain related to the abuse. For months his sexual problems continued. Chuck read sex therapy books and tried the techniques in them to no avail. Finally Chuck went to a urologist for a checkup. He had a low-grade prostate infection. After he took antibiotics, his sex problems disappeared.

Like Wanda and Chuck, many survivors may be too quick to assume that sexual abuse is the sole or primary cause of a sexual problem. A number of factors can combine to create a sexual problem for survivors. It may be hard for you to weed out how much of the problem relates to abuse.

Let's consider Jesse, who has difficulty reaching orgasm. As a child Jesse was taught that masturbation was disgusting and sinful. Because of the messages from her family, Jesse never experimented with touching her own genitals for pleasure. In high school Jesse was raped by a young man she had been dating. During the rape the offender called her a slut. Now in her twenties, Jesse is married and very much in love with her husband. She wants to experience orgasms. For Jesse the combination of sexual abuse and her antisex upbringing lay at the root of her present sexual problem. Becoming orgasmic will require not only her overcoming the sexual trauma experienced in the rape but also her resolving the negative effects of her upbringing.

ANXIETY MAKES SEXUAL PROBLEMS WORSE

Sexual problems may make us worried, guilty, or depressed, further deepening our problem. We may dwell on thoughts like, "I'm not normal," "I'm inferior sexually," "No one would want me for a partner if they knew," "I've failed the partner I have," or, "I'll never be able to change."

Lonnie, a survivor of mother-son incest, made himself sick with worry after experiencing a few days of erection problems. His erection problems began after a horrible nightmare in which his mother stood over his bed laughing at him while he was making love to his girlfriend. Although Lonnie had never had difficulty with erections in the past, after the dream he convinced himself his problem now signalled doom. He worried he'd never get an erection again and that his girlfriend would leave him. His anxiety festered, causing the problem to persist. Lonnie was able to overcome his anxiety by realizing his erection difficulty was a normal, although upsetting, response to the nightmare. As his anxiety went down, his erectile capacity went up.

Barry McCarthy, a Washington, D.C., sex therapist, wrote, "The male who can accept an occasional unsatisfactory experience without it threatening his sexual self-esteem inoculates himself against sexual dysfunction."* Changing how we feel about having a sexual problem is a large part of the solution.

SEXUAL PROBLEMS AND THEIR SOLUTIONS

Let's examine some common sexual problems involving sexual interest, functioning, and relating that may result from sexual abuse. Some problems may apply to you; others will not.

LACK OF SEXUAL INTEREST

Inhibited desire
Fear of sex

DIFFICULTY BECOMING AROUSED AND FEELING SENSATION

Lack of lubrication in women
Lack of erection (impotence) in men

DIFFICULTY EXPERIENCING ORGASM

Lack of orgasm in women
Inhibited ejaculation in men

DIFFICULTY AVERTING ORGASM

Premature ejaculation in men
Rapid orgasm in women

DIFFICULTY WITH INTERCOURSE, FOR WOMEN SURVIVORS

Muscle spasm, pain, and discomfort
Fear of penetration

---

* Barry McCarthy, "Developing Positive Intimacy Cognitions in Males with a History of Nonintimate Sexual Experiences," *Journal of Sex & Marital Therapy*, 13, no. 4 (Winter 1987): 256.

Men and women experience many similar problems. Sexually they are alike in many ways, with similar response patterns and physiological likenesses that can be traced to the womb. At about six weeks' gestation, male hormones influence male embryos to develop a penis and scrotal sac; these organs develop from the same tissues that become a clitoris and the outer vaginal lips in a female. In adults of both sexes, these organs contain sensitive tissues that engorge with blood during arousal as well as muscles that contract at intervals of eight-tenths of a second during orgasm.

When all is working well sexually, women and men both go through the same four stages in the sexual response cycle: excitement (initial building of sexual arousal), plateau (high levels of sexual arousal are maintained and intensified), orgasm (discharging of sexual tension in pelvic floor muscle contractions), and resolution (return to the unaroused state).

Satisfying, healthy intimate relating, of course, involves much more than going through these four stages. Our sexual functioning is a minor part of sexual intimacy. We can soothe and nurture ourselves physically, or cuddle, hug, touch, and whisper sweet words with a partner, regardless of whether we've been functioning in a particular way and whether we feel ready to have sex. *We don't have to let a specific sexual problem we encounter get in the way of warm, enjoyable feelings or interfere with intimacy.*

Sexual functioning problems occur when we choose to have sex and are not able to move through the sexual response cycle with ease and satisfaction, or when we are unable to share our experience with an intimate partner. We become concerned, and even though these problems don't preclude physical intimacy, we still want to improve our ability to feel sexually aroused, have orgasms, or engage in sexual relations and intercourse.

During the past twenty-five years, excellent techniques have been developed to help both men and women successfully overcome their sexual problems. These techniques are based on behavioral methods that reduce anxiety and reshape sexual responses. They were developed on the premise that sexual behavior is learned and therefore can be unlearned and then relearned in a new way.

Sex therapy techniques can be used effectively by survivors but only when the techniques are adapted as they have been in this book—to address survivors' fears and anxieties about sex. Survivors need to modify the techniques to respect their needs to go slowly, feel in control of what's happening, handle automatic reactions, and deal with feelings that might surface that are related to the abuse.* Without these special adaptations, traditional sex therapy techniques can overwhelm survivors, encouraging them to lapse into old, harmful sexual behavior patterns. Survivors whose needs are not met in sex therapy may resume sexual relations before they are ready or may mentally dissociate from the experience. Their healing journey can be interrupted or pushed back.

Overcoming sexual problems takes time, just as relearning touch does. Healing requires a special time and a private, secure environment set aside for doing exercises. You will use new skills—relaxation, active awareness, and creative problem solving (described in chapter 10)—to make changes gradually. You proceed in small, progressive steps, from less challenging to more challenging experiences. Eventually, you will learn sexual responsiveness and functioning in a new way, free from the negative associations of past abuse.

Sexual functioning is *nonvolitional*. This means we can't become sexually aroused or have an orgasm by sheer force of will any more than we can "make ourselves" fall asleep. The best we can do is create situations in which we are likely to have the kind of experiences we want. Then we can let go, relax, and let responses happen.

You may not currently have a specific sexual problem you need to address. Still you will probably find the explanations, stories, and suggestions offered in this chapter helpful in enhancing your sexual experiences.

Let's take a look at specific sexual problems and see how survivors have addressed them effectively.

Lack of Sexual Interest

Lack of sexual interest seems to be the most common specific sexual problem of survivors. Some survivors have an inhibited desire for sex; rarely if ever do they think about wanting to engage in sex. Other survivors may have a lack of sexual interest because of fears of sex or fears of the automatic reactions and responses that may be triggered during sex. Survivors who have been overly interested or preoccupied with sex may find that their interest in sex plummets when they stop compulsive

---

* For detailed descriptions of traditional sex therapy techniques and how they were developed, refer to the books by Barbach, Castleman, Crooks and Baur, Kaplan, McCarthy and McCarthy, Masters and Johnson, and Zilbergeld in the Resources section.

sexual behaviors. An excessive interest in sex can mask underlying inhibitions and fears.

When we consider how much pain and suffering is often caused by sexual abuse, we begin to understand why, after abuse, many survivors lack interest in sex. When sex hurts it's natural to want to avoid it. Turning off one's sexual feelings during abuse is adaptive and protective. We may unconsciously teach ourselves ways to block or muffle awareness of our natural sexual feelings. We may keep ourselves so busy and mentally preoccupied that sexual feelings can't develop.

Continuing this pattern now cheats you of a chance to enjoy intimacy. By now you have learned that healthy sex is different from abusive sex. Perhaps you are in situations in which sex could be safe and pleasurable. Instead of protecting you, a continuing lack of interest in sex now cuts off your pleasure and robs you of the joy of building a special connection with an intimate partner.

To awaken sexual interest, survivors must believe sex is good and that you can feel good about yourself when you are sexual. You also need to know you can handle whatever troublesome reactions are triggered, including fear, discomfort, overexcitement, and flashbacks.

Relationship problems can also diminish sexual desire. Survivors may feel angry or resentful toward a partner because of unpleasant sexual experiences in the past. Some partners communicate the idea that sex is a duty the survivor owes. When this occurs a survivor may get stuck in a power struggle with the partner and hardened to the position that "you can't make me want it!" As long as the partner is seen as an adversary instead of an ally, the lack of desire will probably persist.

Survivors may worry that they will be pounced on by their partners as soon as they show some desire for sex. They may fear the partners will be disappointed if they choose not to act on their desire or that they will expect sex more frequently if they do. Assertiveness and clear communication can help survivors feel safe to explore sexual interest as it emerges and as they feel ready to proceed.

Courtship is also important to people. We tend to forget that we have our own unique mating dances. It's foolish for many of us to think we can go all day without seeing our intimate partner and then expect to get in bed at night and want sex. Sexual desire comes from sharing time, making eye contact, talking, playing, and making nonsexual connections first. You may find your interest in sex increasing as you get in touch with your inner child, build trust with your partner, and practice the relearning touch exercises in chapter 10.

To decrease fear and increase sexual interest, survivors and their partners need to reach an understanding. I believe two ground rules are essential:

1. Expressing interest in sex is not a commitment to sexual activity.
2. Declining sex is not an absolute rejection.

These ground rules about sex are so important that it's worth taking time to learn them in practice. The following exercise can help you and your partner understand and work through issues related to initiating and declining sex. By relieving interpersonal strain and sexual pressure, you can give sexual interest a chance to evolve naturally (see box, pg. 286–87).

Learning skills in initiating and declining sex can increase empathy in couples in which one person has been the initiator more often than the other. A woman survivor who had never initiated sex with her husband was surprised at her reaction when she played the initiator role and her husband declined.

> I didn't expect it, but I felt rejected. I thought I would feel relief when he declined, but I didn't—I felt sad. Now I know how he must feel sometimes.

The survivor's husband enjoyed being in the role of decliner. He liked hearing his wife express her sexual interest in him, something he had never heard her say before. He was pleased to hear her tell him that his smooth skin and warm touch attracted her. It made him feel better about not having sex, just knowing his wife had some positive feelings toward him.

When you do feel ready to have sex, it must be for yourself, not mainly to satisfy your partner. You can allow your interest in sex to emerge by increasing communication with your partner and becoming clear on how sexual possibilities will be pursued, as this survivor explained:

> I talk openly with my partner about the fears that come up when I'm approached romantically—how I worry that I'll be expected to engage in sex. He listens, and then we talk together about how we can be more safe and comfortable. Then we gently touch each other, massage and stroke one another. Sometimes this develops into sex and mutual orgasms, but if it doesn't, that's okay.

PRACTICE INITIATING AND DECLINING SEX EXERCISE

Purpose: To improve communication skills, increase empathy, and reduce pressure regarding expressing interest in sexual activity

In this role-play exercise you and your partner take turns initiating and declining sexual activity. You merely practice these roles. No sexual activity is to take place as a result of the exercise.

Sit in a comfortable position facing your partner, about two or three feet from each other. The survivor chooses which role he or she would like to start out in. There is an "initiator" and a "decliner." You are like actors, playing roles. You do not need to feel the feelings you express just now.

The initiator speaks first for about three minutes. The initiator begins by expressing sexual interest—"I am interested in having sex with you . . ."—and then continues by making at least three statements that express why the initiator wants to have sex.

An initiator might then say, "I respect you and like the person you are. I find you sexually attractive. I appreciate our life together and want to be close with you in a special way. . . ."

The initiator then describes what he or she would like to have happen: "I would like to spend some time cuddling with you and talking. Then I would like us to undress and touch each other gently. Then I would like us to kiss." And so on.

As the initiator speaks the decliner simply listens. It is understood that this is not a "real" initiation but rather a chance to practice. Be honest and specific about what you find attractive in your partner and how you imagine a positive sexual encounter could proceed.

Next it is the decliner's turn to respond for about three minutes. The decliner begins by thanking the initiator for expressing sexual interest. Then the decliner directly declines the invitation. For instance, "I appreciate your interest in having sex with me; however, I am not interested in having sex right now."

The decliner continues by repeating back to the initiator appreciative words for the positive things the initiator expressed, such as "I am glad that you find me sexually attractive. It makes me feel good knowing you respect me and want to show me your love sexually. I like the idea that we would cuddle before undressing." And so on. The initiator listens when the decliner speaks.

The decliner focuses on refusing the sexual initiation in a gracious and respectful manner. The overall message is that you feel fortunate for the invitation, but you're simply not interested at this time.

When the decliner is finished, take a few minutes to notice how each of you feels. When you are ready, switch roles and do the exercise in the opposite role. When this second part of the exercise is complete, spend some time talking together about what you each felt in the roles of initiator and decliner. Which was easier for you to playact? What did you learn about yourself and your partner? When you initiated sex, did you do it as a statement of your feelings—"I am interested in having sex with you"—or did you slip into making a demand—"I want you to have sex with me." Demand initiations tend to increase anxiety in the decliner.

Repeat this exercise several times. You may notice that you feel more comfortable in a role the more you practice playing that role.

Relationships are not the only key to sexual desire. Take time to think about how you view sexual desire. Do you see sexual interest as sharp and urgent, like hunger, or do you view it as fulsome, like the ripening of a fruit on the vine? To develop your interest in sex, I recommend you adopt the second perspective. Sexual interest is something we can learn to cultivate and let ripen. (This becomes especially important as we age. A hormonal rush can't always be counted on to awaken our sexual desires.)

Give yourself permission to cultivate the gentle awareness of your senses. Becoming sensual can naturally lead to becoming sexual. What kinds of sensual experiences do you enjoy? Lying in the sun? Walking on a smooth carpet? Taking a warm bath? Make sensual experiences a priority in your life.

If you want to be more interested in sex, you can take a more direct approach to awakening and developing your sensuality. By engaging in activities that stimulate feelings of sexual arousal or in which you receive and enjoy direct genital stimulation, natural desires are likely to grow.

Here are some suggestions:

1. Do relearning touch exercises.
2. Imagine having sex in a way that you would enjoy.

3. Engage in foreplay such as hugging, kissing, and fondling with your partner.
4. Stimulate your genital area while bathing, resting, or cuddling with your partner.

Sexual interest can be cultivated but not pushed. You need to find a delicate balance between the voice in you saying, "I don't want to do this," and the voice saying, "I'll give it a try." Remember, you can say no at any time, and you can make little steps forward. You have a right to be sexual. Respectful, healthy sex is good.

Difficulty becoming aroused and feeling sensation

Sexual arousal increases our interest in sex, and it helps our bodies to prepare physiologically for intercourse and other sexual activities. When survivors have trouble becoming aroused, it can be very upsetting. Desire can plummet. Women may notice a lack of vaginal secretions that normally lubricate the vagina. The internal walls of their vaginas may fail to expand adequately. Sexual intercourse and other forms of vaginal penetration may be extremely uncomfortable, if not painful. For male survivors arousal difficulties are more externally obvious. A man may have problems getting and maintaining an erection. Under these circumstances, intercourse and other sexual activities may become difficult or even impossible.

There are many reasons why sexual abuse causes arousal difficulties. During sexual abuse, survivors may have learned to cope with confusing, unwanted pleasurable sensations or to endure violence and pain by numbing their sexual areas. This response, while crucial to enduring the abuse, may have become so ingrained and automatic that it cripples sexual responsiveness in the present. To help themselves overcome problems with numbing, survivors need to remember that the sexual abuse is over. They can control their sexual experiences. Practicing new ways of taking care of themselves during sex, such as asserting feelings and needs, setting limits, directing touch, and stopping sexual activity when necessary, can help survivors affirm their sensuality rather than deny it.

For both men and women, problems with numbing can also be approached with a process called *sensation retraining*. Let's say a woman survivor has little or no sensation in her clitoris, even after ten minutes of touching herself. She does, however, experience pleasurable sensations while stimulating her nipples. The woman can retrain her clitoris to feel sensation by spending time first touching her nipples and then simultaneously touching her clitoris. Through this technique she can begin to pair the pleasurable sensations in her nipples with her clitoris—sensation by association. After several sessions like this, the woman may start to notice warm, tingly feelings starting in her clitoris. Eventually these sensations will be noticeable when she touches just her clitoris.

For some survivors their own sexual arousal triggers negative feelings associated with being sexually victimized. As described in chapter 7, these automatic reactions are the result of a crystallizing of the traumatic experiences that occurred during abuse: strong emotional feelings became unconsciously linked with sensations of arousal. Avoiding arousal may be an unconscious attempt to avoid feeling afraid, angry, disgusted, or confused.

Some survivors block arousal because they maintain a negative view of sex and feel guilty for desiring sexual activity, as this survivor described:

> Sometimes when I masturbate to release tension, I lose an erection because I start thinking about how gross sex is and that I shouldn't be doing what I'm doing. I have to make a conscious effort to remind myself that this kind of self-stimulation is healthy and has nothing to do with sexual abuse.

Some survivors believe that becoming aroused will make them similar to the offender. After all, the offender was sexually aroused during the abuse. For these survivors arousal represents a sudden transformation into a person who is bad, out-of-control, or sexually demanding. A survivor of father-son incest told of his problem:

> Sometimes when making love, I lose my erection because I think of how sexually demanding my father was of me. I worry that I'm being sexually demanding toward my wife. It's a very lonely feeling when you think that you're demanding sex and you're unsure it's really desired by your wife. I need a lot of reassurance from my wife that she's enjoying the contact before I can continue.

Survivors may have difficulty mentally separating signs of their own healthy sexual arousal from memories of the offender and the abuse. When this happens, arousal symptoms, such as heavy breathing, warm feelings, increasing pulse, and the swelling of sexual organs, can become more disturbing than enjoyable. A man may be upset by his own erection, a woman by her vaginal secretions or the natural swelling of her clitoris.

Mattie, a survivor of father-daughter incest, noticed that during masturbation, as her clitoris became firm, it would remind her of her father's penis. Immediately she would lose her arousal. Her aroused clitoris had become a trigger for the loss of sexual arousal. Mattie used techniques described in chapter 7 to calm herself, affirm her present reality, and build new associations to her clitoris. She imagined that her clitoris was a button glowing with a pure and healing white light. Its luminescence reflected the love and caring she felt for herself and her partner. By creating her own positive associations, Mattie was eventually able to experience sustained, pleasurable sensations.

It can help to remember that arousal is a healthy human response and in itself has nothing to do with abuse. Sexual arousal represents a desire to feel pleasure and connect in loving ways. Actress Mae West used to tease, "Is that a pistol in your pocket, or are you just happy to see me?"

Survivors can make progress overcoming problems with sexual arousal by paying attention to and challenging their attitudes about sexual arousal. Dennis, a survivor who was upset at the sight of his own erection, said:

> During sex, I remind myself that I am very different from my uncle, the offender. My uncle used his penis as a weapon to exploit and hurt me. I think of my penis as a special part of me that enhances my partner's pleasure as well as my own. I also remind myself that *my arousal is different* than my uncle's arousal. He was aroused to sexually abuse. I'm turned on to having healthy, mutually desired and loving sex.

Survivors can also use progressive exercises, such as the genital awareness and pleasuring exercises described in chapter 10, to help them gradually learn to awaken sensation and experience increasing intensities of arousal. These exercises allow survivors to feel safe and become more comfortable with stronger sensations, one small step at a time. Later, when a survivor feels ready, his or her partner can participate in the exercises as well, so that the survivor can slowly become used to feeling aroused in the partner's presence.

Male survivors can combine the genital pleasuring exercises with other techniques to address impotence and other erectile problems. A man can spend relaxed, private time doing a progressive series of exercises designed to help him tune in to pleasurable sensations and strengthen his erectile capabilities. These exercises include such activities as stroking himself when his penis is flaccid, masturbating until he has an erection and then purposefully stopping until he is flaccid again, and masturbating to fantasies of having sex with a partner, of losing and gaining an erection with a partner, and of having sex in a way that requires no erection at all.

Another approach to solving problems with arousal is to focus on reducing anxiety. Eros is in the mind. If we are physically healthy, our ability to become aroused has more to do with what's going on in our heads than what's happening with our genitals. Worry and anxiety potentiate arousal problems. The more anxious we feel, the less aroused we become. Conversely, the less anxiety we experience, the more aroused we can get.

A male survivor can reduce anxiety by learning to sexually satisfy his partner regardless of whether he has an erection, using methods such as hand, mouth, or vibrator stimulation. When the pressure's off the importance of an erection, a man can create experiences that increase his ability to feel sensations and arousal, and allow him to become more spontaneous in sexual play.

Women survivors can reduce anxiety about vaginal lubrication. While lubrication and relaxation are often signs that a woman is sexually aroused, the absence of lubrication is not an automatic indicator that a woman is not aroused. The amount of lubrication fluctuates throughout a woman's life, decreasing as women age. Lubrication can also vary with a woman's menstrual cycle. It often becomes more pronounced during ovulation.

Since lubrication is not always a reliable measure of arousal, it is best to not make vaginal lubrication a big issue. Use saliva to lubricate the genital area during stimulation and penetration, or keep a safe, commercial lubricant handy and apply it generously before, and several times during, sexual activities that involve vaginal penetration or touching. In deciding whether you are ready to have sex, pay more attention to what you're feeling in your heart and mind than whether you're lubricated.

Learning to feel comfortable becoming sexually aroused opens new doors for self-respect and appreciation. In an atmosphere of safety and support you can enjoy the tingles of sensation and the waves of excitement that your body is naturally capable of experiencing. Allowing yourself to feel sexually aroused is a way of allowing yourself to feel fully alive.

Difficulty experiencing orgasm

Some survivors have difficulty reaching orgasm at all times. Others encounter problems with experiencing orgasm only in certain situations, such as with a partner.

Abuse often inhibits natural curiosity about our genital sensations. We may fail to explore our own bodies and thereby fail to learn how our sexual feelings build to a climax. A survivor said:

> In the past my difficulties with orgasm came from not knowing enough about my sexuality and what stimulation would bring me to orgasm. Because of the abuse, I didn't believe in my right to pleasure and sexual satisfaction, in my right to speak about what I wanted, or in my right to explore and find out what it was I did want in sex. I was depending on my partner to happen to find the right thing to do.

When orgasm problems are due to a lack of self-exploration, survivors can often make great progress by spending time in self-discovery and genital pleasuring exercises.

> I never had an orgasm until a few years ago when I started masturbating for the first time. I read a book about masturbation and thought I'd experiment. Before that I thought sex in any form was gross and disgusting. It's been very healing to have a sexual experience in which I feel satisfied, strong, and sexual. Becoming more comfortable with loving myself in that way helps me know that sex between people can be a nice thing as well.

Because of abuse, some survivors avoided learning about sexual functioning, or they were given false information by the offender. Survivors may fail to reach orgasm because they have been going about it wrong. For example, a heterosexual survivor who has had trouble having orgasm during intercourse may not realize that most women need direct stimulation of the clitoris during intercourse for orgasm to occur. Unless she learns to touch herself, or have her partner stimulate her with his fingers during intercourse, orgasm is not likely to happen. Penile thrusting alone isn't enough for many women.

Survivors may not understand how pelvic muscle strength figures in orgasms. Pelvic floor muscles must be in good condition for a survivor to feel an orgasm when it does occur. Not only do these muscles facilitate orgasm, strong pelvic floor muscles also are directly related to pleasure and enjoyment of orgasm. Whether you are male or female, you can strengthen these muscles using a series of muscle tightening and releasing exercises, known as *Kegel exercises*.* In Kegels, you tighten the same muscles you would need to tighten to stop yourself from urinating in midstream. Tighten hard slowly, pause, then release slowly. Practicing ten minutes of Kegels a day for six weeks is usually sufficient to get these muscles in condition.

Some survivors may have problems reaching orgasm because the sexual abuse damaged their perception of sex and sexual relationships. A survivor told how he solved his inability to have an orgasm:

In the early months of our marriage, I became scared that I couldn't have an orgasm with my wife. It seemed like we were having sex for hours, but I just wouldn't come. Then one day a thought flashed to me: Sex equals power. My thinking went, if I don't have an orgasm, I can prolong sex and be powerful. I realized I didn't want power over the woman I love. That evening's lovemaking was different. With the power element gone I had my orgasm and felt closer to her.

Unresolved feelings toward the offender and the abuse can interfere with orgasmic ability. A survivor with inhibited ejaculation problems realized a connection between his orgasmic difficulty and the fear of abandonment he still felt toward his mother, the offender.

Sex will sometimes start my abandonment issues. I become scared that my lover will abandon me, like my mother did. It's confusing because my lover sometimes enjoys it when I last a long time. But for me it's torture. I become so anxious, I sweat with fear. I feel I'm withholding my coming and myself from my partner to protect myself. Meantime I'm losing out.

Positive self-talk can help survivors overcome distorted beliefs. These beliefs may have developed as a result of the abuse or as means of self-protection. But allowing them to persist now may be inhibiting

* For a more detailed description of Kegel exercises, see *Our Sexuality* by Robert Crooks and Karla Baur, listed in the Resources section.

your ability to experience orgasm. Positive self-talk is a way to separate your attitudes about sexual functioning from the influence of the abuse. Here is an example of how a woman survivor might challenge her negative and inhibiting beliefs about having orgasm:

> *Inhibiting belief*: When my partner is stimulating me, he's trying to make me have an orgasm.
> *Alternative belief*: Regardless of whether I am touching myself or whether my partner is touching me, the arousal I experience is something I'm feeling for myself, not for anyone else.

> *Inhibiting belief*: It's horribly shameful for me to become aroused and have an orgasm in front of my partner.
> *Alternative belief*: My sexual responses are natural and normal. My partner cares for me and enjoys being with me when I'm feeling good.

> *Inhibiting belief*: Having an orgasm is giving in, losing, and getting hurt.
> *Alternative belief*: Sex is something I engage in because I want to. I like the feelings that happen in sex. I am in control of when, where, how, and with whom I have sex. Orgasm is a simple biological response and can't hurt me. It's made up of my feelings and sensations, not some concrete or external object. My orgasms are part of me. They emerge from inside me. Orgasms are an intense expression of my aliveness. The feeling I get from them is a natural way for me to feel pleasure.

Another way survivors can facilitate orgasm is by reducing triggers associated with the original sexual abuse. Have sex in a way that isn't related to what occurred during the abuse. If you were lying down when you were abused and find that climaxing while lying down now is difficult, try having sex while reclining on pillows but still sitting up. If the abuse involved manual stimulation, try oral stimulation instead.

Once you feel confident having orgasms in one way, you can use bridging techniques to have orgasms in other ways. A male survivor who can ejaculate with oral stimulation can bridge to intercourse by fantasizing about intercourse during oral sex. In later sessions he might shift to intercourse once a high level of arousal has been achieved.

Similarly, a woman survivor who can easily have orgasm by touching herself can bridge to becoming orgasmic with a partner by stimulating

herself while being held by her partner and then placing her partner's
hand over her own while she self-stimulates. Later she might alternate
her hand with her partner's hand until she is comfortable having her
partner stimulate her to orgasm alone.

Massage vibrators* can also help in increasing orgasmic potential by
providing a type of stimulation that is different from what occurred in
the abuse. "Using a vibrator has helped me release feelings of guilt associated with receiving pleasure," a survivor said.

Some survivors may have difficulty with orgasm because of the fantasies they rely on to "get them over the hump" and climax. A heterosexual man may feel bad about his homosexual fantasies, a lesbian
survivor may feel bad about her heterosexual fantasies. Many survivors
may feel bad about sexual abuse fantasies. Accepting the fantasy and
learning a technique of switching away from it and back to it can help
you. A survivor who had trouble climaxing with her partner explained
her approach:

> I would use the fantasy to get me near orgasm. Then I'd shift my
> focus to the real situation with my partner right when I reached the
> "point of no return" and during my climax. With each time we had
> sex, I kept shifting earlier and earlier, until I could stay present
> most of the time.†

It's important to keep in mind that while orgasm does involve a surrender to pleasurable sensations, it does not bring about a loss of personal integrity or control. Orgasms can range from a barely noticed
muscle contraction to an intense feeling of release. We no more lose
control in orgasm than we do when we sneeze. We remain ourselves the
whole time. Learning to feel comfortable with the intensity of orgasm is
like learning to enjoy a good, hearty laugh. These are all natural functions that bring pleasant results.

---

* A variety of massage vibrators are available in many drugstores. For more information
on vibrators, you may want to refer to *Good Vibrations: The New Complete Guide to Vibrators*, rev. ed. (2000), by Joani Blank with Ann Whidden, which can be ordered from Good
Vibrations/Down There Press, 938 Howard Street, Suite 101, San Francisco, CA 94103,
(800) 289-8423, e-mail: goodvibe@well.com, web site: www.goodvibes.com.

† Additional exercises designed to reduce dependency on unwanted sexual fantasies can
be found in my book, *Private Thoughts: Exploring the Power of Women's Sexual Fantasies*.
(See the Resources section.)

Difficulty averting orgasm

Some survivors have the opposite problem: orgasms that come too quickly. A survivor may have found a quick orgasm helped in coping with stimulation, tension, or painful emotion felt during abuse. Also, sometimes the abuser left the child alone after orgasm; orgasm was a way to end the abuse more quickly.

As a result of past associations, sexual touch may trigger an early climax. A current situation may remind a survivor of the abuse in some ways. A survivor may feel caught in an intense buildup of anxiety and fear that erupts suddenly in an orgasm, as this survivor experienced:

After our first date I found myself in bed with this woman who wanted sex. We were both aroused. She came onto me, and inside myself I cried a silent cry, "No!" I was paralyzed. I left my body. Before I was inside her I ejaculated. I was crushed. I felt stupid, ashamed. She seemed to ignore what happened. I felt betrayed. I felt demoralized.

Abuse led another survivor to compulsive masturbation that involved rapid ejaculation. The man taught himself to ejaculate quickly to avoid feelings of guilt that accompanied his sexual behavior. "When I'd masturbate, I'd tell myself to hurry up so I won't get caught and get into trouble for what I was doing," he said.

Coming too soon may be related to fears of intimacy. A quick orgasm might allow a survivor to avoid building deeper emotional ties to the partner. A survivor might think that if there are no ties, he or she is protected against feeling betrayed and devastated if the relationship doesn't work out.

Coming quickly may also be an attempt to terminate the sexual experience. Sex in general may be so uncomfortable that the survivor seeks a quick escape. For example, a survivor may want to avoid witnessing the partner's orgasm if it reminds the survivor of the offender's sexual response in the abuse.

Anxiety-reduction techniques, such as relaxation and talking out fears with a partner or therapist, can help survivors overcome problems with rapid orgasm. Using a series of progressive techniques designed to treat premature ejaculation,* survivors can learn how to become more comfortable with increased levels of stimulation, how to recognize sig-

---

* For an excellent little book on this subject, see *How to Overcome Premature Ejaculation* by Helen Kaplan, listed in the Resources section.

nals in their body indicating orgasm is approaching, and how to slow down and postpone the orgasm.

If and when early orgasm does occur, it's best to treat it lightly. Continue with touch and sexual interaction anyway. Don't let the orgasm get in the way of building emotional intimacy with your partner. When you relax and experiment with further touching, over time you may be surprised that new feelings of arousal will surface. These new feelings can sometimes result in a second orgasm that builds more slowly and is more satisfying.

Don't avoid sex. The more you engage in sexual play, the more likely you will be to reduce anxiety and overexcitement tendencies.

Difficulty with intercourse, for women survivors

Women survivors may have difficulty with vaginal penetration because of two sexual problems.

Vaginismus is a reflexive tightening of the muscles in the outer third of the vagina when penetration is attempted. Women with this condition may have difficulty with intercourse as well as with insertion of a finger, dildo, or medical instrument.

Dyspareunia, or painful intercourse, is another dysfunction that can make intercourse difficult. In this condition, a woman experiences pain as burning, cramping, or sharpness that begins sometime during intercourse itself. Both vaginismus and dyspareunia can result from associating fear and pain of past sexual abuse with present intercourse. In some cases painful intercourse may be directly related to actual physical damage to vaginal tissues, nerves, and internal organs done during brutal sexual assault.

A woman who suffers pain during intercourse is likely to avoid sex. This avoidance can lead to further anxiety and discomfort. Natural arousal and lubrication may diminish, and vaginal sensitivity may feel more pronounced during the rare times that intercourse is attempted.

Conversely, some survivors have made matters worse by forcing themselves to endure painful intercourse. The abuse gets reenacted, and negative associations with intercourse are strengthened each time. As one survivor explained:

> I used to feel I had to put up with pain for a man's pleasure. I'd make myself have sex even when it hurt like crazy. I was mad at my partner and myself. It was the rape all over again.

No one should have to tolerate these kinds of pain or prolonged discomfort. But there is much a survivor can do to eventually be able to enjoy sexual experiences involving vaginal penetration. One way is to improve how you think of intercourse and vaginal penetration. If you conceive of intercourse as intrusion and force—something done to you—you may be setting yourself up for a bad experience. (At a seminar I gave for survivors, one woman pointed out that the term *penetration* was upsetting to begin with. She suggests survivors think of *enveloping* instead. A great idea! Imagine that you are enveloping your partner, giving your partner an internal hug. This reduces the sense of threat and reminds you that you are in the driver's seat.)

Changing our thinking can also be a powerful tool in helping relax muscles in the vagina. When you imagine the inside of a vagina, what do you picture? If you see it as a hard little tunnel with a thick steel door, you will approach the possibility of intercourse differently than if you see it as a warm, moist, earthy nook with soft moss and lovely flowers, or a smooth and stretching balloon capable of expanding to many times its size.

Relaxation techniques can be helpful as well. The Kegel exercises described earlier can give a woman a sense of control over the muscles in her vagina. After a woman becomes practiced at Kegels, she can try tightening her vaginal muscles and then relaxing them fully as entry occurs. Slow breathing techniques, commonly used in childbirth, can be incorporated to further facilitate relaxation during intercourse.

I have known survivors to have excellent success using vaginal dilator exercises to overcome problems with intercourse. Vaginal dilators are tube-shaped medical devices that vary in size from about one-half inch in diameter up to the average size of a penis. There are several different kinds: Some are shaped like small rubber penises, some are made of nonbreakable glass, and others are made of smooth white plastic.* Vaginal dilators allow survivors to slowly and progressively feel in control of and comfortable with vaginal penetration.

Here are some suggestions for how to use dilators in a healing program:

---

* Vaginal dilators can be purchased through medical supply stores and pharmaceutical companies. Consult your physician before obtaining and using them. I recommend a white plastic kind manufactured and distributed by Syracuse Medical Devices, Inc., 214 Hurlburt Road, Syracuse, NY 13224, phone: (315) 449-0657, fax: (315) 449-0756.

1. Warm the smallest-sized dilator in a glass of hot water by your bedside. Take a hot, relaxing bath. Dry off and sit back on your bed, reclining on soft pillows.

2. Take the warm dilator, dry it off, and cover the tip with a personal lubricant. Place a large dab of lubricant over your vaginal opening.

3. Relax, breathing fully and steadily. Do a few Kegel exercises to tighten and relax your vaginal opening. When you feel ready, slowly insert the tip of the dilator into the opening of your vagina. Angle the tip downward, toward your tailbone, because this will help steer the dilator comfortably into your vagina and under and around your pubic bone. Insert the dilator only as far as you want to, then rest and continue with relaxation techniques to keep yourself calm and your vaginal muscles loose.

4. Work toward being able to insert the dilator three or four inches inside yourself, and rest it there for about twenty minutes a day every day. The more regularly and routinely you do the insertion, the easier it becomes.

5. Once you are comfortable with resting the smallest dilator inside yourself, experiment with moving it around. Remember, the dilator is helping you slowly stretch the inner muscles of your vagina. Move the dilator up and down, back and forth.

6. Repeat this exercise with the smallest dilator for at least one week. When you feel ready, progress to the next size of dilator. Stay with one size of dilator as long as you need to until you feel relaxed and comfortable with insertion and movement. Master each size before moving on to the next.

7. Continue the exercises until you have mastered the largest dilator. Then you can repeat the exercises guiding your partner's hand as he or she inserts the dilators and moves them around. Eventually, with your partner's cooperation, you can continue the exercises using your partner's fingers or penis.

If you reach a block in inserting a particular dilator, use relaxation, breathing, imagery, and creative problem solving to help. You may want to shift down to an easier size for a longer time, or you can bridge from one size to another slowly during the same twenty-minute period.

Self-stimulation can help survivors through impasses with insertion. Stimulate the clitoris before and during the dilator exercises. Sexual arousal increases natural lubrication and causes vaginal expansion, often making insertion easier. This variation is also useful in helping a survivor associate pleasurable sensations with vaginal fullness. Feeling comfortable with these sensations can eventually facilitate the ability to have orgasms during intercourse.

Once a survivor feels successful with dilator insertion on her own, if she wants she can invite her partner to join her during some sessions. The survivor can teach the partner how to comfortably insert a dilator and move it around. Active and specific communication is essential.

Ginny, a survivor of sibling incest, worked with her husband, Ron, to overcome her problem with vaginal pain and fear of penetration.

GINNY: Once I became comfortable with the dilators myself, I asked Ron to do the inserting. We got to a point where he was leaving the dilator in and also manipulating it a little bit. His participation showed me that he wasn't going to do anything that I didn't want him to do or didn't ask him to do. His helping became a positive thing with me and with him.

RON: I felt involved. Ginny was actually sharing a part of herself with me. Though I was glad, sometimes it was frustrating: I'd wish it was me and not the piece of plastic. The exercises gave us guidelines. We knew what we were to do, for how long, and that it wouldn't go any further. I could relax and Ginny could relax.

Vaginal dilators allow survivors to get used to sensations common in intercourse. Women learn that penetration is not always 100 percent comfortable. Little temporary tugs and pressures are often just part of getting started. If some minor discomfort exists, try moving ahead anyway. If obvious pain persists, however, don't ignore it—stop.

The transition from plastic dilators to a partner's penis is often an exciting step for a couple. The male partner becomes, in essence, "the human dilator." A survivor described her transition:

When we finally did the human dilator exercise, I felt shy, nervous, and embarrassed. There was a conflict going on inside me between wanting to turn off the pleasurable sensations and wanting to experience them. I decided it was okay to enjoy it for myself, and I did!

In the human dilator exercise, a male partner has to learn a passive role, letting the survivor control the insertion and then just resting inside the vagina for a while. One partner was concerned about how to maintain his erection and what would happen if he had an orgasm. I explained in counseling that he could move inside his wife only so much as was necessary to maintain his erection. If he had an orgasm, that was fine, but it would be preferable if he didn't. He said to me, "I think I get the full thrust of what you are saying." To which I replied, "What you need to get is the *half thrust* of what I'm saying." We all had a good laugh.

Over time the human dilator exercise can be expanded to permit insertion by the man of his own penis, clitoral stimulation, some thrusting, and experimentation with different positions. Eventually a couple can apply the skills learned to regular sexual intercourse. A survivor had this to say:

> We go really slowly with intercourse. My boyfriend is very careful to take his time, come into me slowly, a little at a time, and come out if it hurts. I've become used to it, and as a result I am not afraid of possible pain. I like feeling free to move around and change positions. I let him know my needs openly.

As sexual problems become resolved, don't forget this: What's most important is the emotional intimacy, caring, and respect that you and your partner are creating. That is the goal of your healing.

12

Enjoying Sexual Experiences

Sexual healing takes a long time, but gradually it happens.
—ELLEN BASS AND LAURA DAVIS, *The Courage to Heal*

I feel that I have awareness and choice about sex for the first time in my life.
—A SURVIVOR

Yes, sexual healing really does happen. In time survivors learn a new approach to touch and intimacy, return from healing vacations from sex, and engage in pleasurable sexual activities. I like to think of this final stage in sexual healing as being on a *permanent vacation from abusive sex*.

Survivors may be amazed at the many positive changes they are able to make in how they view and experience sex. Several survivors who reached this stage of sexual healing commented on their progress:

Before, I used masturbation to relieve sexual tension and was haunted by memories of my sexual abuse. Now I experience masturbation as a healthy, enjoyable, major part of my sex life. I view sex now as a key, a core aspect of my self-image and self-value.

I have come a long way. I no longer feel sex is dirty or a duty I must perform. I am no longer ashamed to masturbate. I now feel sex is a natural, healthy way of being intimate with my partner and myself.

Sex was something I used to feel trepidation about. Would I be able to perform, deal with feelings, have an orgasm? Or would I be overwhelmed with shame? Now I feel fairly confident I'll have a good time, no matter what happens, and be able to be present.

I am able to stay present with sexual experiences and enjoy them. My husband and I now see each other as friends who appreciate each other, love each other, and want to share pleasure with each other. As a result our sexual life has become more relaxed, easy, and natural.

Partners of survivors make significant changes as well. "I've learned how to make love *with* my wife, not to her," a partner commented. And another partner said, "I no longer feel orgasm is necessary in order to be sexual. I've learned how to be sensual and enjoy touch, regardless of whether we go on to have sex."

When you reach this final stage in sexual healing, the most critical work has been done: You have created a new meaning for sex, improved how you feel about yourself sexually, and gained control of your automatic reactions and sexual behaviors. You've also learned to stay aware, move forward in touch activities, and communicate your feelings and needs to an intimate partner.

Given how past sexual trauma can affect sexuality, you know that for sex to feel okay certain guidelines must be followed. Sex must be your choice, an experience you feel in charge of, and an activity with no expectations, pressure, or demands. You've learned new techniques and skills to enhance sexual intimacy. From here on you'll need to practice what you've learned so you don't forget or slip back into old patterns.

Sexual healing does not have to stop here. As a survivor said:

We've climbed up the big mountain of our sexual healing and gone down the other side. Now we're cruising on even ground. But I think we've still got a few little bumps to go over yet.

FURTHERING SEXUAL HEALING

Survivors often want to go further in their sexual healing, fine-tune what they've learned, and even explore some exciting new territory. Three such ways are:

- Adjusting better to the realities of recovery
- Creating new and more pleasurable sexual experiences
- Allowing intimate partners more freedom to initiate and express themselves sexually.

Adjusting better to the realities of recovery

Sexual healing brings changes in how you experience sex that may take some getting used to. Sex isn't the same for you now as it was before you began healing. While many survivors feel happy about the differences, as with any major change in life, they often experience some disappointments and sadness as well.

Sexual healing can bring with it the loss of some things we enjoyed, even if they were bad for us. If we used to passively withdraw from sex, we may miss how easy it was to avoid sexual situations. It may seem a burden to have to tell a partner directly that we don't want sex. Similarly, if we used to become overexcited by sex and engaged in it compulsively, we may miss the "high" we used to get.

> Sex doesn't fill the same addictive needs it did before. I don't lose myself completely anymore. I still enjoy it a lot, but I am less excited somehow. I know overall I'm better off now. It was self-destructive, but I sometimes do miss the intensity.

We may need to adjust our expectations to match the changes that have come with our sexual recovery. Sexual healing involves making lifelong changes, *for good*. If the progress we have made in healing is to last, we can't revert to old attitudes or behaviors.

At times during lovemaking with her husband, Terry was bothered by images of her brother attempting sex with her. It troubled her that these images came to mind even though she had completed a lot of recovery work. Taking a closer look, Terry discovered that these upsetting images were most likely to occur when she was feeling tired, anxious, or stressed.

> Sometimes the old feelings come back to me, and I get really frustrated by them. I guess that's pretty normal. I used to wish I could just flip a switch and make those bad feelings from the abuse go away forever. It bothers me that I have to face them now and then.

The good news for Terry is that because of sexual healing she has developed effective ways to handle these feelings. She has choices. She knows how to calm herself, affirm her present reality, and talk with her husband. When the old feelings come back, they no longer ruin a sexual experience or interfere with Terry's long-term happiness. "The more I accept my reactions and do what I can do to address them," says Terry, "the less frequent and less intense they are."

Survivors may have some difficulty adjusting to being more aware, to having real, live *feelings*. No longer numb or split off from emotions, we fully experience our anger, sadness, fear, and joy. It's as if we had been blindfolded and now see the light. We sense so much more. Our feelings take on greater importance than they had before. As a result we may become more discriminating about when we want to have sex. A survivor explained the difference sexual healing had made in her approach to sex:

> I experience sex as much more influenced by my emotions. Before,
> I was always ready to make love unless I was sick. Now my desire to
> make love is much more closely tied to my other emotions, and
> affected by them, and therefore is more fragile. But this also means
> I have more emotion to express, and feel, during lovemaking.

Sexual activity is more satisfying when it's congruent with how you feel. While you may be delighted that the quality of your sexual experience has improved, you may feel bad that the frequency is less than you had hoped. This new reality represents a milestone in sexual healing: *Your sexual behavior has become dependent on how you really feel.*

Given these changes, sex may become difficult when you are under certain stresses that relate to past sexual abuse, such as being in the place where the abuse occurred, having contact with the offender, encountering problems in an intimate relationship, or feeling exploited in a work situation. Be aware you will have times like this: Don't be surprised when they occur. Reduce pressure. These times are inevitable and temporary. To help you through them, rely on the skills you learned for creating safety and moving forward in small steps.

Survivors may have trouble adjusting to having to clearly communicate their feelings and needs to a partner. While a survivor may realize that this is important in avoiding problems and disappointments, the constant communication process can seem cumbersome at times. Rita, a survivor, disliked the idea of always having to spell out for her husband, Ian, that she "wanted to be physically intimate and explore touch without there being any expectations for sex." She worried that if she didn't say this, Ian would take her interest in cuddling and massage as meaning she was open to exploring sexual possibilities too. To help herself, Rita invented the term *vanilla touch* to stand for touching that is not expected to lead to sex. Now Rita simply says that she wants vanilla touch, and Ian automatically understands what she means.

Another reality of sexual healing is that permanent changes are made in how sex is approached and experienced. These changes usually mean that significant amounts of time and energy may need to go into preparing for and having sex. It takes time to maintain emotional intimacy with a partner. And it takes time to create safety, trust, and a nondemanding setting for sexual intimacy. "I need to feel appreciated, valued, and related to in other ways than sexual first, before I can even consider sexual relating," a survivor said.

During sex, survivors and partners need to always be prepared to stop, slow down, shift activities, and process old feelings from the abuse. A survivor told of her growth:

> It takes time to deal with the internal voices in me that sometimes whisper, "You're bad, you're bad," when I feel pleasure with a partner or ask for what I want and need sexually. Now when I hear the voices, I pull back from them. I'm more aware of what's going on and give myself space to counter them with positive thoughts.

And a partner talked about the realities of having sex in his relationship:

> We stay in close communication with each other during sex so we can change course if haunting memories of the past should recur. We keep our expectations in harmony with reality. We know that trust and safety come before all else. How do porcupines make love? Very, very carefully!

It can also be very important to end a sexual encounter well. This too takes time. If after sex a partner gets up quickly or rolls over without saying a word, a survivor may be left feeling bad for having had sex. Dina believed that her most emotionally vulnerable times were after sex. It was then that her thinking would start to slide into thinking of herself as a victim and her partner as a perpetrator. Dina was able to mediate these feelings some for herself. She'd remind herself of the chain of events that led up to the sex, that she consented and was able to control her experience. But what seemed to help most was taking time after sex for hugging and holding with her lover. This special time enabled her to break free of old victim-perpetrator ways of evaluating her sexual behavior.

Survivors may create a lot of unnecessary anxiety and upset by comparing their recovered sex life with what they imagine "normal" (nonsurvivor) sexual lives to be. They may berate themselves for not being as sexually free, easygoing, or active as they fantasize others are. Making comparisons like this is unfair and may even damage your progress. When we think this way, we hold onto an overly positive picture of what other people's sex lives are like, forgetting that many nonsurvivors have troubles with sex too. While sexual relating is different and may always be different for survivors than for nonsurvivors, this difference may not be as significant as we may think.

The benefits of sexual healing more than compensate for the losses. We need to keep in mind the positive repercussions of our healing as well: increased self-respect and self-esteem, and the ability to have emotionally intimate relationships, to name a few. A survivor said:

> I wonder if those of us who work on healing might not be more healthy sexually and emotionally in the end than the majority of the population who believe they have "no sexual issues."

Creating new and more pleasurable sexual experiences

As a result of sexual healing, each survivor creates a comfort zone for sexual activity. Within this zone certain behaviors feel okay, while others may not. A survivor might feel fine having sexual relations, but only under the condition that sexual contact is made in the same position every time. Another survivor might feel comfortable with fingers touching genitals but not want oral sex at all.

While establishing limits to sexual behavior and activity is crucial to being able to sexually heal, as time goes on survivors often feel limited by their own restrictions. Then the task becomes one of expanding the outer limits of the comfort zone to make room for new experiences.

Maureen, a survivor who used to withdraw from sex, wanted to know what it would be like to have sexual yearnings and feel "horny" toward her husband.

I want to reach the point when I want sex as much as my husband
does. I'd like to be able to say to him, "Honey, I want to make love
to you right now," rather than, "I think I can, we'll see how it goes."

The range of sexual possibilities is infinite. There are many kinds of
sexual activities and many ways of doing them.* Lovemaking can be
playful, passionate, intense, or spiritual. When we stick within a certain
range of activities, our sexual life may start to feel predictable and bor-
ing, eventually limiting our sexual pleasure and sense of aliveness. Sex
has been compared to eating dinner. Sometimes you joke about the
dishes. Sometimes you take the meal seriously. It's good to know we can
be open to having many different types of sexual "dinners."

How do you expand your sexual comfort zone? You can trust the
progress you've already made and slowly challenge yourself to take some
new risks. Remember all the skills for staying relaxed and aware: stopping when needed, creating steps to bridge from one experience to
another, and communicating your feelings and needs with a partner.
These can all be used to conquer new areas in sexual enrichment.

Consider a new sexual experience you might want to explore.
Make sure that it would not be harmful or abusive to you in any way.
Sexual behaviors associated with sexual abuse, such as sadomasochism,
dominant-submissive relationships, and physically dangerous activities,
must always remain off-limits. These behaviors are incompatible with
the principles of healthy sexual intimacy.

Ask yourself: Is there anything I need to learn about this sexual
activity before I do it? What are my worst fears about this activity?
What do I need to do to ensure this activity will go well?

Kathryn had always been afraid of having sex in a position where she
sat up, straddling and facing her partner. She realized that this fear
stemmed from past abuse, when her uncle would force her onto his lap
and fondle her. She talked with her current partner, Jeff, about exploring new positions gradually. To expand her comfort zone, Katheryn
decided to create bridges between touch activities with which she
already felt comfortable and the woman-on-top position during sex.

To begin making changes, she and Jeff used the hand clapping exercise they had already learned during their healing work on relearning
touch (presented in chapter 10). They went through the exercise several times, making changes with each variation: first with both partners

---

* See the Resources section for books and tapes on sexual enrichment.

fully clothed, sitting on the floor; then sitting on the bed; then with clothes off, sitting on the bed; then in the woman-on-top position with clothes on; and finally in the woman-on-top position with clothes off. During the exercises Katheryn and Jeff would stop, rest, and talk whenever she felt anxious or ready to stop.

Katheryn enjoyed the exercise and associated it with fun, pleasure, and playful contact with Jeff. Her ability to relax and be comfortable with Jeff in the exercises gave her a bridge for transferring these good feelings into the sexual position. Surprisingly for Katheryn, this new position has become one of her favorites. "The only problem now," jokes Katheryn, "is that Jeff and I keep wanting to clap when we're done!"

Brad, a survivor of childhood molestation, wanted to explore the area of spiritual sexuality. Now that he was comfortable with his sexual functioning and was feeling good about his relationship with his partner, he wanted to see how sex could express a connection with life and nature. First he realized he needed to learn more. He found a book about spiritual sexuality at a local bookstore that specialized in personal growth and psychology books. In his readings he discovered an activity he wanted to try with his partner. The activity involved intercourse with little or gentle thrusting, slow breathing, and focusing mentally on how deeply united they were at that moment. Brad had concerns that his partner, Emily, wouldn't want to do the activity or would find it silly. To ensure that the activity would go well, he first discussed it with Emily and made sure she was interested in trying it. They agreed to try it for a few minutes as part of regular lovemaking. Although it was awkward at first, Brad and Emily did the exercise and agreed to try it a little longer the next time they made love. Months later Brad said, "My enjoyment of sex has grown beyond the physical sense. It involves sharing in an intimate, spiritual way as well."

Another way that survivors can improve sexual experiences, whether alone or with a partner, is by becoming more able to receive pleasurable sensations. As part of sexual healing, survivors are encouraged to direct a sexual experience and stay in charge. But you can learn to relax and let yourself be receptive to what is happening in the moment. This type of surrender to sensation is a skill you can learn, not a defeat or a loss of power. You increase your power by being able to receive more sensually. You learn to let go of muscle tightness that may be restraining and inhibiting sexual pleasure. To develop skills for this healthy type of surrender, Stella Resnick, a Gestalt therapist who specializes in treating sexual problems, advises practicing the following exercise during the course of each day:

> Stop for a few minutes: Close your eyes, inhale deeply, all the way to the top of your chest, and blow the air out in a complete exhale. Imagine that you are also blowing out any tension or unpleasant feelings you've picked up along the way. Then rotate your head a few times, stretch your neck, your arms, and back. Yawn and relax your jaw, and reconnect to your senses—scanning your environment slowly with your eyes, smelling the air, hearing distant sounds, feeling the objects that touch your skin, the tastes in your mouth.
>
> Practicing little moments of surrender makes big surrenders easier. As resistance and angst diminish, softness and trust grow, as so too grow feelings of love and tenderness. When we surrender, we become more loving, and in the process, we end up showing more of what there is in us to love.*

I recommend first trying this sensual surrender exercise as part of the safe nest and safe embrace exercises described in chapter 10. Eventually, you can use this skill of sensual surrender to help you let go of muscle tension, breathe fully, and feel more sensations during your sexual experiences. Increasing movement and breath is an excellent way to increase arousal and pleasurable intensity in lovemaking.

The rewards of expanding sexual horizons make the efforts worthwhile, as this survivor explained:

> Sex is good and fun. It's never been like this for me before. I'm more open and expressive during sex. I laugh. I can be intense.

As survivors we can give ourselves permission to experiment and feel good with lots of different kinds of sexual experiences. "I've learned that feeling the pleasure of sex is nothing to be ashamed about," a survivor said. "It's okay to feel good and enjoy sex. In fact, I deserve to feel good."

Allowing intimate partners more freedom in sex

Recently I received a call from Marla, a former client whom I had last seen for sex therapy with her husband, Rhett, two years before. Marla

* Stella Resnick, "Sweet Surrender," *The New Age Journal,* 1980 (November): 41–45.

had been sexually abused by her father and had suffered sexual problems in her marriage as a result. On the phone Marla said she was feeling depressed and needed to come back into counseling again. I wondered what was causing her problems. My last contact with her had been several months ago on the phone when she told me things were going well, she and Rhett were having sexual relations about once a week, she enjoyed the experiences and had even felt strong urges that led to her initiating sex with Rhett on several occasions.

Sitting in my office, Marla explained what was troubling her now. The other night in bed Rhett had turned to her and asked, "So is this how it's always going to be? Is our sex life going to be like this for the rest of our lives? Am I always going to have to wait until you say you want to have sex before I can touch you sexually? Will you always be the one controlling what we can and can't do? I just want to know so I won't expect something more than can really happen."

His words hit hard. Marla was upset. "Why can't Rhett be satisfied with all the positive changes I've made? We had such trouble with sex before. Isn't it enough that I'm able now to be sexual and enjoy it?" As she talked out her feelings and her anger went down, Marla herself began to wonder about the limits of her sexual healing.

Marla could understand that Rhett felt as if his hands were tied. He wasn't free to express his sexual urges and desires freely. Their sex life was out of balance and lacked spontaneity. Marla wanted to find ways to loosen her need for so much control and to allow Rhett more freedom to take the initiative sexually, without her sliding back into old feelings of fear and resentment.

This is a common dilemma couples may encounter in the final stages of sexual healing. Some of the things survivors do to ensure their safety and comfort—such as be the one to initiate and control all the sexual activity—inhibits and limits the partner. Partners may feel sexual encounters have become *overcontrolled* by the survivor.

The fact that partners begin to risk stating their needs more directly is a measure of the sexual healing progress that has taken place. A partner in a similar situation asked, "Can there ever be an unscripted sexual encounter?" And another partner said:

> I'd like to be able to compliment my wife on her looks, flirt with her, and get into my sexual energy without her thinking I'm pressuring her to have sex.

In a long-term relationship, partners need room to express their sexual interests and energy, and to receive validation and support.

In counseling I asked Marla if she was able to express her limits and needs before and during sex. She said yes. Then I asked if she was confident that Rhett could stop what he was doing at any time if she asked him. Again yes. Assertiveness, trust, respect, and communication were well established. Marla realized that at this time perhaps her need for so much overt control of their sexual experiences was no longer necessary. Still it was frightening for her to consider loosening up.

For this next step in healing to work, the survivor and partner must agree that, at all times, the survivor's needs for safety come first. The survivor does not "give up" control but rather feels the control is always present, on an underlying level. From this orientation, survivors can begin to challenge themselves to let the partner be freer in expressions of passion and sexual activities. Remember, you can stop at any time. Honest communication, respect, and emotional intimacy are still understood as more important than what goes on sexually.

Denise and Robert, another couple, invented a system for initiating sex that felt more balanced and was comfortable for both of them. They decided to take turns with initiating. Denise is responsible for initiating sex, then the next time it's Robert's turn. When an initiation is made, regardless of whether the other person accepts, it counts as a turn. As Denise explained:

> Alternating like this helps me to feel safe and able to keep out of my "here he comes *again*" and "that's all he ever wants" trap. Once Robert has initiated, I know that nothing will happen again unless I want it to. This arrangement gives me the opportunity to have proactive power over my own pleasure—I don't get to have any fun unless I choose it. So I get to practice choosing to have pleasure. And it gives Robert a sense of having some control finally.
>
> In our long abstinence period nobody initiated anything. In the relearning touch exercises, the process was still guided by my pace and comfort level. Now Robert also gets opportunities to express his desire.

As survivors challenge themselves to go along and explore sexual experiences that partners initiate, something wonderful can start to happen. You may find that you enjoy the new energy that your partner brings into the sexual experiences. Your partner may introduce you to something new that you like! And you may enjoy experiencing your partner feeling freer and more alive. "I'm learning to think of his sexual energy as *his delight*, not my obligation," a survivor said.

Eventually, even with the conditions necessary for continued sexual healing, intimate relationships can feel more balanced and equal.

> Sex is something my partner and I share when we both want to. We communicate now and take our time. We're responsible and playful with each other. Sex is beautiful and fun.

As survivors feel more relaxed and confident during sex, they may find themselves enjoying sex in ways they never thought possible before.

> Lately when my partner and I have sex, it feels like we're creating a dance together. We touch each other gently and easily. We move to the same rhythm. Neither of us pulls back or presses forward for the next step. We stay in the moment with each other. I'm open to the whole experience. Since I've let go of fear, I've been able to feel more love for my partner during sex.

THE JOYS OF SEXUAL HEALING

It's a wonderful feeling to overcome hurts from the past and to reclaim sexuality as good and healthy for ourselves. It's amazing how flexible and resilient survivors can be. "Through all the fear, horror, and hard work, I've gained tremendous strength, hope, and serenity," a survivor said.

Sexual healing may be painful, confusing, and challenging. It can take a long time. But the rewards make all the effort worth it.

> It's been an extremely difficult row to hoe. I may never "get it" fully. But my taste of real, true sexuality reminds me how worth it the struggle is. Sex is wonderful, exciting—a gift of the universe. Any of us would be foolish not to learn how to accept it, experience it, and appreciate it. As a survivor, I've been cheated from this gift most of my life, but I am changing that dynamic: I've taken control of my sexuality for myself.

As you move forward in your sexual healing, remember you are not traveling alone. A large and growing number of survivors and intimate partners of survivors are on this journey as well. Therapeutic and social support exists to help you. Together we all are learning to separate the pain and sadness of sexual abuse from the incredible pleasure and joy of healthy sexuality. Each of us along this path is creating our own new, individual meaning for sex, healthy and enjoyable enough to last the rest of our lifetimes.

Resources

The following list contains books, articles, videotapes, and audiotapes that may be of help to you in sexual healing. These resources present information on sexual abuse, sexuality, and other relevant topics. Because sexual healing is a special focus in recovery from sexual abuse, few references address it directly or in much detail. You will need to pick and choose relevant material from what you read.

BOOKS

Sexual Abuse Recovery

Adams, Caren, and Jennifer Fay. *Free of Shadows: Recovering from Sexual Violence.* Oakland, Calif.: New Harbinger, 1990.
  Guidance for rape victims, family, and friends.

Bass, Ellen, and Laura Davis. *Beginning to Heal: A First Book for Survivors of Child Sexual Abuse.* New York: HarperCollins, 1993.

―――. *The Courage to Heal: A Guide for Women Survivors of Child Sexual Abuse.* New York: HarperPerennial, 1994.
  Section on intimacy and sexuality.

Bear, Euan, and Peter Dimock. *Adults Molested as Children: A Survivor's Manual for Women and Men.* Orwell, Vt.: Safer Society Press, 1988.
  An excellent 70-page booklet, especially helpful for survivors and partners just starting out in recovery. Safer Society Press, P.O. Box 340, Brandon, VT 05773, (802) 247-5141.

Butler, Sandra. *Conspiracy of Silence: The Trauma of Incest.* San Francisco: Volcano Press, 1996.

Caruso, Beverly. *The Impact of Incest*. City Center, Minn.: Hazelden Information Education, 1987.
> *General information about incest and a short section on sexuality concerns.*

Davis, Laura. *Allies in Healing: When the Person You Love Was Sexually Abused as a Child*. New York: HarperPerennial, 1991.
> *A support book for partners. Section on sexuality.*

Davis, Laura. *The Courage to Heal Workbook: For Women and Men Survivors of Child Sexual Abuse*. New York: HarperCollins, 1990.
> *Section on sexuality.*

Dolan, Yvonne. *One Small Step: Moving Beyond Trauma and Therapy to a Life of Joy*. Available at http://www.iUniverse.com., 2000.

Engel, Beverly. *The Right to Innocence: Healing the Trauma of Childhood Sexual Abuse*. New York: Ivy Books, 1991.
> *Brief mention of sexuality concerns.*

Estrada, Hank. *Recovery for Male Victims of Child Abuse: An Interview with Hank Estrada, Incest Survivor*. Santa Fe: Red Rabbit Press, 1990.
> *One man's journey from recognition to recovery. Brief mention of sexuality concerns.*

Evert, Kathy, and Inie Bijkerk. *When You're Ready: A Woman's Healing from Childhood Physical and Sexual Abuse by Her Mother*. Walnut Creek, Calif.: Launch Press, 1987.
> *Poignant story; some graphic detail of abuse and sexual effects.*

Forward, Susan, and Craig Buck. *Betrayal of Innocence: Incest and Its Devastation*. New York: Penguin, 1988.
> *Case descriptions illustrating different types of incest.*

Gil, Eliana. *Outgrowing the Pain: A Book for and About Adults Abused as Children*. New York: Dell Books, 1988.

———. *Outgrowing the Pain Together: A Book for Spouses and Partners of Adult Survivors*. New York: Dell Books, 1992.

———. *United We Stand: A Book for Individuals with Multiple Personalities*. Walnut Creek, Calif.: Launch Press, 1990.

Hagans, Kathryn, and Joyce Case. *When Your Child Has Been Molested: A Parent's Guide to Healing and Recovery*. San Francisco: Jossey-Bass Publishers, 1998.
> *Helpful general suggestions.*

Hansen, Paul. *Survivors and Partners: Healing the Relationships of Sexual Abuse Survivors*. Longmont, Colo.: Heron Hill Publishers, 1991.
> *Paul Hansen, 7548 Cresthill Drive, Longmont, CO 80501.*

Hunter, Mic. *Abused Boys: The Neglected Victims of Sexual Abuse.* New York: Fawcett Columbine, 1991.
> *Brief section on sexual concerns.*

King, Neal. *Speaking Our Truth: Voices of Courage and Healing for Male Survivors of Childhood Sexual Abuse.* New York: HarperPerennial, 1995.

Lew, Mike. *Leaping Upon the Mountains: Men Proclaiming Victory over Child Sexual Abuse.* Jamaica Plain, Mass.: Small Wonder Books, 1999.

————. *Victims No Longer: Men Recovering from Incest and Other Sexual Child Abuse.* New York: HarperCollins, 1990.
> *General discussion about sexual effects; helpful section on sexual orientation confusion.*

Maltz, Wendy, and Beverly Holman. *Incest and Sexuality: A Guide to Understanding and Healing.* Lexington, Mass.: Lexington Books, 1991.
> *The first publication to specifically address the sexual effects of incest. Special sections on family dynamics, self-concept, sexual repercussions, intimate partners, and finding therapeutic help.*

Oksana, Chrystine. *Safe Passage to Healing: A Guide for Survivors of Ritual Abuse.* New York: HarperCollins, 1994.

Parrot, Andrea. *Coping with Date Rape and Acquaintance Rape.* New York: Rosen Publishing Group, 1999.

Poston, Carol, and Karen Lison. *Reclaiming Our Lives: Hope for Adult Survivors of Incest.* Boston: Little, Brown and Company, 1989.
> *Some mention of sexual concerns.*

Sanford, Linda. *Strong at the Broken Places: Overcoming the Trauma of Childhood Sexual Abuse.* New York: Random House, 1990.

Spear, Joan. *How Can I Help Her? A Handbook for Women Sexually Abused as Children.* City Center, Minn.: Hazelden Information Education, 1991.
> *A good booklet for partners wanting to understand sexual abuse, its effects, and how they can help healing. To order a copy, contact The Hazelden Foundation: (800) 328-9000.*

Thomas, T. *Men Surviving Incest: A Male Survivor Shares on the Process of Recovery.* Walnut Creek, Calif.: Launch Press, 1989.
> *Brief section on sexuality.*

Warshaw, Robin. *I Never Called It Rape: The Ms Report on Recognizing, Fighting and Surviving Date and Acquaintance Rape.* New York: HarperPerennial, 1994.
> *Brief section on sexual consequences.*

Sexual Addiction and Compulsivity

Carnes, Patrick. *Contrary to Love: Helping the Sexual Addict*. Minneapolis, Minn.: CompCare Publications, 1989.

———. *Don't Call It Love: Recovering from Sexual Addiction*. New York: Bantam, 1992.

———. *Out of the Shadows: Understanding Sexual Addiction*. City Center, Minn.: Hazelden Information Education, 1992.

Earle, Ralph, and Gregory Crow. *Lonely All the Time: Recognizing, Understanding, and Overcoming Sexual Addiction, for Addicts and Co-dependents*. New York: Pocket Books, 1998.

Kasl, Charlotte. *Women, Sex and Addiction: A Search for Love and Power*. New York: HarperCollins, 1990.

Mura, David. *A Male Grief: Notes on Pornography and Addiction*. Minneapolis, Minn.: Milkweed Editions, 1987.
  Convincing thesis on the negative effects of using pornography. Milkweed Editions, Post Office Box 3226, Minneapolis, MN 55403.

Schneider, Jennifer. *Back from Betrayal: Recovering from His Affairs*. Ballantine Books, 1990.

Stoltenberg, John. *Refusing to Be a Man: Essays on Sex and Justice*. Portland, Ore.: Breitenbush Books, 1989.
  Has several excellent chapters on the negative influences of pornography and its relationship to rape.

Sex Education and Enrichment

Anand, Margo. *The Art of Sexual Ecstasy: The Path of Sacred Sexuality for Western Lovers*. Los Angeles: Jeremy Tarcher, 1991.

Barbach, Lonnie. *For Each Other: Sharing Sexual Intimacy*. New York: New American Library, 1984.

———. *For Yourself: The Fulfillment of Female Sexuality*. Garden City, N.Y.: Anchor Books, 1976.

Castlemen, Michael. *Sexual Solutions: A Guide for Men and the Women Who Love Them*. New York: Touchstone, 1989.

Crooks, Robert, and Karla Baur. *Our Sexuality*. Pacific Grove, Calif.: Brooks/Cole Publishers, 1998.

Gilles, Jerry. *Transcendental Sex: A Meditative Approach to Increasing Sensual Pleasure*. New York: Holt, Rinehart, and Winston, 1978.

Heiman, Julia, and Joseph LoPiccolo. *Becoming Orgasmic: A Sexual and Personal Growth Program for Women.* New York: Simon and Schuster, 1988.
   Some mention of sexual abuse.

Henderson, Julie. *The Lover Within: Opening to Energy in Sexual Practice.* Barrytown, N.Y.: Barrytown Ltd., 1999.

Kaplan, Helen. *How to Overcome Premature Ejaculation.* New York: Brunner/Mazel, 1989.

Kennedy, Adele, and Susan Dean. *Touching for Pleasure: A 12-Step Program for Sexual Enrichment.* Chatsworth, Calif.: Chatsworth Press, 1988.

Lee, Victoria. *Soulful Sex: Opening Your Heart, Body & Spirit to Lifelong Passion.* Berkeley, Calif.: Conari Press, 1996.

Loulan, Jo Ann. *Lesbian Sex.* Minneapolis, Minn.: Spinsters Ink, 1984.

Love, Patricia, and Jo Robinson. *Hot Monogamy: Essential Steps to More Passionate, Intimate Lovemaking.* New York: Plume Books, 1999.

Maltz, Wendy. *Intimate Kisses: The Poetry of Sexual Pleasure.* Novato, Calif.: New World Library, 2001.
   A highly praised anthology of poetry celebrating the joys of healthy sexual pleasure. The poems describe various aspects of sexual pleasure, from anticipation, arousal, and ecstasy to remembrance.

————. *Passionate Hearts: The Poetry of Sexual Love.* Novato, Calif.: New World Library, 1996.
   An award-winning anthology that celebrates the joys of healthy sexual sharing throughout the life of a relationship, from early courtship to mature love. Very educational and healing for survivors and their intimate partners.

Maltz, Wendy, and Suzie Boss. *Private Thoughts: Exploring the Power of Women's Sexual Fantasies.* Novato, Calif.: New World Library, 2001.
   This book was formerly published under the title In the Garden of Desire: The Intimate World of Women's Sexual Fantasies. *It contains chapters on how sexual abuse influences the formation of sexual fantasies, how to evaluate fantasy problems, and how to heal unwanted sexual fantasies caused by past abuse.*

Masters, William, Virginia Johnson, and Robert Kolodny. *Masters and Johnson on Sex and Human Loving.* Boston: Little, Brown and Company, 1988.

McCarthy, Barry, and Emily McCarthy. *Couple Sexual Awareness: Building Sexual Happiness.* New York: Carroll & Graf, 1990.

Montagu, Ashley. *Touching: The Human Significance of the Skin.* New York: HarperCollins, 1986.

Moore, Thomas. *The Soul of Sex: Cultivating Life as an Act of Love*. New York: HarperCollins, 1998.

Ogden, Gina. *Women Who Love Sex: An Inquiry into the Expanding Spirit of Women's Erotic Experience*. Cambridge, Mass.: Womanspirit Press, 1999.
   These women's stories affirm the heart-felt, healing, and self-affirming possibilities in sexual relationship.

Stanway, Andrew. *The Art of Sensual Loving: A New Approach to Sexual Relationships*. New York: Carol & Graf, 2000.

Zilbergeld, Bernie. *Male Sexuality: A Guide to Sexual Fulfillment*. Boston: Little, Brown and Company, 1978.

Zoldbrod, Aline. *Sex Smart: How Your Childhood Shaped Your Sexual Life and What to Do About It*. Oakland, Calif.: New Harbinger Publications, 1998.

Intimacy

Covington, Stephanie. *Leaving the Enchanted Forest: The Path from Relationship Addiction to Intimacy*. San Francisco: HarperSanFrancisco, 1988.

Hendrix, Harville. *Getting the Love You Want: A Guide for Couples*. New York: HarperPerennial, 1990.
   Conscious loving skills for couples healing from past hurts.

Lerner, Harriet. *The Dance of Intimacy: A Woman's Guide to Courageous Acts of Change in Key Relationships*. New York: HarperCollins, 1990.

Scarf, Maggie. *Intimate Partners: Patterns in Love and Marriage*. New York: Ballantine, 1996.

Woititz, Janet. *Struggle for Intimacy*. Deerfield Beach, Fla.: Health Communications, 1986.

General Interest

Beattie, Melody. *Codependent No More: How to Stop Controlling Others and Start Caring for Yourself*. New York: HarperCollins, 1996.

Black, Claudia, and Laurie Zagon. *It's Never Too Late to Have a Happy Childhood: Inspirations for Adult Children*. New York: Ballantine, 1989.

Bradshaw, John. *Healing the Shame That Binds You*. Deerfield Beach, Fla.: Health Communications, 1988.

Bruckner-Gordon, Fredda, Barbara Kuer Gangi, and Geraldine Urbach Wallman. *Making Therapy Work: Your Guide to Choosing, Using, and Ending Therapy*. New York: Harper & Row, 1988.

Davis, Martha, Matthew McKay, and Elizabeth Robbins Eshelman. *The Relaxation & Stress Reduction Workbook*. Oakland, Calif.: New Harbinger, 1998.

Ford, Clyde. *Compassionate Touch: The Body's Role in Emotional Healing and Recovery*. Publishers' Group West, 1999.

Fossom, Merle A., and Marilyn J. Mason. *Facing Shame: Families in Recovery*. New York: W. W. Norton, 1989.

Gannon, Patrick. *Soul Survivors: A New Beginning for Adults Abused as Children*. New York: Prentice Hall, 1989.
  Includes a helpful section for partners.

Kaufman, Gershan. *Shame: The Power of Caring*. Rochester, Vt.: Schenkman Books, 1992.

Klausner, Mary Ann, and Bobbie Hasselbring. *Aching for Love: The Sexual Drama of the Adult Child*. San Francisco: Harper/Hazelden, 1990.
  Presents healing strategies for women who are adult children of alcoholics. Contains direct discussion of sexuality issues.

Kushner, Harold. *When Bad Things Happen to Good People*. New York: Avon Books, 1992.

Lerner, Harriet. *The Dance of Anger: A Woman's Guide to Changing the Patterns of Intimate Relationships*. New York: HarperCollins, 1997.

Mellody, Pia, with Andrea Miller and J. Keith Miller. *Facing Codependence: What It Is, Where It Comes From, How It Sabotages Our Lives*. San Francisco: HarperSanFrancisco, 1989.

Miller, Alice. *The Drama of the Gifted Child: The Search for the True Self*. New York: Basic Books, 1996.

———. *For Your Own Good: Hidden Cruelty in Child-Rearing and the Roots of Violence*. New York: Noonday Press, 1990.

NiCarthy, Ginny. *Getting Free: You Can End Abuse and Take Back Your Life*. Seattle: Seal Press, 1986.

Potter-Efron, Ronald, and Patricia Potter-Efron. *Letting Go of Shame*. City Center, Minn.: Hazelden Information Education, 1996.

Sonkin, Daniel Jay, and Michael Durphy. *Learning to Live Without Violence: A Handbook for Men*. San Francisco: Volcano Press, 1997.

Whitfield, Charles. *Healing the Child Within: Discovery and Recovery for Adult Children of Dysfunctional Families*. Deerfield Beach, Fla.: Health Communications, 1989.

PROFESSIONAL BOOKS AND ARTICLES

Bachman, Gloria, Tamerra Moeller, and Jodi Benett. "Childhood Sexual Abuse and the Consequences in Adult Women." *Obstetrics & Gynecology* 71, no. 4 (1988): 631–642.

Becker, Judith, et al. "The Incidence and Types of Sexual Dysfunctions in Rape and Incest Victims." *Journal of Sex & Marital Therapy* 8, no. 1 (Spring 1982): 65–74.

Briere, John, et al. "Sexual Fantasies, Gender, and Molestation History." *Child Abuse & Neglect* 18, no. 2 (1994): 131–137.

Briere, John. *Therapy for Adults Molested as Children: Beyond Survival.* New York: Springer, 1996.

Cooper, Al, et al. "Online Sexual Compulsivity: Getting Tangled in the Net." *Sexual Addiction & Compulsivity* 6, no. 2 (1999): 79–104.

Courtois, Christine. *Healing the Incest Wound: Adult Survivors in Therapy.* New York: W. W. Norton, 1996.

Cunningham, Jean, et al. "Childhood Sexual Abuse and Medical Complaints in Adult Women." *Journal of Interpersonal Violence* 3, no. 2 (1988): 131–144.

Dimock, Peter. "Adult Males Sexually Abused as Children: Characteristics and Implications for Treatment." *Journal of Interpersonal Violence* 3, no. 2 (June 1988): 203–221.
    An excellent article for treating men with compulsive sexual disorders.

Dolan, Yvonne. *Resolving Sexual Abuse: Solution-Focused Therapy and Ericksonian Hypnosis for Adult Survivors.* New York: W. W. Norton, 1991.

Finkelhor, David. *Child Sexual Abuse: New Theory and Research.* New York: Free Press, 1984.

Finkelhor, David, and Angela Brown. "The Traumatic Impact of Child Sexual Abuse: A Conceptualization." *American Journal of Orthopsychiatry* 55, no. 4 (October 1985): 530–541.

Garnets, Linda, et al. "Violence and Victimization of Lesbians and Gay Men: Mental Health Consequences." *Journal of Interpersonal Violence* 5, no. 3 (September 1990): 366–383.

Gelinas, Denise. "The Persisting Negative Effects of Incest." *Psychiatry* 46, no. 3 (1983): 312–332.

Gil, Eliana. *Treatment of Adult Survivors of Childhood Abuse.* Walnut Creek, Calif.: Launch Press, 1988.

Gilbert, Barbara, and Jean Cunningham. "Women's Postrape Sexual Functioning: Review and Implications for Counseling." *Journal of Counseling and Development* 65 (October 1986): 71–73.

Herman, Judith. *Trauma and Recovery.* New York: Basic Books, 1997.

Hindman, Jan. *Just Before Dawn: From the Shadows of Tradition to New Reflections in Trauma Assessment and Treatment of Sexual Victimization.* Ontario, Ore.: Alexandria Associates, 1989.

Jehu, Derek. *Beyond Sexual Abuse: Therapy with Women Who Were Childhood Victims.* Chichester, England: John Wiley and Sons, 1988.
   A rich resource for clinicians specializing in treating sexual effects.

———. "Sexual Dysfunctions Among Women Clients Who Were Sexually Abused in Childhood." *Behavioral Psychotherapy* 17 (1989): 53–70.

Kleinplatz, Peggy. *New Directions in Sex Therapy: Innovations and Alternatives.* Philadelphia, Penn.: Brunner/Mazel, 2000.
   Contains a chapter written by Wendy Maltz on sex therapy with survivors of sexual abuse.

Koop, C. Everett. "Report of the Surgeon General's Workshop on Pornography and Public Health." *American Psychologist* 42, no. 10 (October 1987): 944–945.

Koss, Mary, and Mary Harvey. *The Rape Victim: Clinical and Community Approaches to Treatment.* Lexington, Mass.: The Stephen Greene Press, 1987.

Lieblum, Sandra, and Raymond Rosen. *Sexual Desire Disorders.* New York: Guilford Press, 1999.

Maltz, Wendy. "Identifying and Healing the Sexual Repercussions of Incest: A Couples Therapy Approach." *Journal of Sex and Marital Therapy* 14, no. 2 (Summer 1988): 142–170.

———. "The Maltz Hierarchy of Sexual Interaction." *Sexual Addiction and Compulsivity* 2, no. 1 (1995): 5–18.

Masters, William. "Sexual Dysfunction as an Aftermath of Sexual Assault of Men by Women." *Journal of Sex & Marital Therapy* 12, no. 1 (Spring 1986): 35–45.

Mathews, Ruth, Jane Mathews, and Kathleen Speltz. *Female Sexual Offenders: An Exploratory Study.* Orwell, Vt.: Safer Society Press, 1989.

McCarthy, Barry, and Susan Perkins. "Behavioral Strategies and Techniques in Sex Therapy." In R. A. Brown and J. R. Field, eds., *Treatment of Sexual Problems in Individual and Couples Therapy.* Costa Mesa, Calif.: PMA Publishing, 1988.

Miller, William, Ann Marie Williams, and Mark Bernstein. "The Effects of Rape on Marital and Sexual Adjustment." *The American Journal of Family Therapy* 10, no. 1 (Spring 1982): 51–58.

Porter, Eugene. *Treating the Young Male Victim of Sexual Assault: Issues and Intervention Strategies.* Syracuse, N.Y.: Safer Society Press, 1986.

Russell, Diana. *The Secret Trauma: Incest in the Lives of Girls and Women.* New York: Basic Books, 1999.

Sarrel, Philip, and William Masters. "Sexual Molestation of Men by Women." *Archives of Sexual Behavior* 11, no. 2 (1982): 117–131.

Schepp, Kay Frances. *Sexuality Counseling: A Training Program.* Muncie, Ind.: Accelerated Development, 1986.

Sprei, Judith, and Christine Courtois. "The Treatment of Women's Sexual Dysfunctions Arising from Sexual Assault." In R. A. Brown and J. R. Field, eds., *Treatment of Sexual Problems in Individual and Couples Therapy.* Costa Mesa, Calif.: PMA Publishing, 1988.
    Helpful discussion of sexual healing techniques and strategies.

Stuart, Irving, and Joanne Greer. *Victims of Sexual Aggression: Treatment of Children, Women and Men.* New York: Van Nostrand Reinhold, 1984.

Weeks, Gerald, and Larry Hof, eds. *Integrating Sex and Marital Therapy: A Clinical Guide.* New York: Brunner/Mazel, 1987.

Westerlund, Elaine. *Women's Sexuality After Childhood Incest.* New York: W. W. Norton, 1992.

VIDEOTAPES AND AUDIOTAPES

Partners in Healing: Couples Overcoming the Sexual Repercussions of Incest. Produced by Wendy Maltz, Steve Christiansen, and Gerald Joffee. Moderated by Wendy Maltz. A forty-three-minute videotape of three couples, one with a male survivor, discussing sexual healing. Especially helpful to partners understanding the impact of abuse on their relationship and how they can work with the survivor to heal. Distributed by InterVision, 261 E. 12th Avenue, Suite 100, Eugene, OR 97401, (800) 678-3455, (541) 343-7993.

Relearning Touch: Healing Techniques for Couples. Produced by Wendy Maltz, Steve Christiansen, and Gerald Joffee. A forty-five-minute videotape, moderated by Wendy Maltz, sensitively demonstrates the relearning touch techniques. Includes interviews with three couples who have used the techniques to improve communication, deepen emotional intimacy and create positive sexual experiences. Beneficial to non-survivor couples, as well. Distributed by InterVision, 261 E. 12th Avenue, Suite 100, Eugene, OR 97401, (800) 678-3455, (541) 343-7993.

Healing Sexual Abuse: The Recovery Process. A one-hour video that sensitively interviews survivors and talks about the healing process. Varied Directions, 18 Mt. Battie Street, Camden, ME 04843, (800) 888-5236, fax (207) 236-4512, e-mail: Joyceb3955@aol.com.

To a Safer Place. An award-winning fifty-eight-minute video covering one woman's recovery journey from incest. Brief mention of sexual repercussions. Produced and available from the National Film Board of Canada, P.O. Box 6100, Station Centre-ville, Montreal, Quebec, Canada H3C 3H5, (800) 267-7710, fax: (514) 283-7564.

Relaxation/Affirmation Techniques and *Relax-Quick* by Nancy Hopps. These two helpful audiotapes (also available in CD) offer a variety of straightforward ways to facilitate relaxation and strengthen body/mind connection. Synergistic Systems, P.O. Box 5224, Eugene, OR 97405, (541) 683-9088, (541) 302-2671.

Letting Go of Stress: Four Effective Techniques for Relaxation and Stress Reduction produced by Emmett E. Miller, M.D. and Steven Halpern, Ph.D. A popular classic. Source, P.O. Box W, Stanford, CA 94309, (800) 52-TAPES, (415) 453-9800.

Opening the Heart of the Womb by gifted teacher, Stephen Levine. A two-cassette meditation tape created especially for women who have experienced sexual trauma and other wounds to their sexuality to help them reclaim body and spirit and awaken to joy. Sounds True, P.O. Box 8010, Dept. BP98, Boulder, CO 80306-8010, (800) 333-9185.

Enhancing Sensual Pleasure by Steven Halpern. Relaxing and uplifting music for couples making love. Sound Rx, Dept. ESP, P.O. Box 2644, San Anselmo, CA 94979, (800) 876-8637.

ORGANIZATIONS, PROGRAMS, AND WEB SITES

Many of the organizations listed here provide referral services for obtaining professional therapy. In considering a therapist, support group, or treatment program, you may want to consult physicians, mental health referral agencies, and sexual assault centers for more information about the services in your area. Interview therapists and learn details about program philosophy and operations before making your choice.

Inclusion on this list does not indicate a recommendation or endorsement by the author. Use your own judgment when contacting any of these organizations and web sites. Many organizations suggest that you enclose a self-addressed stamped envelope with written inquiries.

Adult Survivors of Child Abuse (ASCA), web site: http://www.ascasupport. org. On-line information to assist survivors of child abuse. Publishes a newsletter.

Alternatives to Fear, 2811 E. Madison, #208, Seattle, WA 98112, (206) 328-5347, web site: http://www.boutell.com/alternatives-to-fear/index.html. Acquaintance rape education for adults and teens; self-defense information.

American Association for Marriage and Family Therapy (AAMFT), 1133 15th St., NW, #300, Washington, D.C. 20005-2710, (202) 452-0109, fax: (202) 223-2329, web site: http://www.aamft.org. A national organization with information on relationship sexuality problems, adolescent behavior problems, and referral service.

American Association of Sex Educators, Counselors, and Therapists (AASECT), P.O. Box 238, Mount Vernon, IA 52314, fax: (319) 895-6903, e-mail: AASECT@worldnet.att.net, web site: http://www.aasect.org. A national certifying organization that, upon your request, provides you with a list of counselors, psychologists, clinical social workers, and physicians who are certified sex therapists in your region.

American Social Health Association (ASHA), P.O. Box 13827, Research Triangle Park, NC 27709, (919) 361-8400, fax: (919) 361-8495, web site: http://www.ashastd.org. Information on STD support groups and prevention.

American Women's Self Defense Association (AWSDA), 713 N. Wellwood Ave., Lindenhurst, NY 11757, (888) STOP-RAPE, web site: http://www.awsda.org. Information and referrals regarding rape prevention and self defense.

Bay Area Women Against Rape (BAWAR), 357 MacArthur Blvd., Oakland, CA 94610, 24-hour crisis line: (510) 845-7273. A national organization dedicated to rape prevention and providing services to ritually abused survivors and their therapists.

Campus Outreach Services, web site: http://www.campusoutreachservices.com. Provides approaches to dealing with the issue of sexual assault on college campuses, in high schools, and in the military.

Childhelp USA, 15757 N. 78th St., Scottsdale, AZ 85260, (480) 922-8212, fax: (480) 922-7061, web site: http://www.childhelpusa.org. Provides training consultation, and resources for child victims and adult survivors. For referrals and information call their National Child Abuse Hotline at (800) 4-A-CHILD.

Codependents of Sexual Addiction (COSA), 9337-B Katy Fwy., #142, Houston, TX 77024, (612) 537-6904. A national service organization for partners, relatives, friends, and employees of people with sexual addictions. It offers twelve-step recovery support groups in many communities across the country, as well as literature, audiotapes, and information on conferences.

Family Violence and Sexual Assault Institute (FVSAI), 7120 Herman Jared Dr., Fort Worth, TX 76180, (817) 485-2244, fax: (817) 485-0660, e-mail: fvsai@cspp.edu, web site: http://www.fvsai.org. A clearinghouse of information and networking, with special information for countering the backlash against sexual abuse awareness.

HealthySex.com, web site: http://www.HealthySex.com. Developed by Wendy Maltz, this site provides information on healthy sexuality. It includes articles, check-lists, comparison charts, and resources to help individuals and couples understand and develop skills for healthy sexual intimacy. In addition, the site offers information on Wendy Maltz's books, videos, healthysex products, and speaking presentations.

Incest Survivor Information Exchange, P.O. Box 3399, New Haven, CT 06515. Produces a newsletter for adult survivors.

Incest Survivors Resource Network International, Inc., P.O. Box 7375, Las Cruces, NM 88006-7375, (505) 521-4260, fax: (505) 521-3723, e-mail: isrni@ zianet.com. Provides education resources and information on national and international conferences.

Interfaith Sexual Trauma Institute (ISTI), Saint John's Abbey and University, Collegeville, MN 56321-2000, (320) 363-3931, e-mail: isti@csbsju.edu, web site: http://www.csbsju.edu/isti/archive/newsltrs.html. Helpful information for survivors recovering from sexual abuse perpetrated by clergy and other religious leaders.

International Society for the Study of Dissociation (ISSD), 60 Revere Dr., Suite 500, Northbrook, IL 60062, (847) 480-0899; e-mail: issd@issd.org, web site: http://www.issd.org. A membership-based professional organization for therapists who work with dissociative disorders, including multiple personality.

King County Sexual Assault Resource Center, P.O. Box 300, Renton, WA 98057, (425) 226-5062. Provides publications, books, programs, and counseling for sexual assault prevention and treatment.

The Linkup, 1412 West Argyle, #2, Chicago IL 60640, (773) 334-2296, e-mail: ilinkup@aol.com, web site: http://www.ilinkup.org. A national organization of survivors of clergy abuse.

Men Assisting, Leading, and Educating (M.A.L.E.), P.O. Box 460171, Aurora, CO 80040-1716, (303) 693-9930, National Support Hotline: (800) 949-MALE, fax: (303) 693-6059, e-mail: male@malesurvivor.org. An organization for non-offending male survivors of child sexual abuse. Publishes the newsletter *Men's Issues Forum* and provides seminar, workshop, and referral information.

Men Can Stop Rape, web site: http://www.mrpp.org. A pro-feminist organization of men working to end men's violence against women through school classes, college workshops, and community action.

Mental Health Net, web site: http://www.mentalhelp.net. An on-line mental health guide and directory. Includes articles, information, and links for sexuality concerns.

National AIDS Hotline, (800) 342-AIDS, web site: http://www.ashastd. org/nah/nah.html. A national organization providing both over-the-phone and on-line information, support, and referrals for AIDS testing and treatment.

National Center for Redress of Incest and Sexual Abuse, 1858 Park Road, NW, Washington D.C. 20010, (202) 667-1160. Provides information to address the legal needs of survivors.

National Child Abuse Hotline, (800) 4-A-CHILD, web site: http://www.child-helpusa.org. A 24-hour crisis line for abuse reporting and referrals.

National Council on Sexual Addiction and Compulsivity, e-mail: ncsac@mindspring.com, web site: http://www.ncsac.org. A nonprofit organization promoting education and understanding of sexual addiction. Includes articles, member directory, resources, and annual conference information.

National Self-Help Clearinghouse, Graduate School, City University of New York, 365 5th Ave. #3300, New York, NY 10016, (212) 817-1822, e-mail: info@selfhelpweb.org, web site: http://www.selfhelpweb.org. A nonprofit organization providing listings of self-help groups throughout the United States. Publishes an on-line newsletter.

National Sexual Violence Resource Center (NSVRC), 123 N. Enola Dr., Enola, PA 17025, (717) 909-0710, fax: (717) 909-0714, e-mail: resources@ nsvrc.org, web site: http://www.nsvrc.org. Coordinates information, organizations, and services for sexual assault survivors on national, state, and local levels. Provides resources for the intervention and prevention of sexual violence.

One Voice: The National Alliance for Abuse Awareness, P.O. Box 27958, Washington, D.C. 20038-7958, (202) 667-1160, e-mail: OVoiceDC@aol.com. An advocacy group for child and adult victims of sexual abuse. Highly recommended for survivors and professionals wanting to become politically active in preventing and curbing child abuse.

Parents United International, 615 15th St., Modesto, CA 95354, (209) 572-3446, e-mail: parents.united@usa.net, web site: http://members.tripod.com/ ~Parents_United/Chapters/PUI.htm. A national self-help organization providing an on-line directory of self-help groups for offenders, victims, and non-offending partners.

Rape, Abuse, and Incest National Network (RAINN), 635-B Pennsylvania Ave., SE, Washington, D.C. 20003, National Hotline: (800) 656-HOPE, fax: (202) 544-3556, web site: http://www.rainn.org. A national organization providing a 24-hour hotline for survivors of sexual assault. Referral service and on-line counseling.

Rape Recovery Help and Information, web site: http://raperecovery.terrashare.com. A large internet inventory of organizations and programs to assist victims of rape.

Safer Society Foundation, P.O. Box 340, Brandon, VT 05733, (802) 247-3132, referral line (802) 247-5141, web site: http://www.safersociety.org. A national research, advocacy, and referral center on the prevention and treatment of sexual abuse.

Sex Addicts Anonymous (SAA), P.O. Box 70949, Houston, TX 77270, (800) 477-8191, (713) 869-4902, e-mail: info@saa-recovery.org, web site: http://www.sexaa.org. Information on sexual addiction and twelve-step recovery programs in your area.

Sex and Love Addicts Anonymous (SLAA), P.O. Box 338, Norwood, MA 02062-0338, (781) 255-8825, e-mail: fwsoffice@slaafws.org, web site: http://slaafws.org. Provides twelve-step recovery programs for survivors with compulsive sexual problems.

SexHelp.com, web site: http://www.sexhelp.com. Dr. Patrick Carnes's on-line sexual addiction recovery information site. Provides a wealth of resources and links for people with sexual addictions. It offers an interactive questionnaire that can help assess whether or not a person has a sexual addiction or compulsion, and to what extent.

Sexual Health Network, 3 Mayflower Lane, Huntington, CT 06484, (203) 924-4623, e-mail: info@sexualhealth.com, web site: http://www.sexualhealth.com. An excellent site that provides sexuality information, on-line counseling, and referrals. It features questions on sexual recovery for survivors with answers by Wendy Maltz, M.S.W.

Survivors & Friends, web site: http://www.oz.net/survivor. Recovery support for survivors of sexual abuse and their partners, parents, and other loved ones.

Survivors Healing Center, 2301 Mission St., # C-1, Santa Cruz, CA 95060, (831) 423-7601, fax: (831) 469-8315, e-mail: shc@cruzio.com, web site: http://www.cruzio.com/~shc. Information, referrals, and workshops for adult survivors of sexual abuse.

Survivors of Incest Anonymous, P.O. Box 21817, Baltimore, MD 21222-6817, (410) 282-3400, web site: http://www.siawso.org. Offers self-help support groups based on personal experiences, twelve-steps, and other information.

Survivorship, web site: http://www.survivorship.org. An on-line organization with resources for survivors of ritualistic and sadistic abuse.

Trauma Information Pages, P.O. Box 11143, Eugene, OR 97440, web site: http://www.trauma-pages.com. This award-winning web site, created by psychologist David Baldwin, Ph.D., offers free access to treatment resources and extensive research focused on emotional trauma and posttraumatic stress disorder.

Twelve-step recovery programs: Alcoholics Anonymous, Narcotics Anonymous, Al-Anon, Adult Children of Alcoholics, and others (some of which have been listed separately in this Resources section) are national organizations that provide free and confidential self-help meetings throughout the country. For information on meetings in your area, check the phone book for local chapter agencies or visit http://www.12steps.org for links to various self-help organizations.

VD National Hotline, (800) 227-8922. Provides information and referrals for the identification and treatment of sexually transmitted diseases.

VOICES in Action, Inc., P.O. Box 148309, Chicago, IL 60614-8309, (773) 327-1500, fax: (773) 327-4590, e-mail: voices@voices-action.org, web site: http://www.voices-action.org. A national network for incest survivors and pro-survivors (partners and other support people). Publishes a newsletter, organizes an annual conference, has special interest groups, and provides referrals. Annual membership fee.

Welcome to Barbados web site: http://www.welcometobarbados.org. A Tori Amos–inspired web site for rape and sexual abuse survivors, including survivor stories, a chat room, mailing list, and more.

RESIDENTIAL TREATMENT CENTERS

Inpatient hospital and residential treatment programs, specifically designed for treating adult survivors of sexual abuse, are scattered throughout the United States. The focus of these programs varies but may include treatment for sexual trauma, sexual dependency, drug and alcohol dependency, and dissociative disorders. These programs vary in approach, length of stay, and cost. Contact your local physicians, hospitals, and public health departments for information on other existing programs. The following are several nationally recognized centers.

Del Amo Hospital, 23700 Camino del Sol, Torrance, CA 90505, (800) 533-5266, (310) 530-1151, web site: http://www.delamohospital.com. Inpatient treatment for men and women sex addicts, trauma survivors, and sexual offenders.

The Meadows, 1655 N. Tegner St., Wickenburg, AZ 85390, (800) MEADOWS, web site: http://www.themeadows.org. Residential treatment for numerous addictions, including sexual addictions.

River Oaks Hospital, 1525 River Oaks Road West, Harahan, LA 70123, (504) 734-1740, (800) 366-1740. Provides intensive inpatient treatment for adolescents and adults suffering from sexual trauma and sexual compulsions.

Sierra Tucson, 16500 N. Lago del Oro, Tucson, AZ 85737, (800) 842-4487, web site: http://www.sierratucson.com. Special focus given to addictions, codependency problems, sexuality, intimacy and family problems, and issues related to adult children of dysfunctional families.

Index

About the Author

Wendy Maltz, M.S.W., is a nationally recognized psychotherapist and expert on healthy sexuality and sexual healing. A frequent lecturer, she is coauthor of *Private Thoughts: Exploring the Power of Women's Sexual Fantasies* and *Incest and Sexuality: A Guide to Understanding and Healing,* and editor of two poetry anthologies, *Passionate Hearts: The Poetry of Sexual Love* and *Intimate Kisses: The Poetry of Sexual Pleasure.*

A licensed clinical social worker, licensed marriage and family therapist, and certified sex therapist, Wendy has more than twenty-five years of clinical experience treating sex, intimacy, and relationship concerns. She has written and narrated two highly acclaimed video productions for couples: *Partners in Healing* and *Relearning Touch.* An experienced media presenter, her work has been featured in many national magazines, such as *Cosmopolitan, New Woman, Ladies Home Journal, Glamour, Parents,* and *Mademoiselle.* Wendy is codirector, with her husband Larry, of Maltz Counseling Associates in Eugene, Oregon. Her web site is: www.HealthySex.com.